To Dr Wexler

A superior competent physician.
It is a pleasure to work with you

Earl Brewer

Other Monographs in the Series, Major Problems in Clinical Pediatrics:

> Avery: *The Lung and Its Disorders in the Newborn Infant.* Second Edition.
>
> Cornblath and Schwartz: *Disorders of Carbohydrate Metabolism in Infancy.*
>
> Markowitz and Kuttner: *Rheumatic Fever—Diagnosis, Management and Prevention.*
>
> Oski and Naiman: *Hematologic Problems in the Newborn.*
>
> Rowe and Mehrizi: *The Neonate with Congenital Heart Disease.*
>
> Smith: *Recognizable Patterns of Human Malformation*—to be published in 1970.

JUVENILE RHEUMATOID ARTHRITIS

By

Earl J. Brewer, Jr., M.D.

Assistant Professor, Department of Pediatrics,
Baylor College of Medicine;
Chief, Arthritis Clinical Research Center,
Texas Children's Hospital, Houston, Texas

Volume VI in the Series
MAJOR PROBLEMS IN CLINICAL PEDIATRICS

ALEXANDER J. SCHAFFER
Consulting Editor

W. B. Saunders Company, Philadelphia, London, Toronto

W. B. Saunders Company: West Washington Square
Philadelphia, Pa. 19105

12 Dyott Street
London W.C.1

1835 Yonge Street
Toronto 7, Ontario

Juvenile Rheumatoid Arthritis

© 1970 by W. B. Saunders Company. Copyright under the International Copyright Union. All rights reserved. This book is protected by copyright. No part of it may be duplicated or reproduced in any manner without written permission from the publisher. Made in the United States of America. Press of W. B. Saunders Company. Library of Congress catalog card number 69-12875.

To

DR. MAY OWEN

*A great physician and teacher.
A continuing inspiration to students of
medicine and the community.*

**GUERIR QUELQUEFOIS,
SOULAGER SOUVENT,
CONSOLER TOUJOURS.**
  —*15th century folk saying.*

Contributors

ELIZABETH BARKLEY, B.S., R.N., P.T.

    Formerly Physical Therapist, Arthritis Clinical Research Center, Texas Children's Hospital, Houston, Texas.

EARL J. BREWER, Jr., M.D.

    Assistant Professor, Department of Pediatrics, Baylor College of Medicine; Chief, Arthritis Clinical Research Center, Texas Children's Hospital, Houston, Texas.

SIDNEY E. CLEVELAND, Ph.D.

    Professor of Psychology, Department of Psychiatry, Baylor College of Medicine, Houston, Texas.

W. MALCOLM GRANBERRY, M.D.

    Clinical Instructor, Baylor College of Medicine; Orthopedic Consultant, Arthritis Clinical Research Center, Texas Children's Hospital, Houston, Texas.

DAN G. McNAMARA, M.D.

    Associate Professor, Department of Pediatrics, Baylor College of Medicine; Director of Pediatric Cardiology, Texas Children's Hospital, Houston, Texas.

EDWARD B. SINGLETON, M.D.

    Associate Professor of Radiology, Baylor College of Medicine; Director of Radiology, St. Luke's and Texas Children's Hospitals, Houston, Texas.

Foreword

Children who suffer from chronic illness often present problems that are difficult to solve—medical, social, and emotional. Despite the inherent difficulties, it is a real challenge to those of us dedicated to the well-being of young patients to make special efforts to seek solutions.

One of these problems stands out above all the rest: that of meeting the basic need for excellent and effective over-all care without forgetting that the patient himself is a developing human being who needs the emotional security provided by a family group, an assured place in the family circle, and a healthy attitude toward a prolonged and often capricious malady.

Children with rheumatoid arthritis present many complex and poorly understood problems. In this volume the author has made every effort to assemble known facts and to make them available for the use of the practicing physician.

The section on pathogenesis is provocative, and the section on management presents a number of practical solutions for the therapeutic dilemmas which often confront the physician and the family. Of particular interest is the home-care program, in which he has outlined management of the patient within the framework of an enlightened home environment, supplemented by intelligent supervision. In this plan of management, the patient is guided along the road to recovery primarily as an outpatient.

The author has presented a difficult subject in a practical and intelligent manner. He recognizes and anticipates advances in medical knowledge, advances which are greatly needed in this important and little understood medical condition.

RUSSELL J. BLATTNER, M.D.
Professor and Chairman,
Department of Pediatrics,
Baylor College of Medicine;
Physician-in-Chief,
Texas Children's Hospital

Preface

The purpose of this monograph is to present to the clinical physician a concise discussion of current knowledge regarding manifestations, course, differential diagnosis, and therapy of juvenile rheumatoid arthritis. The author has, in particular, tried to present a continuing home care treatment program that has proved to be successful in the arthritis unit of the Junior League Outpatient Department at the Texas Children's Hospital.

I wish to express deepest appreciation to Dr. Milton Markowitz who conceived the idea for a monograph concerned with juvenile rheumatoid arthritis and through his interest and encouragement made it possible for me to be the author.

The preparation of the manuscript would never have been possible without the devoted and superbly competent help of Mrs. Violet Cromar. To the other secretaries who aided with the work in various stages I offer my sincerest thanks.

To the Administration of Texas Children's Hospital who so cooperatively provided the physical requirements for research and preparation, and their skilled photographer, Mr. Manfred Gygli, I extend my deep appreciation.

Dr. Don B. Singer and Dr. Leon Librik were most kind to review portions of the monograph concerned with pathology and corticosteroid physiology respectively.

Dr. Russell J. Blattner kindly consented to write the Foreword for this book and appropriately so, for he was the physician who first interested me in the problems of chronic illness in childhood and, in particular, rheumatoid arthritis.

EARL J. BREWER, JR., M.D.

Contents

Chapter One
MANIFESTATIONS OF DISEASE.. 1

Chapter Two
CARDITIS WITH RHEUMATOID ARTHRITIS....................................... 48
    Dan G. McNamara, M.D., and Earl J. Brewer, Jr., M.D.

Chapter Three
RADIOGRAPHIC DIAGNOSIS OF RHEUMATOID ARTHRITIS IN THE
PEDIATRIC PATIENT 59
    Edward B. Singleton, M.D.

Chapter Four
LABORATORY DATA 68

Chapter Five
DIFFERENTIAL DIAGNOSIS 80

Chapter Six
PSYCHOLOGICAL ASPECTS OF JUVENILE RHEUMATOID ARTHRITIS...... 116
    Sidney E. Cleveland, Ph.D., and Earl J. Brewer, Jr., M.D.

Chapter Seven
HOME TREATMENT PROGRAM 132
    Elizabeth Barkley, B.S., R.N., P.T., and
    Earl J. Brewer, Jr., M.D.

Appendix—Exercise Program with Illustrations 144

Chapter Eight
Orthopedic Management of Juvenile Rheumatoid Arthritis.. 156

W. Malcolm Granberry, M.D., and Earl J. Brewer, Jr., M.D.

Chapter Nine
Drug Therapy 180

Index 223

Chapter One

MANIFESTATIONS OF DISEASE

THE CLASSIC PICTURE

An active and happy four-year-old girl was observed by her mother to move a little more slowly in the mornings. Over a period of time, she noticed that her daughter's knees had almost imperceptibly become enlarged. In a short time, there followed further enlargement of the knees and also the wrists with limitation of motion of the cervical spine. Significant pain did not seem to be present, but wasting of the muscles about the knees and wrists was marked, and restriction of joint motion was rapid. When seen by the physician, the lymph glands had enlarged to the size of a hazelnut in the supratrochlear, brachial artery, axillary, inguinal, and posterior triangular areas of the neck. Similarly, the spleen had enlarged to one or two fingerbreadths below the left costal margin. A slight prominence of the eyes was noted along with profuse perspiration unrelated to temperature. Recording of the temperature revealed that periods of pyrexia occurred lasting several days followed by longer intervals of apyrexia and, at times, a more or less continuous slight pyrexia. Examination of the blood revealed only anemia. A remarkable feature in this child's illness was the general arrest of physical development resulting in dwarfing without arrest of mental development. The course of this patient was protracted with periods of improvement followed by progressive deterioration until eventually joint disease became generalized. No valvular heart disease was found but physical signs suggestive of an adherent pericardium appeared on one occasion.

This vignette is a composite case history of the prominent findings listed by Dr. George F. Still in 1896. Dr. Still at the time was Medical Registrar and Pathologist at the Hospital for Sick Children, Great Ormond Street, London. The purpose of his paper was to show that there were at least three distinct joint afflictions that had been previously included under one heading, rheumatoid arthritis in children. Twelve of 22 cases reported were of the type just described. The second type presented the same general enlargement of the joints with subsequent bony thickening, lipping, and bony grating, but no enlargement of lymph glands or spleen and no evidence of pericarditis. Six cases were of this nature.

The third type was seen in a child whose fingers suddenly became stiff secondary to the formation of fibrous nodules over the tendons.

The elbows and wrists slowly became enlarged with limitation of motion, accompanied by stiffness of the neck. Marked limitation of motion occurred over the next one and one-half years with the elbows and wrists showing firm thickening and none of the fusiform elastic enlargement peculiar to the first type described. This condition was equated with that described by Jaccoud as chronic fibrous rheumatism (Still, 1897).

Dr. Still's lucid description of what are now considered to be various types of rheumatoid arthritis in children served to bring this condition to the attention of the medical profession. The description remains a classic one for seriously involved cases.

Unfortunately, over the years, the term Still's disease has acquired a variety of meanings. Clinicians often describe a Still's type of onset with high fever, rash, lymphadenopathy, and absent or minimal arthritis. Although this type of onset certainly does occur and is the mode of onset most frequently associated with the disease in the clinician's mind at the present time, this was not the type of case noted by Still in his clearly written description.

Rheumatoid arthritis in the pediatric age group, like its adult counterpart, is a chronic, destructive arthritis often accompanied by systemic manifestations. The etiology is unknown and the clinical course is capricious, often unpredictable in severity as well as duration.

The purpose of this monograph is to present in as clear and concise a manner as possible the current concepts regarding manifestations, course, diagnosis, and therapy.

INCIDENCE AND PREVALENCE

Age at Onset

The age at onset varies considerably throughout the pediatric age group (Fig. 1-1). The average and the median ages at onset in our series of 100 patients were 6.4 years and 6 years respectively, with a range of one week to 15 years of age. Two peaks of incidence seem to occur: between 2 and 4 years, and between 8 and 11 years.

Sex

Rheumatoid arthritis in the pediatric age group affects girls more frequently than boys. The incidence reported has varied from 1.5:1 (Pickard, 1947) to 5:1 (Coss and Boots, 1946). Our own group included 61 girls and 39 boys, an approximate ratio of 1.6:1.

Prevalence

Accurate data regarding the prevalence of rheumatoid arthritis are not available. The percentage of children among all patients with rheumatoid arthritis has varied in reports from 4 to 7 per cent (Barkin, 1952; Kuhns and Swaim, 1932; Coss and Boots, 1946; Edström, 1958).

Manifestations of Disease

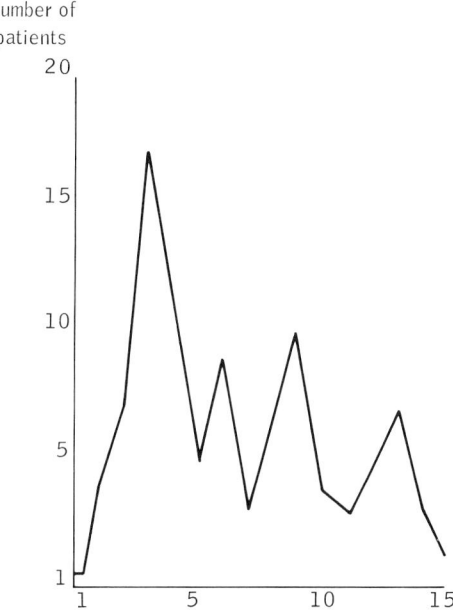

Figure 1-1 Age at onset of disease.

In England, Lawrence estimated that 2.7 per thousand of the adult population developed polyarthritis during childhood, and an incidence of 100,000 patients has been reported in the United Kingdom (Ansell and Bywaters, 1963).

Season

In adults there is thought to be a seasonal difference in onset, with more cases occurring between October and April; however, in our group of children there seemed to be no significant difference in the month or season of onset (Fig. 1-2).

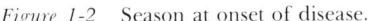
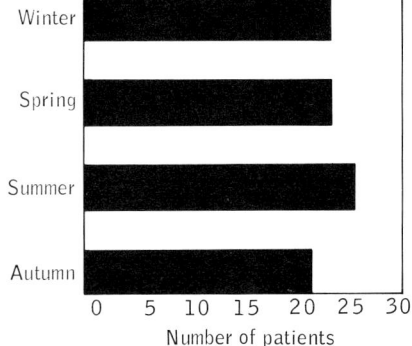

Figure 1-2 Season at onset of disease.

ASSOCIATED CONDITIONS

Any disease of unknown etiology may lead a physician to speculate almost endlessly about possible preceding conditions of importance. Such is the case with juvenile rheumatoid arthritis; infection, climatic changes, allergy, genetic predisposition, trauma, surgery, and endocrine malfunction have all been implicated as associated preceding conditions.

Infection

Authors have noted preceding infection in 19 to 57 per cent of patients, (Edström, 1958; Norcross et al., 1958; Barkin, 1952; Coss and Boots, 1946; Pickard, 1947). In the initial group of 100 patients reported at the Texas Children's Hospital, preceding infection of some type occurred in 45 children. The infections were usually respiratory in nature, but many other types of infection have been noted within one month of onset of disease. Early authorities were intrigued with the relationship between rheumatoid arthritis and respiratory disease caused by beta-hemolytic streptococcal infection. A review of some of this material in recent years has shown that laboratory contamination by a streptococcal carrier possibly accounted for the large number of patients reported infected with beta-hemolytic streptococci (Vaughan, 1966).

Lockie reported that 31 per cent of 80 patients had antecedent upper respiratory infections with beta-hemolytic streptococci (Norcross et al., 1958). Elevated streptococcal agglutination reactions have been reported in a significant number of patients with rheumatoid arthritis. This phenomenon is now thought to be related to the activity of antigammaglobulin antibodies composing the rheumatoid factors. Significantly high agglutination titers against other bacteria have also been seen (Vaughan, 1966).

Most rheumatologists feel that focal infection does not play a significant role in the adult patient with rheumatoid arthritis. A significant number of children, however, do have exacerbation of disease manifestations with infections, usually respiratory in nature. Considerable interest continues in the possibility that rheumatoid arthritis is an infectious disease.

Trauma

The relationship of trauma as a precipitating factor in juvenile rheumatoid arthritis is tenuous at best. Local trauma may bring to focus arthritis of a joint or joints not previously noticed because of an insidious onset. The physician caring for a patient must always search for a possible specific etiology, and retrospective search can more often than not elicit a history of significant trauma in almost any child. In the Texas Children's Hospital group, a significant traumatic incident had preceded the onset of disease in 11 per cent of the children, including falls with injury to knees, ankles, shoulders, and toes. One child had a bee sting prior to onset. All these patients had trauma within one month of the onset of illness.

Surgery

Surgical procedures of many types have been associated with the onset of rheumatoid arthritis in children. The surgical procedure may involve the same relation that trauma appears to have. Ten per cent of the Texas Children's Hospital study patients had had surgery of some type within one month of onset; six had had tonsillectomies and adenoidectomies and four, other minor procedures.

Diet

The possibility that rheumatoid arthritis may be the result of certain dietary deficiencies or excesses has been considered over the years. Low carbohydrate diets, high doses of vitamins A, B, C, D, and E, cranberry juice, garlic, canteloupe juice, watermelon juice, sea water, radishes, and various sugar and molasses mixtures have all been advocated at one time or another by laymen or physicians. All the many dietary replacement regimes have fallen into disuse after an adequate trial. Such nostrums and dietary additions gain some prominence because remissions are often quite sudden, and whatever happens to be at hand in the way of therapy or dietary excess or omission seems relevant to the patient who has experienced improvement.

A proper diet will be discussed later in the book, and the discussion contained here should not be construed in any way to mean that an adequate, proper, and nutritious diet is not essential for maintenance of good health.

Social and Economic Factors

Social and economic factors seem to have no specific relation to the incidence of rheumatoid arthritis in children. In the Junior League Outpatient Department of Texas Children's Hospital approximately one half of patients are so-called private patients and one half are so-called clinic patients. This simply means that one half of the patients are from families with incomes that exceed $5000 per year. The disease does not seem to follow along economic or social lines. The quality of nutrition, however, does affect the severity of the disease in the individual. A lack of protein in the diet will place any child on the brink of disaster almost daily in his life. For this reason patients in the lower income brackets often have more serious disease than members of the upper income strata. This is true also for many other chronic diseases, however, and the severity of the disease is related directly to the level of nutrition and the ability and interest of the parents in obtaining adequate medical care.

Climatic Conditions Associated with Rheumatoid Arthritis

Adult rheumatoid arthritis patients are well known to be intolerant of certain changes in the weather. Children with rheumatoid arthritis have the same problem. The patient develops increased pain in his involved joints, and actually has an increase in swelling, tenderness, and limitation of motion in many instances. All juvenile rheumatoid arthritis patients do not exhibit this manifestation or have exacerbation of disease with alteration of the climate.

Edström (1948) maintained a group of patients for as long as three months in a controlled, warm, dry climate, using an insulated area in which the humidity was maintained at 35 per cent and the temperature at 84° F. In this controlled atmosphere the majority of patients improved with regard to joint function and pain.

Hollander (1961) constructed an elaborate, controlled climate chamber that could control and measure temperature, barometric pressure, humidity, air flow, and ionization constants. Patients who subjectively showed exacerbation of arthritis with changes in the weather were placed in the climate chamber for several weeks. Elaborate consideration had been given to comfort and facilities, with medical care continuing as before. The various modalities mentioned were then altered after suitable control periods, and later the modalities were changed in combination. No single change in weather modality produced an exacerbation of arthritis in a significant number of patients. By rapid increase of humidity and rapid decrease of barometric pressure simultaneously, exacerbation of arthritis was produced clinically in the majority of these patients, but by no means were all patients affected. This observation, that change in barometric pressure and humidity is important, correlates with the observation that flare-up will occur most often prior to cold rain or snowfall. A persistently high humidity and persistently low barometric pressure do not produce exacerbation, but rather it is the change that seems to be important.

The studies discussed show very well that there is some basis in fact for the weather-sensitive individual with arthritis, whether he has rheumatoid arthritis or osteoarthritis. A significant number of juvenile rheumatoid arthritis patients have this same capacity to detect certain changes in the weather because of exacerbations.

Geographic Distribution

The geographic distribution of rheumatoid arthritis has not been studied in detail. It has been reviewed by both Hill (1939) and Ragan (1962). Lawrence (1963) has postulated that rheumatoid arthritis has the highest incidence in temperate zones between latitudes 50 and 60 degrees north. Studies in Puerto Rico (Mendez-Bryan et al., 1963) reveal a greatly diminished incidence when compared to that of the United States and the United Kingdom. Detailed studies of equatorial points of the earth remain to be done, but such studies would be influenced by lack of long-term medical care in these areas, plus reduced average longevity of the population.

Family History

For many years physicians have been intrigued with the seemingly increased number of patients' relatives evidencing rheumatic disease.

Every arthritis clinic has one or more families who seem to exhibit increased evidence of the disease. As many as 20 or 30 relatives in one family have been known to have rheumatoid arthritis. The incidence of rheumatic disease in relatives of patients with rheumatoid arthritis has varied from 2.35 to 16 per cent (Masi and Shulman, 1965; Lawrence, 1963; Mikkelsen, 1966). Early studies were based on historical data with no examination of the relatives, but revealed a high incidence. More recent studies have centered around two areas of investigation: twin studies for concordance or discordance, and incidence of disease among relatives of known patients.

Twin studies are of special interest for two reasons. The study of monozygotic and dizygotic twins can demonstrate possible genetic etiology, either dominant or recessive. In addition, genetic studies of monozygotic and dizygotic twins can give evidence of a predisposition to the disease even if the etiology is environmental in nature. This method of study of genetically controlled constitutional susceptibility to a disease was implemented by Herndon and Jennings in studying poliomyelitis (1951). Previous observations in 1934 and 1942 had shown heavy familial aggregation of paralytic poliomyelitis, not only with given sibship, but in related sibships widely separated geographically and in different generations. The point was raised that such pedigrees were especially selected and perhaps could be expected to occur by chance alone. In another study of poliomyelitis, Addair and Snyder (1942) collected all cases of paralytic poliomyelitis with residual paralysis in an isolated section of McDowell County, West Virginia, over a period of 50 years. All 29 patients were shown to be related to one another. In Herndon and Jennings' study of 3890 reported cases of poliomyelitis from 1940 to 1948 classified regarding twinning, 56 patients were found to be of plural birth, with 55 being members of twins and one being a member of triplets (Table 1-1). The 45 sets of twins in the study included 14 sets of monozygous twins, 31 sets of dizygous twins, and one set of triplets. The observed number of monozygous and dizygous twins corresponds with the expected random rate (one-third monozygous, two-thirds dizygous).

Paralytic poliomyelitis was found in both monozygotic twins in 35 per cent of the cases, but only 6 per cent of the dizygotic pairs had concordant poliomyelitis. The difference was statistically significant, and the existence of a genetic factor, affecting in some manner the incidence of a known infectious disease, was concluded.

Table 1-1 Incidence of Twins in Poliomyelitis (3890 Reported Cases, 1940–1948)*

With poliomyelitis	Members of twins—55	Members of triplets—1
Included in study	Sets of twins—45	Sets of triplets—1
Monozygous	Sets of twins—14 (31%)	
Dizygous	Sets of twins—31 (69%)	

*Adapted from Herndon, C. N., and Jennings, R. G.: A twin study of susceptibility to poliomyelitis. Amer. J. Hum. Genet., 3:17, 1951.

Such studies in rheumatoid arthritis have not been done, and need to be done. Jacox and Meyerowitz have carefully studied 11 sets of monozygotic twins in whom at least one member had definite or classic rheumatoid arthritis. None of these twins have been concordant for rheumatoid arthritis. All twins affected had rheumatoid arthritis for at least two years and the age range was 11 to 68 years (Meyerowitz et al., 1968; Jacox, personal communication).

Moesmann (1959) summarized the available literature on monozygotic twins with rheumatoid arthritis, and reviewed 50 twins, including eight patients of his own. Concordance was present in 36 per cent. This figure is of interest because it corresponds to the concordance present in the carefully performed poliomyelitis study (Herndon and Jennings, 1951). Moesmann's study, being a report of the literature rather than a direct examination of patients, leaves in question the status of the twins with regard to monozygosity or dizygosity, and the diagnosis of rheumatoid arthritis. If the disease were caused by a genetically dominant or recessive single gene with total penetrance, the incidence of concordance should approach 100 per cent in monozygotic twins. In dizygotic twins, a recessively transmitted condition should approximate 25 per cent concordance, and in the case of a dominant single gene, inheritance should approach 50 per cent concordance.

However, as in most inheritable diseases, the genetic structure is recessive and multifactoral, in that environmental circumstances alter the clinical appearance of the disease.

Baum and Fink (1968) have reported the occurrence of juvenile rheumatoid arthritis in both members of monozygotic twins and reviewed the available literature (Table 1-2). Of the ten monozygotic twin sets reviewed, three were concordant, an incidence of 30 per cent.

Another report concerning the incidence of twins with juvenile rheumatoid arthritis, by Ansell et al. (1963), shows that among 316 definite cases of juvenile rheumatoid arthritis, there were four monozygotic and four dizygotic twins. Two concordant pairs were found in the four monozygotic twins. A period of five years intervened between onset of symptoms in one pair, and one year in the other pair.

In 1961, Burch, O'Brien, and Bunim began a controlled survey among the Blackfeet and Pima Indians (Table 1-3). The advantage of choosing these two groups located in Montana and Arizona was that

Table 1-2 Monozygotic Twins with Juvenile Rheumatoid Arthritis*

Author	Number of Twin Sets	Sex	Age at Onset	Number Concordant	Number Discordant
Ansell	4	?	Under Age 16	2	2
Brandt and Weihe	1	M	8-9	—	1
Moesmann	1	F	15	—	1
Jacox	3	F	7, 11, 14	—	3
Baum and Fink	1	F	2	1	—

*From Baum, J., and Fink, C. W.: Juvenile rheumatoid arthritis in monozygotic twins: A case report and review of the literature. Arthritis Rheum., *11*:35, 1968.

Table 1-3 Incidence of Rheumatoid Arthritis in Blackfeet and Pima Indians*

	Number	Incidence (Per Cent)
Blackfeet	1102	4.1
Pima	968	5.4

*Data from Bunim, J., Burch, T. A., and O'Brien, W.: Influence of genetic and environmental factors on the occurrence of rheumatoid arthritis and rheumatoid factor in American Indians. Bull Rheum. Dis., 15:349, 1964.

most of the relatives of any one Indian lived in the same area. A total of 2070 Indians were included in their survey. In another study of the Blackfeet Indians, among 275 married couples rheumatoid arthritis was not observed in either spouse of 254 couples; 20 cases were encountered involving one spouse of a couple; and in only one instance were both spouses involved (Burch et al., 1964).

This incidence closely corresponds with the incidence of rheumatoid arthritis of 4 per cent, the computation of expectancy based on Hardy-Weinberg-Law. Rheumatoid factor, measured by the Bentonite flocculation test, was present in neither spouse of 218 couples; however, in 32 cases it was present in single spouses, and in two cases both spouses had positive rheumatoid factor. Again, the expected frequency was virtually the same. The conclusion of this carefully performed study is that multiple cases of rheumatoid arthritis, in a given population, can be explained on the basis of chance alone.

Bywaters studied 277 living relatives of 93 probands with juvenile rheumatoid arthritis; 9 of 120 male relatives, and 13 of 157 female relatives examined, had active polyarthritis. The expected calculated number would be 4 males and 8 females. Four of the males were found to have spondylitis, and 1 male had gout. The remainder of the patients, including the females, had rheumatoid arthritis. Erosive arthritis of the hands was found by roentgenogram four times as frequently in the female relatives as in the control group of identical age distribution. Sacroiliitis was three times more common in the male relatives than in the controls. None of the juvenile rheumatoid arthritis seropositive probands' relatives had positive rheumatoid factor. The incidence of rheumatoid factor was lower in relatives than in a random sample (Ansell and Bywaters, 1962).

In view of the several studies that seemed to point toward a lack of genetic relationship with an increased familial incidence, the possibility of exogenous environmental factors as an etiological agent must be seriously considered.

MODE OF ONSET

The onset of juvenile rheumatoid arthritis is capricious as its course and prognosis. In the beginning, symptoms may be limited

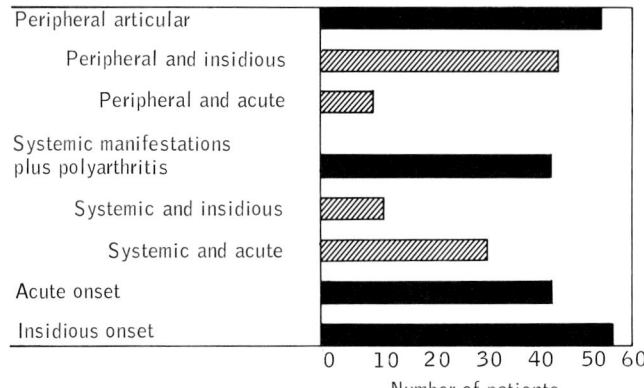

Figure 1-3 Type of onset of disease in 100 patients.

entirely to the peripheral joints with few or no symptoms of systemic disease. Other patients have prominent manifestations of systemic involvement with arthritis. Some patients have a sudden onset with immediate appearance of symptoms, and other patients have an insidious onset with symptoms appearing almost imperceptibly over a period of time (Fig. 1-3).

Peripheral Articular Onset

In children with this type of onset arthritis is almost the only sign of involvement. Articular symptoms and signs noticed by the parent usually include swelling of the joint over a period of time. The swelling may be quite sudden or slowly progressive over a period of many months. Pain is not usually a prominent feature in those patients in whom initial swelling increases gradually over a long period of time. On the other hand, patients who have had sudden articular swelling often complain of significant pain. Tenderness occurs more often than subjective pain. Some limitation of motion is usually manifest by the time swelling is noted. Redness of the skin overlying the joint is not often present. Mild warmth to the touch is often noted by astute and careful observers, and usually may be elicited by carefully comparing the opposite members; extreme heat about the joint is unusual. The weight-bearing joints, such as knees and ankles, are most frequently involved initially. A significant number of patients begin with monarticular arthritis.

Fifty-six of the first 100 patients followed at the Texas Children's Hospital had a peripheral articular type of onset. In 46 of these patients the onset was insidious, but ten children had a sudden and explosive onset.

Monarticular Onset

About 30 per cent of patients have, as the initial episode of juvenile rheumatoid arthritis, only one joint involved. Within a few weeks

Manifestations of Disease

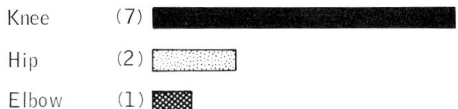

Figure 1-4 Monarticular joint involvement in 10 per cent of 100 patients studied.

or months many more joints are usually involved, but about 10 per cent persist with only one joint affected in a significant manner. This involvement is usually in the knee, but the hip, elbow, or other joints are occasionally involved (Fig. 1-4).

Occasionally the onset of disease is heralded by polyarthritis, with or without systemic manifestations, proceeding subsequently to monarticular disease of the knee or hip with no further involvement of other joints. In cases of monarticular onset in our series the average age at onset was 5.5 years, ranging from 2.5 years to 14 years in the group of six girls and four boys. The age and sex data are the same as in the general group. The vast majority (80 per cent) of the ten patients with persistent monarticular arthritis had a peripheral and insidious type of onset. Only two patients had an acute onset, with one presenting peripheral articular manifestations; the other patient was acutely ill with systemic disease (Fig. 1-5).

The clinical course of monarticular arthritis will be discussed under clinical manifestations, but it is appropriate to note here that later in the course of disease many patients have signs of systemic disease. In addition, in many of these patients, at some time during the course of disease, one or two other joints are involved in very minor and transient episodes.

Systemic Onset with Polyarthritis

The disease often begins with polyarthritis or monarticular arthritis accompanied by such systemic manifestations as fever, rash, malaise, pallor, lymphadenopathy, hepatomegaly, splenomegaly, subcutaneous nodules, or pericarditis. The onset of systemic symptoms is more often sudden and explosive in nature. Forty-four of the 100 patients recently reviewed displayed this type of beginning. Thirty-three of these patients had a sudden and explosive onset, and 11 developed manifestations insidiously over a period of several weeks or months.

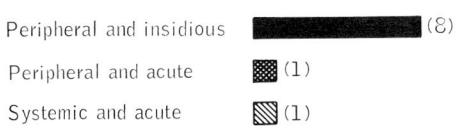

Figure 1-5 Monarticular onset in 10 per cent of 100 patients studied.

PATTERNS OF DISEASE

A wide spectrum of disease patterns exists with regard to joints in juvenile rheumatoid arthritis. Although no useful purpose is served by subdividing juvenile rheumatoid arthritis into empiric types for descriptive purposes, an understanding of disease patterns is worthwhile to the clinician in caring for the patient.

The majority of patients who have a sudden onset of polyarthritis with systemic manifestations pursue a clinical course of acute exacerbations lasting from one week to several months, followed by partial remission in the form of reduction of joint swelling. The partial remission may last from a few weeks to several years with intermittent sudden exacerbations of joint swelling, pain, or tenderness.

In patients who exhibit a sudden onset of polyarthritis with systemic manifestations, only rarely does the disease continue with the same degree of severity. These patients generally have severe disease and become rapidly debilitated. An occasional patient will have sudden and severe polyarthritis with pain or tenderness lasting a few weeks to a few months, followed by a total clinical remission and subsequent exacerbations at intervals of several months to several years.

Patients who have an insidious onset of peripheral articular arthritis, with no systemic manifestations, also usually have periods of partial remission with minimal joint involvement interspersed with acute exacerbations.

In general, in children with monarticular rheumatoid arthritis one or two other joints eventually become involved to a lesser degree than the one major joint. Most often the knee is the site of monarticular involvement, and the ankles and hips are the sites of minimal joint

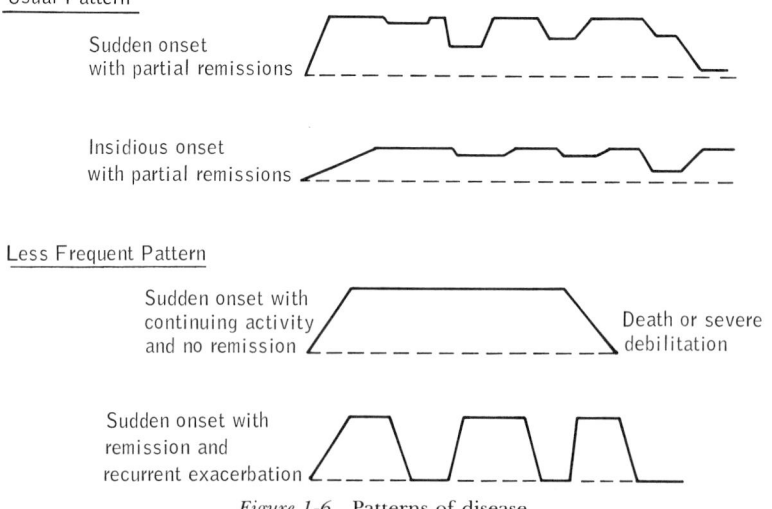

Figure 1-6 Patterns of disease.

involvement accompanying monarticular arthritis. The pattern of joint involvement is usually that of continuing monarticular disease for the course of the illness. The patient usually has the disease for a period of two to three years.

Green has described a pauciarticular arthritis that is mild with an excellent prognosis and minimal or no permanent joint deformity (Griffin et al., 1963). Patients in this category undoubtedly include children with mild rheumatoid arthritis, but no useful purpose is served by omitting this type of patient from the category of juvenile rheumatoid arthritis.

Patterns of Pain and Tenderness

Four main patterns of pain are apparent when children with rheumatoid arthritis are closely observed over a period of years.

1. Pain on motion with tenderness to palpation is the most common pattern. This pain is usually not exquisite or totally incapacitating. Instead the child must be questioned directly regarding the pain, and in the younger age group a noticeable limp may be the only indication that pain is indeed present. The tenderness elicited by palpation is customarily mild and at times found only at the extreme ranges of motion.

2. Tenderness to palpation alone with no subjective pain is frequently the pattern of a patient's disease. Such definite but mild tenderness to palpation accompanied by swelling may be the only indication of disease. Tenderness alone of some joints, in patients who have definite swelling of other joints, may be the only manifestation of involvement. Swelling in the tender joint may or may not occur later. In some joints, such as the hip, swelling cannot be readily recognized; in such joints, tenderness must be carefully elicited.

3. Swelling of the joint, with no pain or tenderness, is not as frequent but definitely occurs. Although, in general, patients exhibit the same type of response, different joints will manifest all of the patterns at one time or another. The wrist and occasionally the metacarpal and proximal interphalangeal joints are excellent examples of this type of involvement.

4. Acute episodes of intense pain with exquisite tenderness occur rarely but deserve mention. In patients who exhibit this manifestation, the disease often begins with an acute episode of pain and tenderness lasting from one or two days to two or three weeks. The initial episode may be the only time this occurs. At least three of our patients had episodes of sudden exquisite pain and tenderness lasting a few days, with just as sudden a remission to a more chronic state of the disease with minimal or no pain and tenderness.

Patterns of Response in Certain Age Groups

The developing pediatric subject from infancy through teen-age years necessarily varies in response to the same disease. Infants (less than two years of age) cannot effectively provide documentation of symptoms, and observation of disease becomes essential. An example is morning stiffness. Some infants are unable to move upon arising after rest, and only after a half hour or more does effective locomotion take place. The phenomenon of morning stiffness may be inferred to have occurred. Again, pain as a symptom may not be directly observed but withdrawal and tenderness to palpation and range of motion can serve adequately as clues. The normal pudgy obesity of this age group makes difficult the accurate observation of minimal joint swelling, particularly of knees, ankles, and metacarpal joints.

Speech in the two- to six-year-old age group is, of course, markedly improved and careful questioning should reveal the same information obtained in older age groups. Again, observation of the patient often means more than questioning. A limp more often than not is the only indication of pain in a joint. Two- to six-year-old children do not usually spontaneously complain of pain. The variance of figures in some studies relating to the lack of pain in children with rheumatoid arthritis may well relate more to the age group than to the absence of pain (Grokoest et al., 1962).

Teen-age Group

There are many studies available regarding the emotional lability of the normal teen-ager. Moods in this group are often either extremely buoyant or extremely depressed. The reaction of teen-agers to rheumatoid arthritis is colored by this sensitivity. In particular, tenderness seems to be distressing to the point that even light touch can evoke considerable response. This particular age group has a great concern over self and body image, and any alteration or imperfection disturbs them much more than it does younger children or adults.

CLINICAL MANIFESTATIONS

Morning Stiffness

Morning stiffness in the adult patient with rheumatoid arthritis is a well-known symptom, helpful in diagnosis of the disease. Adults with rheumatoid arthritis objectively feel a difficulty in moving muscles after a period of rest. This is most prominent early in the morning after a night's sleep. The stiffness is not the result of pain and, with activity, completely disappears during the day; its duration ranges from a few minutes to several hours. Few other diseases exhibit this manifestation.

Children with rheumatoid arthritis have the same experience after periods of inactivity and sleep. Morning stiffness in children must be regarded as a phenomenon to be elicited by the physician and not simply a symptom to be reported by the patient as in the adult. Observation, therefore, becomes important in ascertaining the presence or absence of stiffness. Marked morning stiffness occurs sometimes to the point that children are simply unable to rise from bed spontaneously and must be carried to the morning bath. After a few minutes in the tub with moist heat and activity, the stiffness disappears and the child is able to move about more freely, with complete disappearance of stiffness later in the morning. To a lesser degree, the phenomenon may occur in the same child after an afternoon nap or after sitting in a classroom for an hour. Moving about the room occasionally for a minute or so during an hour in class will often prevent occurrence.

At times, morning stiffness must be ascertained entirely by observation. After inactivity, the patient will move his entire head, neck, and shoulders as a unit rather than turning his head alone. After an hour or so of activity, normal head motion will return spontaneously. Some observers believe this is mainly due to pain that is reduced with activity. Whether inactivity or pain is responsible for morning stiffness is difficult to determine and may not be significant. Other children will have difficulty in gait for a period of time after inactivity, with subsequent disappearance of stiffness in a few minutes to a few hours. This response differs from the pain that may occur after excessive activity and fatigue, in that improvement occurs with use.

Gibson prefers to think of stiffness as a "jelling" that disappears after activity. When considered as a phenomenon to be elicited in several ways, morning stiffness is a useful clinical manifestation in the diagnosis of rheumatoid arthritis in children.

Rash

A variety of rashes and papular eruptions occur in juvenile rheumatoid arthritis. Rheumatoid rash is considered to be a specific finding and was observed at one time or another in 44 per cent of our patients. Other authors have reported a frequency varying from 20 to 70 per cent (Grossman et al., 1965; Isdale and Bywaters, 1956; Johnson and Dodd, 1955). Rheumatoid papule is a rare but nonspecific condition observed in one of our patients. Children with rheumatoid arthritis hyperreact to many agents, and urticarial rashes are common. Erythema marginatum is known to occur only rarely in rheumatoid arthritis; erythema multiforme has sometimes also been noted.

Rheumatoid Rash. Rheumatoid rash is an evanescent, salmon-pink, usually circumscribed macular rash varying in size from 2 to 6 mm. in greatest diameter for individual lesions (Fig. 1-7). The larger lesions may have a pale center with extreme paleness of the skin immediately to the periphery of the outer border of the rash. The rash tends to become confluent and may be as large as 8 or 9 cm. in rare instances. Occurrence is predominantly on the chest, axilla, thighs, and upper arms, but the face is also involved at times. The rash is usually intermittent, and may be present for a few minutes to more than four years (Isdale and Bywaters, 1956).

The rash may appear at any time during the course of the disease and is associated in particular with fever, splenomegaly, and lymphadenopathy. The time of appearance can precede onset of arthritis by six months to three years (Isdale and Bywaters, 1956).

Histologic examination reveals edematous collagen fibers, perivascular cellular infiltration in the upper portion of the corium with polymorphonuclear leukocytes, and, to a lesser extent, lymphocytes, plasma cells, and histiocytes (Schlesinger et al., 1961).

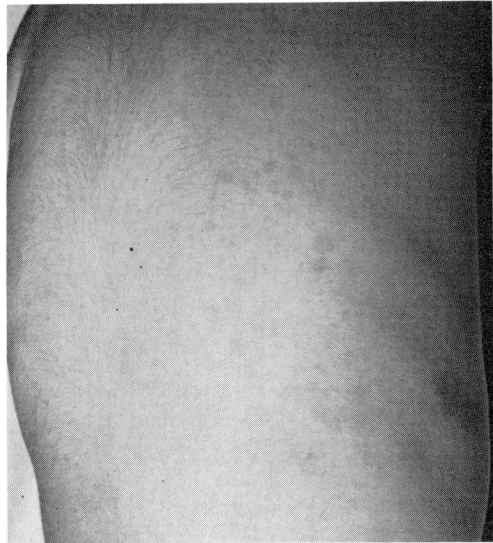

Figure 1-7 Rheumatoid rash.

Rheumatic Papules. Rheumatic cutaneous papules are rare occurrences in juvenile rheumatoid arthritis, only one such case having been seen in Texas Children's Hospital (Fig. 1-8). In this patient rheumatoid papules occurred at age four and three-fourths years. The

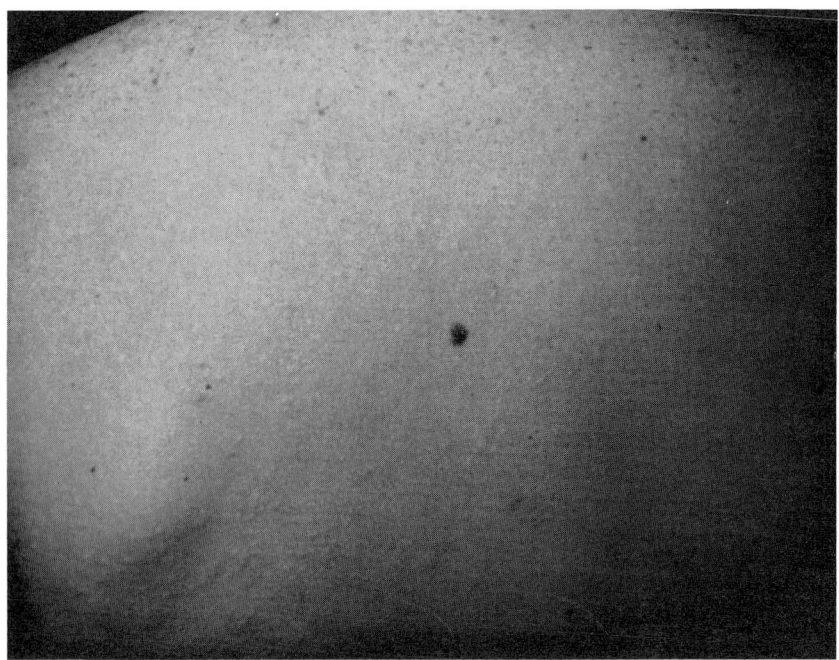

Figure 1-8 Rheumatic papules.

papular lesions were raised, yellowish white with very slight erythema at the base; they blanched on pressure. The papules were located on the back and proximal upper extremities principally, and lasted over a period of five and one-half years. The lesions fluctuated in size slightly over a period of many months. Biopsy revealed that the epidermis was slightly hyperkeratotic and very slightly acanthotic. The main change occurred in the dermis where there was a poorly circumscribed, diffusely nodular infiltration of histiocytes in the middermis. Some of these were around small blood vessels and some were scattered diffusely in the dermis. A few lymphocytes were also present. Examination of many sections failed to reveal any evidence of necrobiosis or other changes that would be distinctive for rheumatoid nodules.

Rheumatoid papules have been previously reported by Burns et al. (1964) in a patient with rheumatic fever. The lesion, therefore, does not appear to be specific for rheumatoid arthritis, and occurs in at least one related disease.

Other Rashes. Children with rheumatoid arthritis have rashes other than the previously described rheumatoid rash and rheumatoid papule. Patients often have urticarial rashes and erythema multiforme; these rashes are nonspecific. Obviously any child may have the myriad of other rashes afflicting children, such as contact dermatitis, heat rash, and various viral exanthems.

Subcutaneous Nodules

Subcutaneous nodules occur in about 10 per cent of children with rheumatoid arthritis at some time during the course of the disease. The incidence has ranged from 2 to 12 per cent in a total of 1116 cases of juvenile rheumatoid arthritis reviewed (see Table 1-5). The nodules occur subcutaneously and vary in size from a few millimeters to several centimeters in greatest diameter. On palpation, a nodular mass of cystic consistency is found, with no attachment to the overlying skin as a rule, but the nodules are often not freely mobile because the base is attached to tendon sheaths or periarticular structures. The nodules are not tender and are customarily found near the olecranon process of the elbow, the extensor tendon sheaths of the fingers and wrist area, and the distal phalangeal areas of the fingers and toes. In the areas of fingers and toes, subcutaneous nodules are only a few millimeters in size because of the tightness of the skin and may appear to have some attachment to the skin. Nodules are also seen along the anterior border of the tibia.

Care must be taken to differentiate bursal swelling near joints from enlarged lymph nodes. Epitrochlear lymph nodes have been known to be confused with subcutaneous nodules, and bursal swelling of the tendon sheath can resemble subcutaneous nodules. Aspiration or biopsy often is the only way to be sure.

Subcutaneous nodules are associated with severe exacerbation of disease but are not related to prognosis. Fifty per cent of Bywaters' 12 juvenile patients with subcutaneous nodules had a positive rheumatoid factor test (Bywaters et al., 1958).

Table 1-4 Comparative Histological Features of Subcutaneous Nodules*

	Rheumatic	Juvenile Rheumatoid	Adult Rheumatoid
Necrosis	0	0	+
Palisade	0	0	+
Edema	+	+	0
Fibrinoid lattice	+	+	±
Vascular islands	+	+	0
Fibrosis	0	+	+

*Modified from Bywaters, E. G. L., Glynn, L. E., and Zeldis, A.: Subcutaneous nodules of Still's disease. Ann. Rheum. Dis., 17:278, 1958.

Subcutaneous nodules occur in juvenile rheumatoid arthritis, in rheumatic fever, and in children with no discernible disease. Histological examination of subcutaneous nodules in adults with rheumatoid arthritis reveals a classic pattern of central necrosis surrounded by palisading fibroblasts with an outer zone of fibrosis. Classic rheumatic fever nodules are characterized by lack of definite zoning with much fibrinoid lattice in which chronic inflammatory cells and histiocytes are distributed. Little necrosis or palisading of fibroblasts is apparent. Vascular islands are prominent in the edematous connective tissue.

The subcutaneous nodules seen in rheumatoid arthritis in children appear histologically to be a mixture of those associated with classic rheumatic fever and those of adult rheumatoid arthritis. Table 1-4 is a chart of the characteristics usually described in the subcutaneous nodules of the three disease states.

In an extensive study, Bywaters found that in 12 patients with juvenile rheumatoid arthritis and subcutaneous nodules, characteristically the nodules were more compatible with those of rheumatic fever than with those of rheumatoid arthritis (Bywaters et al., 1958). Sokoloff (1966), in reviewing subcutaneous nodule biopsies in juvenile rheumatoid arthritis, found that the histologic appearance differs from both the adult rheumatoid nodule and the nodule of rheumatic fever, in that the nodules consist largely of fibrous tissue containing irregularly disposed aggregates of proliferated fibroblasts in relatively small numbers and irregular areas of fibrinoid aggregation. Neither geographic areas of necrosis nor palisade formation was in evidence.

Subcutaneous nodules are also found in children who have no obvious rheumatoid arthritis or other rheumatic disease; trauma or the presence of a foreign body may be possible causes. The usual location has been on the lower extremities in the area of the tibia. One patient has been followed for four years at the Texas Children's Hospital Arthritis Clinic and biopsy on two occasions showed the histologic appearance of a classic adult rheumatoid arthritis subcutaneous nodule (Figs. 1-9, 1-10). In all of the 11 patients with no discernible disease and subcutaneous nodules who have had biopsies at Texas Children's Hospital,

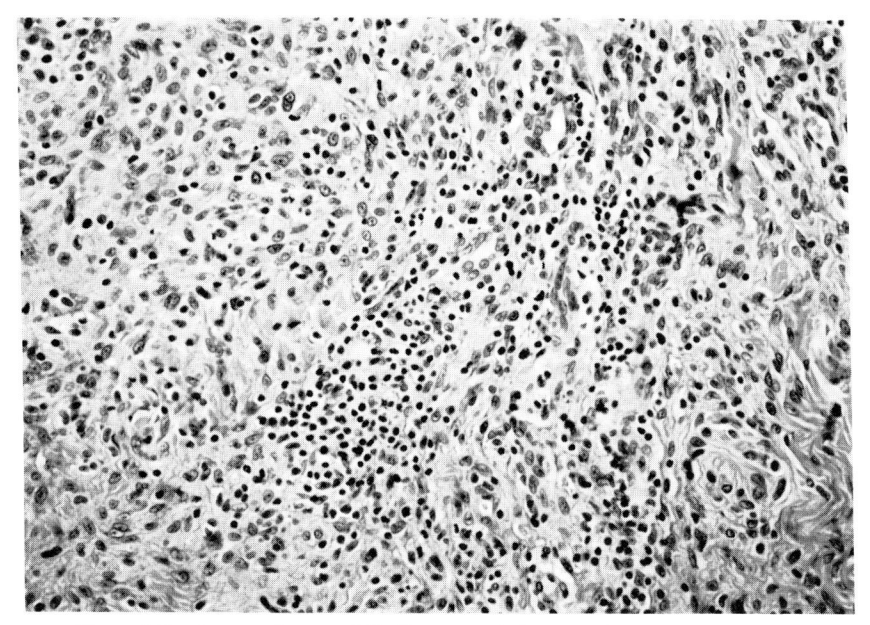

Figure 1-9 A central zone of fibrillar necrosis is seen, with surrounding histiocytes palisading along the edges of the necrotic zone. A few lymphocytes participate in the reaction. (Hematoxylin and eosin, original magnification 100 ×.)

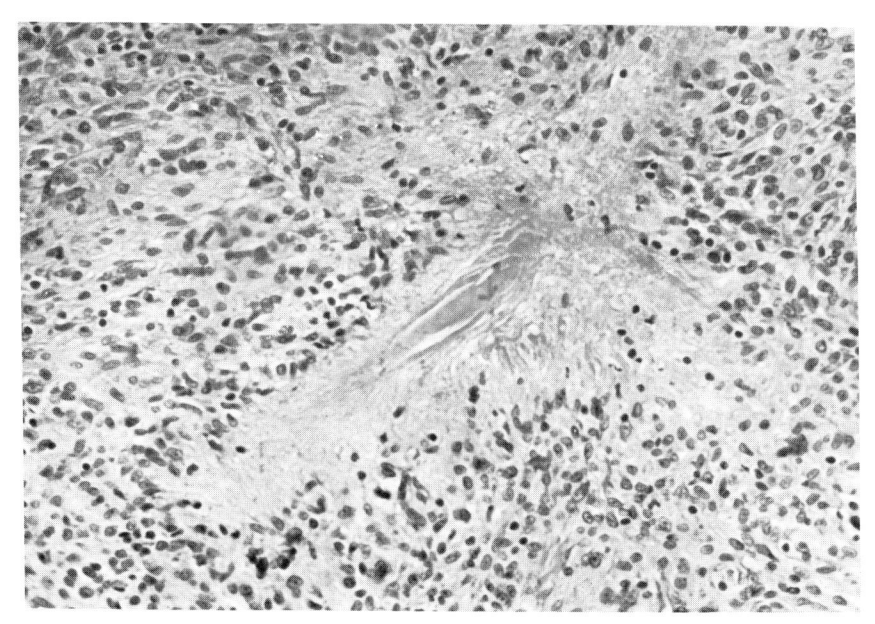

Figure 1-10 In same specimen shown in Figure 1-9, a more cellular deposition is seen, composed of large clusters of lymphocytes with surrounding, palisading histiocytes and fibroblasts. This lesion is more vascular, with multiple capillaries and venules. (Hematoxylin and eosin, original magnification 100 ×.)

there were histologic features of both rheumatoid arthritis and rheumatic fever nodules, but the findings were not specific.

Fever

Fever occurs in three of four children with rheumatoid arthritis, the incidence varying from 62 to 90 per cent in various series (Rawson et al., 1965; Kelley, 1960; Calabro and Marchesano, 1967). Seventy per cent of the Texas Children's Hospital group were febrile at some point of the disease. Fever was reported as a first symptom in 24 to 37 per cent of adults with rheumatoid arthritis by Short et al. (1957).

Patients with fever generally have more severe systemic episodes of disease with rash, lymphadenopathy, splenomegaly, pericarditis, leukocytosis, elevated sedimentation rate, and anemia occurring more commonly (Calabro and Marchesano, 1967). Fever usually accompanies acute exacerbations of disease. A major concern to the physician is the patient whose fever precedes the onset of arthritis, leaving the diagnosis obscure.

Calabro and Marchesano (1967) reported that 18 of 50 patients with juvenile rheumatoid arthritis had fever antedating the onset of articular manifestations. Twelve of these patients had fever higher than 102° F. with a median duration of three and one-half months and a range of three weeks to nine years. Six additional patients had fever lower than 102° F. antedating articular manifestations, with a median duration of two and one-half weeks, and a range of one to 13 weeks. This is the first documented quantitation of fever preceding the onset of articular disease. The experience at Texas Children's Hospital has shown that careful examination of joints usually reveals early articular manifestations within a few weeks after the onset with fever. Undoubtedly there are a few patients with fever preceding the onset of objective joint manifestations for varying periods of time.

Patients with monarticular rheumatoid arthritis seldom have high fever and other manifestations of systemic disease. This is probably related to severity of illness.

All types of febrile responses occur in juvenile rheumatoid arthritis. The fever curve that is most frequently associated with the disease in the clinician's mind is the daily diurnal swing of fever from normal to higher than 102° F., with return to normal or subnormal. This type of fever is often called hectic, spiking, septic, or intermittent. This same febrile response occurs in other diseases such as sepsis or leukemia. This type of fever is the most troublesome to the clinician, especially when present prior to the onset of objective articular manifestations.

Another febrile response is fever higher than 102° F. with daily remissions to a lower level, but not to normal. This type of curve may occur in the same patient with intermittent fever, and has also been termed spiking, septic, remittent, and hectic.

A low grade fever, lower than 101 or 102° F., with daily rise and fall to normal, or even continuous fever, is probably more common than the high spikes of intermittent fever, and it occurred in 25 of 100 patients reviewed. Continuous fever higher than 101° F. is an uncommon type of febrile response.

MANIFESTATIONS OF DISEASE 21

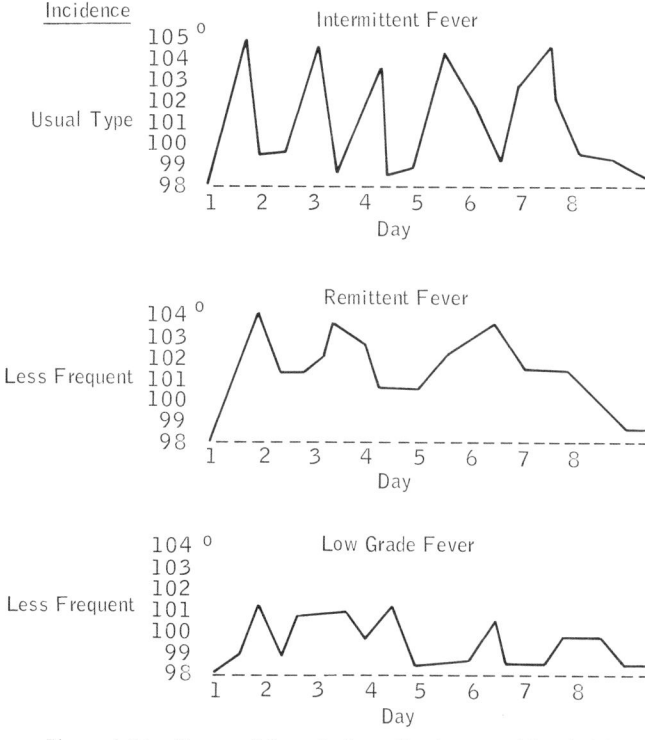

Figure 1-11 Types of fever in juvenile rheumatoid arthritis.

The recrudescence of fever in response to salicylate administration has been cited by many as a helpful tool in differentiating rheumatic fever from rheumatoid arthritis. A significant number of patients with rheumatoid arthritis have prompt remission of temperature after proper salicylate administration, and febrile response cannot be used as a differential diagnostic tool. The response of fever to salicylates, steroids, and indomethacin is discussed in another chapter.

Lymphadenopathy

Generalized lymphadenopathy is associated with severe exacerbation of systemic disease and occurs at one time or another in perhaps 25 per cent of all patients. In the series reported, the average has been about 23 per cent with a range of 9 to 60 per cent in a total number of 1017 patients (Table 1-5). Lymphatic enlargement may occur at any location but is most often seen in the axillary, cervical, inguinal, and epitrochlear regions. The enlarged nodes are nontender and well circumscribed, and the duration of enlargement may be a few days to several months. Protracted enlargement of the lymph nodes over a period of years is known, but is unusual. There is always difficulty in assessing localized lymph node enlargement and its relation to rheumatoid arthritis, particularly in the cervical region of a child with a

Table 1-5 Clinical Manifestations of Rheumatoid Arthritis in a Series of Studies

	Number of Patients	Nodules	Spleno-megaly	Hepato-megaly	Lymph-adenopathy	Fever	Rash	Ocular Manifesta-tion	Cardiac Involve-ment
Grokoest et al.	110	2 (2%)	11 (10%)	12 (11%)	28 (25%)	48 (44%)	10 (9%)	2 (2%)	—
Norcross, Lockie, and MacLeod	62	—	9 (15%)	5 (8%)	10 (16%)	26 (40%)	—	5 (7%)	12 (19%)
Lockie	28	—	4 (14%)	3 (11%)	5 (18%)	12 (43%)	—	1 (4%)	2 (7%)
Ansell and Bywaters	316	22 (7%)	79 (25%)	—	—	79 (25%)	79 (25%)	25 (8%)	22 (7%)
Lindbjerg	75	6 (8%)	7 (9%)	3 (4%)	29 (39%)	35 (47%)	15 (20%)	8 (11%)	3 (4%)
Toumbis	50	6 (12%)	13 (26%)	12 (24%)	20 (40%)	37 (74%)	7 (14%)	—	19 (38%)
Grossman	229	21 (9%)	29 (13%)	—	48 (21%)	—	46 (20%)	5 (2%)	8 (3%)
Laurin and Fauvreau	31	—	1 (3%)	3 (10%)	3 (10%)	17 (55%)	11 (35%)	5 (15%)	—
Martel et al.	80	8 (10%)	14 (18%)	—	7 (9%)	—	15 (19%)	3 (4%)	10 (13%)
Schlesinger	100	7 (7%)	—	—	—	—	40 (40%)	5 (5%)	6 (6%)
Edström	161	—	7 (4%)	7 (4%)	7 (4%)	—	—	12 (7%)	—
Coss and Boots	56	2 (4%)	17 (30%)	13 (23%)	35 (60%)	—	—	—	7 (13%)
Kelley	100	10 (10%)	33 (33%)	33 (33%)	33 (33%)	—	—	—	—
Pickard	35	—	5 (14%)	6 (17%)	1 (3%)	—	—	1 (3%)	2 (6%)

Clinical Manifestations in 100 Patients at Texas Children's Hospital

Manifestation	Yes	No	Not known
Morning stiffness	83	16	1
Initial hepatomegaly	19	81	
History of preceding infection	46	52	2
History of preceding surgery	10	90	
History of preceding trauma	12	88	
Family history of rheumatoid arthritis	41	58	1
Family history of rheumatic fever	15	83	2
Family history of allergy	36	61	3
Fever (low grade, 26; spiking, 44)	70	29	1
Rash	44	56	

Manifestation	Yes	No	Not known
One joint involved first	51	47	2
Bilateral joint involvement at any time	80	20	
Monarticular joint involvement	10	90	
with other minor joint involvement	7	3	Data incomplete
Nodules	27	59	14
Abdominal pain	26	58	16
Lymphadenopathy (first exam)	24	75	1
Hepatomegaly (at any time)	5	79	16
Splenomegaly (first exam)			

high incidence of local respiratory infection. In the epitrochlear region, care must be exercised not to confuse an enlarged lymph node with a subcutaneous nodule.

Splenomegaly

Splenomegaly occurs in perhaps one fourth of all patients, with an average frequency of 16 per cent, ranging from 3 to 33 per cent in a total of 1333 patients (Table 1-5). The spleen is usually moderately firm in consistency, nontender, freely mobile, and not nodular on physical examination. It usually extends 2 to 4 cm. below the left costal margin in the midclavicular line. Massive enlargement of the spleen is unusual and, when present, plasma cell hepatitis must be ruled out. Bywaters has found that when patients manifest splenomegaly, amyloidosis must be considered later in the course of the disease (Ansell and Bywaters, 1963).

Portal hypertension does occur as a complication of juvenile rheumatoid arthritis, and enlargement of the spleen to the iliac crest is known. In patients with massive enlargement of the spleen, studies for esophageal varices should be undertaken and bleeding secondary to esophageal varices has occurred in at least one of the Texas Children's Hospital patients.

Hepatomegaly

Hepatomegaly (greater than 2 cm. below the right costal margin in the midclavicular line) occurred in 18 of 67 patients in our study who were specifically evaluated and followed over a period of years. The usual incidence reported is 16 per cent, with a range of 4 to 33 per cent in a total of 708 patients reviewed (Table 1-5). The liver, when enlarged, usually extends 2 to 5 cm. below the right costal margin in the midclavicular line, and is nontender, soft in consistency, and smooth in outline. The usual duration of hepatomegaly is a few days to one or two months. Prolonged and persistent hepatomegaly is unusual.

When massive hepatomegaly is present, with enlargement to the iliac crest and with associated ascites, plasma cell hepatitis must be ruled out.

Liver function tests were performed in those patients with hepatomegaly, and no abnormalities were detected other than an increase in the gamma globulin measured by serum electrophoretic methods. The prothrombin times were increased only in those patients receiving large doses of aspirin. When salicylate dosage was significantly reduced, return to normal levels occurred. The cephalin flocculation, thymol turbidity, bilirubin, serum glutamic oxaloacetic transaminase, and serum glutamic pyruvic acetic transaminase were all normal.

Three needle liver biopsies have been performed in patients with hepatomegaly, and periportal round cell infiltration was the only abnormality noted. The architecture and cellular histology were completely normal. Two patients revealed changes consistent with plasma cell hepatitis and associated massive hepatosplenomegaly, peritoneal effusion, and elevation of the gamma globulin greater than 2.5 gm. per ml. Plasma cell hepatitis will be discussed in Chapter Five. There is some concern that this entity may well be a part of the spectrum of severe juvenile rheumatoid arthritis.

Ocular Involvement

Rheumatoid arthritis in children may involve the iris, ciliary body, lens, cornea, and, rarely, the sclera or choroid. The incidence of ocular involvement varies from 2 to 15 per cent in the reported series (Table 1-5). The simplest, but least common, lesion is acute iritis, detected principally by asymmetry of the pupil. In pure form, the lesion is often acute and responds well to corticosteroid drops when administered in early stages. The insidious onset of iritis, with subsequent involvement of the ciliary body, is followed at times by a band-like keratopathy or the development of cataracts. The lesion may be unilateral but is more often bilateral (Smiley et al., 1957). Bilateral involvement is not necessarily present at the same time.

Ocular inflammation usually begins several years after the onset of juvenile rheumatoid arthritis. Occasionally polyarthritis and inflammation of the eye occur within months of each other. Only rarely does isolated iridocyclitis occur several years prior to the onset of rheumatoid arthritis (Smiley et al., 1957; Blegvad, 1941; Vesterdal et al., 1950; Franceschetti et al., 1951; Hatherley, 1951).

The insidious onset of iridocyclitis is usually found by the patient or physician noticing asymmetry of the pupil or diminution of vision. Rarely there is acute onset of pain, conjunctivitis, or obvious leukocytic aggregation with cellular precipitation into the anterior chamber of the eye. Slit lamp examination in early involvement reveals a nongranulomatous fibrinous inflammation of the iris, and synechiae present from the anterior surface of the iris to the anterior lens capsule. Cellular debris may be found in the anterior chamber fluid. The anatomic pathology is not well documented (Sokoloff, 1966).

Band keratopathy consists of fibrosis of the cornea complicating iridocyclitis. This complication developed in nine of 18 eyes with iridocyclitis in Bywaters' series (Smiley et al., 1957). Cataract formation secondary to iridocyclitis is not common. When present, involvement is severe with rapid progression and serious interference with vision.

Unusual sequelae of ocular involvement include phthisis bulbi and secondary glaucoma. Ophthalmologists see patients who have recurrent or persistent attacks of acute iridocyclitis, with serious interference with vision, but no arthritis. Although rheumatoid arthritis does occur with increasing frequency in this type of patient, a significant number fail to ever manifest arthritis.

Posterior subcapsular cataracts have been reported in patients receiving corticosteroid therapy but this complication has not been of importance in children.

Ocular inflammation in the United States has not been reported with the frequency found elsewhere (Smiley et al., 1957). The disparity in incidence may be related to the length of time the patients have been

Manifestations of Disease

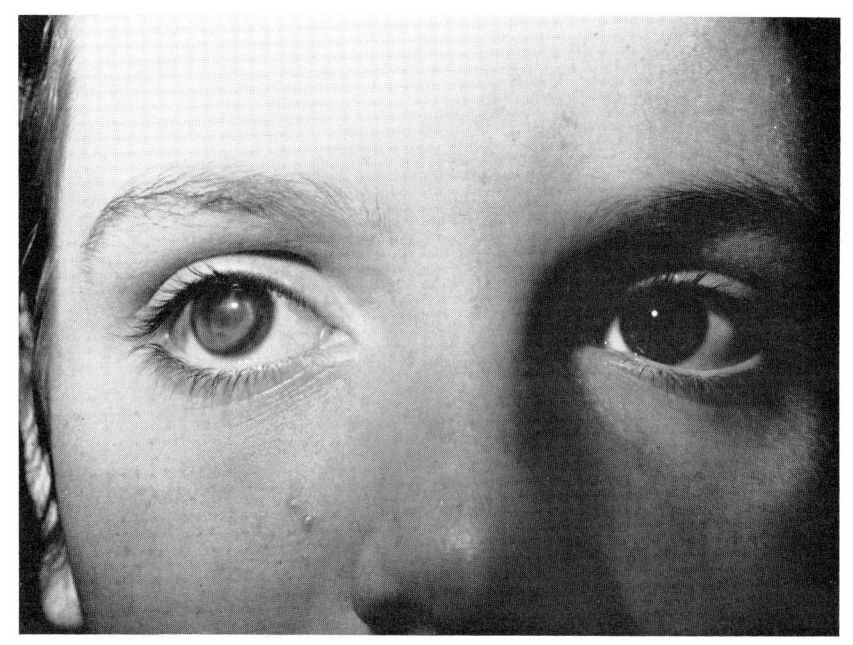

Figure 1-12 Iridocyclitis with severe iritis and secondary keratitis, right eye. Cornea opacification required corneal transplantation.

systemically followed. Children with rheumatoid arthritis should have a slit lamp ophthalmological examination each year.

Nonspecific Abdominal Pain

Nonspecific abdominal pain occurs in about one fourth of children with juvenile rheumatoid arthritis at some time during the course of the disease. The symptom is of concern to the physician, and the many causes of abdominal pain must be considered carefully each time it occurs. In addition, many children, at one time or another, have significant abdominal pain for which no cause is ever found. The incidence of peptic ulcer also seems to be increased in patients with rheumatoid arthritis. Even beyond the usual organic and emotional causes of abdominal pain found in any child, patients with juvenile rheumatoid arthritis seem to have episodes of nonspecific abdominal pain. There has been no characteristic location of the pain; it varies from epigastric or periumbilical areas to areas designated by diffuse complaints. The pain may be mild and constant or acute and cramping and may last an hour to several days. The frequency of episodes, as a rule, is limited to an occasional attack.

When abdominal pain occurs, one must be careful to rule out gastritis associated with salicylate medication, peptic ulcer, gastroenteritis, or emotional stress. Other causes, including surgical diseases, must also be ruled out.

Peptic Ulcer

Peptic ulcer occurs with increasing frequency in adults with rheumatoid arthritis, but the incidence had increased even before the advent of steroid therapy. Medications used in the treatment of rheumatoid arthritis enhance the likelihood of peptic ulcer, the corticosteroid derivatives being the leading precipitating factor. Salicylates can cause gastritis and are ulcerogenic. Phenylbutazone and indomethacin also can precipitate peptic ulcer in patients with rheumatic diseases.

Peptic ulcer in children with arthritis also seems to occur with increasing frequency and is aggravated by several of the medications used in therapy. Peptic ulcer has occurred in seven of our patients, almost all of whom were on steroids at the time of the occurrence. The onset of peptic ulcer in these patients is usually heralded by epigastric abdominal pain that is at times dull and aching with no radiation, interspersed with periods of acute and severe cramping.

Physical findings are usually limited to tenderness in the epigastric region and right upper quadrant. Auscultation usually reveals no alteration in peristalsis. Distention may be prominent in children during acute episodes. The child is often acutely ill with pain but more often than not merely has subjective complaints.

The pain is not necessarily related to meals, nor is it alleviated with food or milk. Nausea has not been a prominent symptom in these children. Melena can be the initial manifestation and, indeed, hemorrhage can be massive. The following case history presents some of the problems encountered.

N. D. was a nine-year-old white female who was admitted to the hospital October 27, 1963, with a history of rheumatoid arthritis for two and three-fourths years. The patient previously had had high fever; polyarthritis involving the wrists, elbows, shoulders, and knees; rheumatoid rash, hepatomegaly, and splenomegaly. Seven months prior to admission the patient had been hospitalized for pneumonia and severe systemic symptoms of rheumatoid arthritis for which prednisone was given orally in dosages of up to 15 mg. daily.

On the day of admission, the patient complained of nausea and abdominal pain. Massive hematemesis occurred four times immediately prior to admission.

Physical examination revealed a temperature of 99.4° F. The heart rate/minute was 130, the respiratory rate/minute 35, and the blood pressure 108/92. The patient was acutely ill and pale. The pertinent physical findings were limited to the abdomen, with epigastric tenderness and increased peristalsis to auscultation. The liver was enlarged 2 to 3 cm. below the right costal margin; the spleen was 2 to 3 cm. below the left costal margin. Initial laboratory data revealed the hemoglobin to be 8.7 gm. per 100 ml.; hematocrit 29 per cent; W.B.C. 25,200; and platelets "adequate." The differential count was 74 per cent polymorphonuclear leukocytes, 22 per cent lymphocytes, 3 per cent monocytes, and 1 per cent eosinophils. Upper gastrointestinal roentgenographic examination on October 23, 1963, prior to admission had revealed no abnormality of the esophagus and no evidence of varices. The stomach appeared normal but the pyloric canal revealed two ulcers, one of which was posterior and inferior, with extension of contrast material into what may have been a perforation. A similar small ulcer was seen on the lesser curvature with no evidence of perforation (Fig. 1-13).

Course in Hospital. The patient pursued a febrile course with fever at one time over 106° F. Blood cultures were negative. She was treated with suction initially, followed by a milk and cream diet, an antispasmodic, an antacid, and intravenous hydrocortisone. Bleeding persisted intermittently and the patient

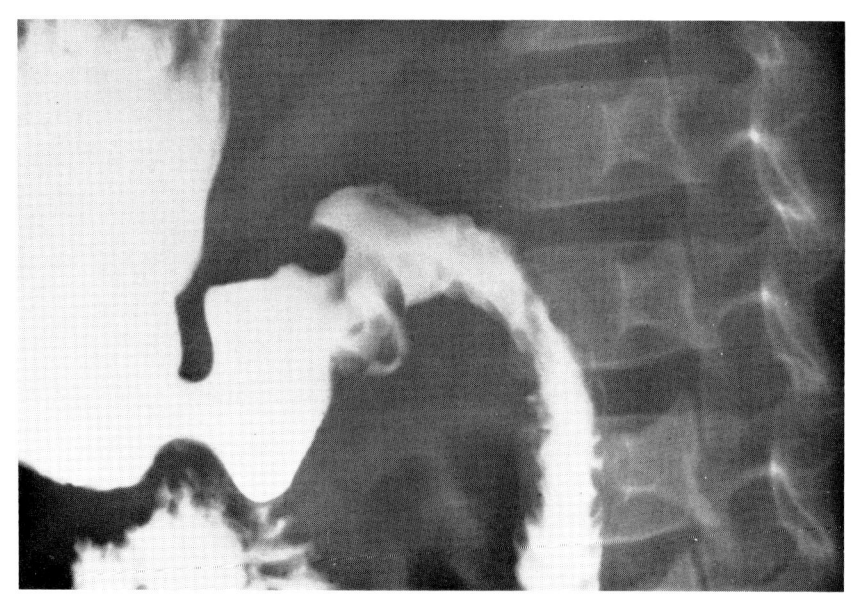

Figure 1-13 Gastric ulcers: A shallow crater is seen on the lesser curvature of the antrum, and a large ulcer with distention of the mucosal folds is seen on the greater curvature side of the antrum, with involvement of the proximal portion of the pyloric canal.

required over 4000 ml. of whole blood transfusion from admission on October 27 to November 12. Because of persistent bleeding and the possibility of ulcer perforation with dissection into the pancreas, exploration was performed on November 14. On exploration, enlargement of the liver and spleen was noted and a large posterior pyloric peptic ulcer was found. Half of the ulcer was in the stomach and half in the duodenum; it measured about 1.5 cm. at the greatest diameter, with penetration into the pancreas. A partial gastrectomy (20 per cent) was performed along with vagotomy and gastrojejunostomy. The stump of the duodenum was placed in the pancreatic defect. The patient improved dramatically following surgery, but with almost immediate recrudescence of the 106° F. fever. The patient was never hypertensive, but maintenance of normal blood pressure was difficult because of blood lost prior to the operation.

The patient recovered uneventfully after surgery with stabilization of the hemogram, and was dismissed on the twenty-sixth postoperative day in satisfactory condition. She had no subsequent recurrence of ulceration or symptoms, even though steroid therapy continued to be necessary to reduce the fever of 105 to 106° F. to a more nearly normal level.

The prognosis for these peptic ulcers is excellent and healing occurs with proper medication even while steroid medication is continued at a reduced dosage of less than 10 mg. per day of prednisone, or the equivalent. A detailed discussion of therapy is found in Chapter Nine.

GROWTH FACTORS

Alterations in body growth depend primarily on the severity of the disease. As the disease process becomes more severe, growth alterations occur. The degree of growth alteration depends also on the duration of

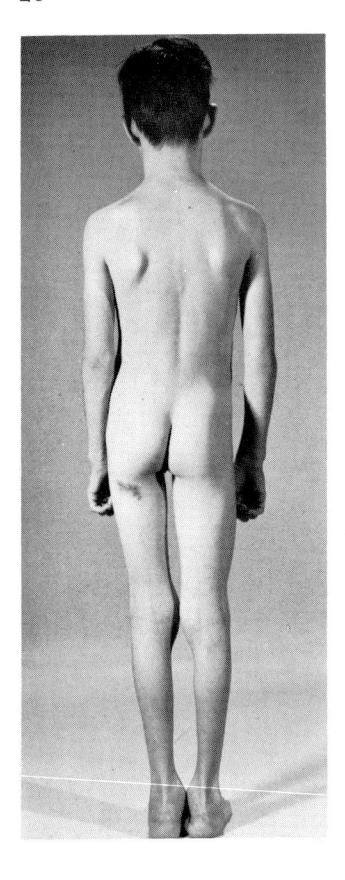

Figure 1-14 A 10-year-old boy had had rheumatoid arthritis of the left knee and both ankles for three and one-half years. Overgrowth of the affected left lower extremity is evident.

activity. The longer serious disease activity is present, the more significant growth alteration becomes. Disturbances of growth are both generalized and local. Generalized growth failure can result from inadequate nutrition as well as from the active disease process. Diminution of growth can result from retardation of epiphyseal development or from premature fusion of epiphyses. In the same patient who has generalized undergrowth, local alterations of growth may occur causing actual overgrowth of a given joint, such as the knee, unilaterally, resulting in variation in leg length (Fig. 1-14). Undergrowth of the joint is manifest by either retardation of epiphyseal development or by premature epiphyseal fusion.

Generalized Growth Disturbance

Even before the advent of steroid therapy, stunting of growth had been well documented in juvenile rheumatoid arthritis (Ansell and Bywaters, 1956; Still, 1897). Radiologically, inhibition of growth can be shown by growth disturbance lines in the metaphyses of the bones of the major extremities (Harris, 1933; Hewitt et al., 1955). The lines are horizontal bands of calcific density of varying widths depending on the duration of the growth inhibition secondary to the disease state. The lines probably represent deposits of calcium in the absence of orderly growth. They are nonspecific and occur in any disease process inhibiting growth.

The majority of patients with mild juvenile rheumatoid arthritis do not exhibit significant growth failure in either height or weight. However, in severe disease, growth failure exceeding 25 per cent is common even with no steroid therapy (Fig. 1-15).

Cortisone and its derivatives are definitely known to inhibit growth. Apparently growth inhibition results from pituitary suppression of growth hormone resulting in retardation of the orderly development of the epiphyses and of normal growth and length. After the cessation of steroid administration, many patients do exhibit a rapid return toward normal height and weight over a period of about a year or two. Whether the patients ever recover total height lost during the inhibition of growth resulting from the administration of steroids is difficult to determine. Patients who receive steroid preparations always have severe disease; the inhibition of growth due to disease and that due to steroid administration cannot be separated clearly.

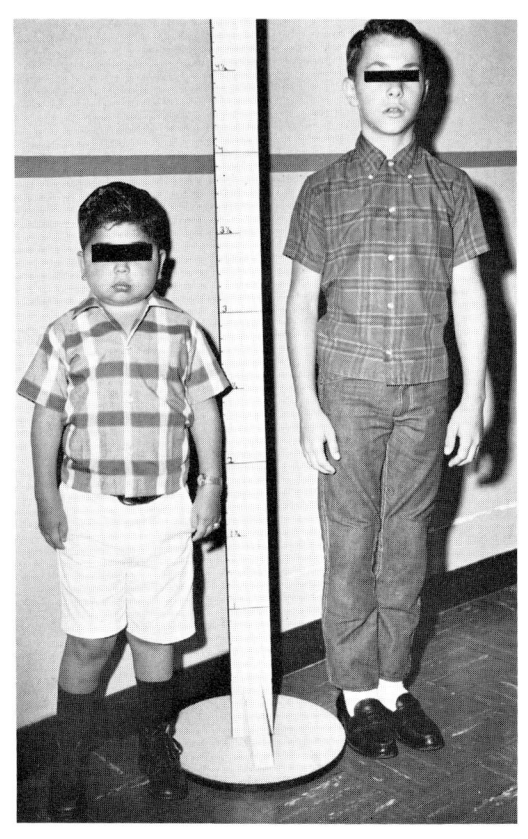

Figure 1-15 Undergrowth shown with normal child for comparison.

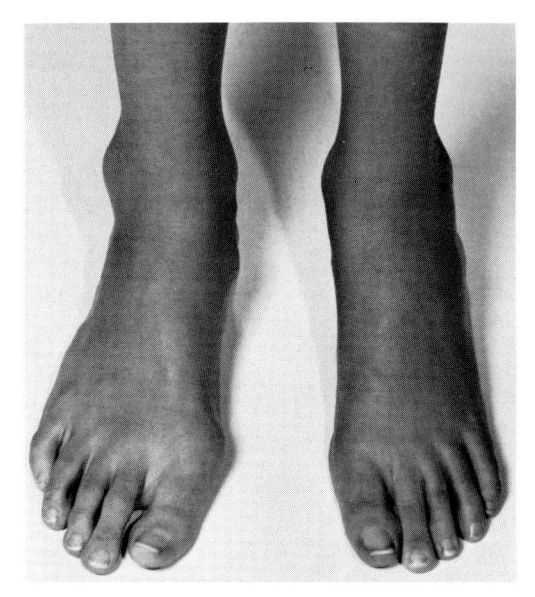

Figure 1-16 Partial undergrowth of foot.

Testosterone and its many analogues were popular for a few years in attempts to increase the growth of children with rheumatoid arthritis. Rapid growth over a period of months is possible with testosterone and its derivatives but as an unfortunate later effect, it causes premature closure of the epiphyses, ultimately further stunting total adult growth. For this reason, this product and its derivatives are no longer recommended.

Localized Growth Alteration

An interesting paradox of juvenile rheumatoid arthritis is that while the total body growth may be inhibited, simultaneous local overgrowth of an extremity may occur. Various reasons are given, including increased vascularity causing excessive and enhanced growth of the epiphyses. Some observers have reported increased hirsutism and perspiration in the extremities with overgrowth (Ansell and Bywaters, 1956).

Undergrowth of a particular joint may cause an actual shortening of the part (Fig. 1-16). Entire extremities may suffer from total growth failure.

EXAMINATION OF THE JOINTS

Examination of the joints in the pediatric age group has the added dimension of providing knowledge of changes in the growing child. An appreciation of the normal appearance of joints in each age group becomes important. The techniques of examination, to elicit valid information concerning inflammation, vary in different age groups. Joint examination should begin by observing the patient walking a considerable distance. In this manner, a limp becomes apparent, the quality of posture is noted, the angle at which joints are held can be readily seen, and functional limitation of motion of the extremities and neck is observed. The symmetry of the shoulders and hips while walking should be noted. Weakness of the upper back muscles or shoulder can often be demonstrated by shoulder drop. Scoliosis of the lumbar spine caused by a difference in leg length can also be observed by watching the patient during walking.

Erythema

Examination of the individual joints begins with observation of the skin for redness. Significant erythema is unusual in juvenile rheumatoid arthritis. In fact, if it is present, one must carefully consider pyogenic arthritis or other etiologies.

Heat

The skin overlying the involved joints is often slightly warm to the touch when compared with the other side or other areas, but extreme heat is unusual.

Swelling

Inflammation of the synovium is not the sole cause of joint swelling or enlargement. Usually periarticular swelling or edema also occurs. Periarticular swelling is a diffuse inflammatory swelling extending beyond the limits of the synovium. Synovial thickening itself can be detected by rubbing the fingers over a bony prominence. A thickened synovium has a compressible, almost spongy, texture to palpation or pressure. Effusion in the joint is often best demonstrated by ballottement or manually forcing fluid from one part of the joint to another and palpating the change in location of the swelling. Bursal swellings about the joint often connect with the synovial lining of the joint itself and must be distinguished from subcutaneous nodules. Distortion of bony architecture can sometimes be detected by palpation. Such distortion usually consists of expansion of the width of the joint.

Tenderness

Tenderness is usually not severe in children with rheumatoid arthritis but may occasionally be almost exquisite in character. A few patients have tenderness of the overlying skin.

Limitation of Motion

Limitation of motion is an important aspect of joint examination, for it not only helps in establishing joint involvement but is essential in following the progress of disease; improvement is a major goal of therapy. The extent of limitation of motion must be established in all ranges of normal motion of the joint—in particular, the weight-bearing joints in extension and flexion. The limitation must be established by active motion (motion performed by the patient himself) or passive motion (motion performed by the examiner). Quite early in the disease, children with rheumatoid arthritis have a marked limitation of active motion and less restriction of passive motion.

Crepitation

Many patients and parents note unusual sounds when the joints are moved. This is crepitation and is related either to synovial surface alterations or, at times, to the rush of fluid from one part of the joint to another with movement.

Muscular Atrophy

The muscles must be observed carefully for early evidence of atrophy or wasting. Weakness is a prominent early finding in muscles around the involved joints. Spasm of the muscles as a reaction to pain can also be prominent.

Specific Joint Involvement

Knee

Examination of the knee should begin by observing the patient for a limp while he is walking. The child should be checked for knock-knee deformity, which is gauged by measuring the distance between the malleoli of the ankles. Minimal swelling of the joint is best observed by noting the bony landmarks and the concavities on various sides of the patella. Loss of concavity, with convexity causing bulging, is often the only sign of minimal knee involvement. Atrophy of the muscles (the quadriceps and the posterior tibial group) may be observed and measured by comparison with the circumference of the opposite member. It is important to remember that all features of the disease may be bilateral, and a knowledge of the normal becomes essential. Palpation will detect the nature of knee swelling. Synovial thickening is best ascertained by rolling the synovial tissue between the finger and a bony prominence. Periarticular soft tissue swelling is distinguished in this manner also. Effusion can often be detected by ballottement or forcing fluid to the upper part of the joint and then gently pushing the fluid back into the anterior bulging surfaces.

Swelling is the most prominent finding in involvement of the knee; periarticular swelling is the usual type. Synovial thickening is often a prominent finding. Effusion is usually moderate in amount; massive effusion is unusual.

Another method of demonstrating the presence of fluid in the knee is to flex the knee to force fluid from the anterosuperior portion.

The knee is then extended and the hand placed over the kneecap area. A palpable thrill occurs as the fluid rushes back to the anterior part of the knee.

A striking early finding in patients with knee involvement is the rapid atrophy of the quadriceps muscle group. Atrophy of other muscles about the knee, above and below, is also present. Weakness accompanies this rapid atrophy and contributes to the limitation of motion.

Limitation of motion, when present, is usually about 15 to 30 degrees of flexion contracture and is commonly caused by swelling rather than pain or tenderness. There is often restriction of motion on extreme flexion from the normal 120 degrees to only 80 or 90 degrees of flexion. Patients who are placed in cylinder casts for several weeks often develop stiffness at the angle the knee is placed. The angle often precludes normal gait later. Some patients do not have this problem, but in the author's experience the majority sustain some flexion contracture with prolonged cylinder casting. In the knee, this particular fixation of movement can be corrected with adequate physical therapy and orthotic devices. Tenderness is elicited by direct palpation and by motion of the joint.

Bursae may be located at the points of attachment of the medial and lateral collateral ligaments of the knee, the tibial tuberosity, and the prepatellar area. The motion of the knee varies from 0 degrees full extension to 120 or 130 degrees of flexion. There is little, if any, lateral or medial movement of the knee joint. This can be checked by exerting pressure inward and outward with the femur fixed. Subluxation can be checked by exerting force on the tibia anteriorly and posteriorly with the femur fixed.

In juvenile rheumatoid arthritis, erythema is unusual. Tenderness is usually not severe and marked limitation of motion is, more often than not, iatrogenic. If left to their own devices, children seem to maintain a reasonable range of motion in the knee.

Later manifestations of the disease include overgrowth and undergrowth of the affected joint. Widening of the epiphysis and metaphysis can also occur with narrowing of the joint space. Actual destruction of the joint with erosion of the cortex and secondary inflammatory tissue invasion can occur. Bony ankylosis is rare in this joint. Posterior subluxation of the tibia has been reported but one cannot discount the iatrogenic effects of various forms of traction (in particular, Buck's traction) (Griffin et al., 1963).

Because of the normal irregularity of growing epiphyses, an evaluation of bony erosion is frequently difficult. This is particularly true regarding the knee.

Ankle

Observation of a child with ankle involvement often reveals a duck-like, flat-footed gait, much like that of a one- to two-year-old, as a result of limitation of motion. Minimal swelling of the ankle is best observed by noting convex bulging of the internal and external retromalleolar sulci, anterior to both malleoli, lateral to the tendon of the peroneus tertius, and medial to the tibialis anterior tendon. At these two points the ankle joint is most superficial, and palpation of the synovial tissue is best accomplished here. Periarticular soft tissue swelling is best distinguished in this area also. Effusion is difficult to ascertain with certainty, but tension of the capsule and ballottement are helpful guides. Atrophy of the muscles of the lower leg is often a prominent associated finding. Periarticular swelling accompanied by synovial thickening and some effusion are the usual findings in the ankle joint of children with rheumatoid arthritis (Fig. 1-17). Massive effusion is seen on occasion.

Tenosynovitis of the tendon sheaths associated with the retinaculum surrounding the ankle joint must be differentiated from ankle joint involvement itself. The two often occur together but may occur singly. The extent of tenosynovitis is determined by palpation to differentiate from ankle joint involvement alone. Bursae in the area can be confused with tenosynovitis; such bursae often connect with the ankle joint itself. A frequent site of bursitis is at the Achilles tendon attachment to the os calcis. Clinically, pain on walking occurs especially with the foot in dorsiflexion, and pain anterior to the tendon is present.

Plantar flexion of the ankle joint up to 45 degrees from neutral position is normal, and dorsiflexion to 20 degrees from neutral position is considered normal. Normally there should be no lateral or medial motion of the ankle joint itself.

As with other joints, erythema is unusual and tenderness is usually

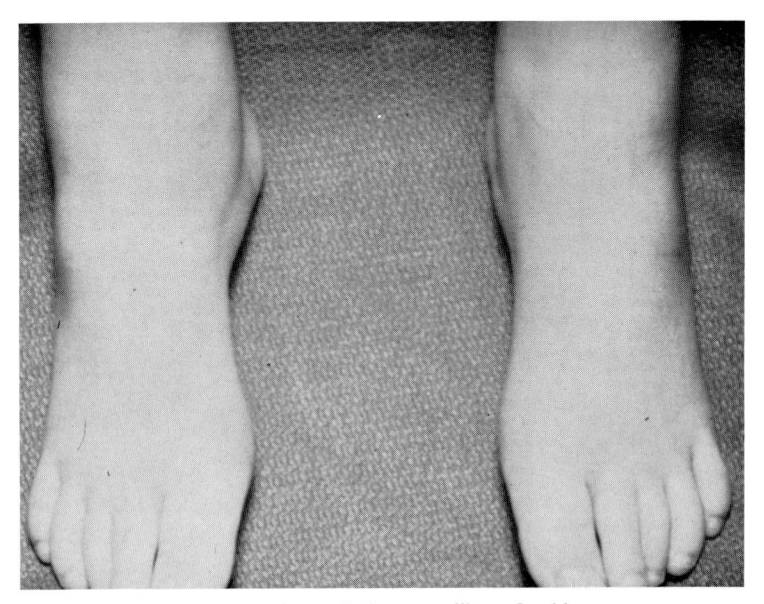

Figure 1-17 Soft tissue swelling of ankle.

not severe. Limitation of motion most often occurs in dorsiflexion, usually as a result of tightening of the Achilles tendon.

Later manifestations of the disease in the ankle joint again involve overgrowth and undergrowth of the part with a reduction of joint space. Juxta-articular osteoporosis is seen along with soft tissue swelling early in the disease. Bony ankylosis is extremely rare.

Foot

Examination of the foot must be conducted with the child bearing weight and also sitting. Pronation of the feet with attendant valgus of the calcaneus is a frequent finding. Pes planus (flattening of the long arch) is an accompanying feature. A cock-up deformity of the metatarsal phalangeal joints may be present. Local tenderness, particularly of the talonavicular and the metatarsophalangeal joint areas, often is the only objective physical finding. In the growing child, swelling is difficult to detect in these areas. Areas of callus or abrasions should be noted because many children have been subjected to poorly fitted shoes; variations in the size of the foot due to swelling may cause local pressure. The foot normally moves 20 to 40 degrees from neutral position in inversion, and 20 degrees from neutral position in eversion. Limitation of motion, when present, usually occurs in dorsiflexion of the ankle.

Later manifestations can occur as a flattening of the foot with rigidity caused by flattening of the longitudinal arch; talonavicular joint involvement leading to peroneal muscular spasm, accompanied usually by significant involvement of the ankle with narrowing of the joint space; and flattening of the entire posterior foot. A cavus foot deformity can occur with a cock-up toe deformity.

Wrist

Rheumatoid involvement of the wrist presents one of the most troublesome and restricting problems in children. Swelling and limitation of motion are the two most prominent features. The wrist should extend to about 70 degrees from neutral position and flex to about 80 degrees from neutral position. Lateral medial motion should have a range of about 65 degrees from neutral position. When the wrist is involved, a striking early feature is limitation of extension. Both active and passive motion are often restricted, followed later by restriction of flexion and lateral medial motion. Swelling of the joint is usually periarticular, accompanied by synovial thickening. Massive effusion of the wrist is not a usual finding. Tenosynovitis of the extensor tendon sheath is a frequent manifestation and can be differentiated by palpating the extent of the sheath, and by location of tenderness along the tendon sheath. Bursal swelling frequently accompanies tenosynovitis and arthritis of the wrist.

Muscular weakness about the wrist is often noted early and one is hard pressed to decide whether limitation of motion is caused by synovial involvement, tenosynovitis of associated tendon sheaths, or muscu-

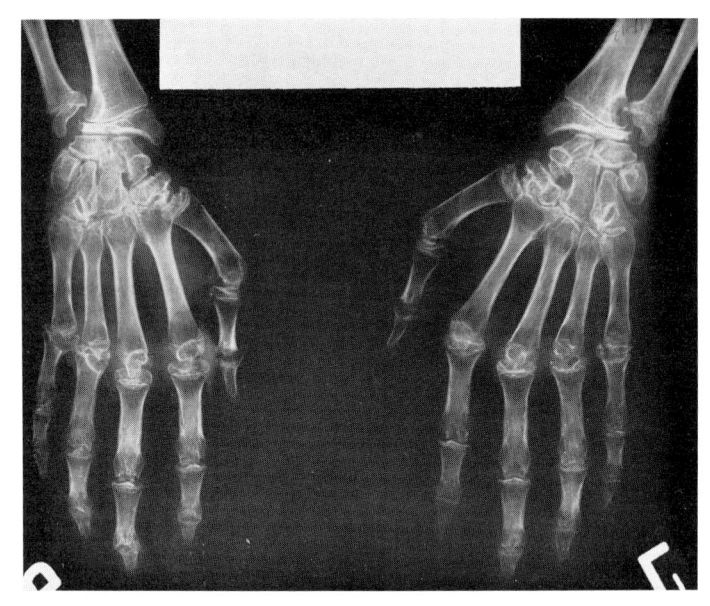

Figure 1-18 Radiographs of the hands, showing advanced changes of rheumatoid arthritis involving the metacarpophalangeal joints, the interphalangeal joints, and the carpal joints. Extensive destruction of articular cartilage is evident with associated ulnar deviation of the phalanges. Marked erosive changes are seen at the distal ulnoradial articulation.

lar atrophy and weakness. A combination of all of these causes is probably more common.

In particular, the wrist is prone to ankylosis as a late manifestation. This is accompanied by destructive changes, as shown by x-ray, with actual fusion of carpal bones, reduction of joint space in the wrist, local erosions, and cystic changes within the bones themselves (Fig. 1-18). Ulnar deviation of the wrist, with swelling and tenderness on the radial side, can occur later in the course of the disease.

The synovial sheath of the extensor tendons is often involved in a striking manner and contributes a great deal to limitation of motion of the wrist. Early tenosynovectomy of the extensor tendon sheath has not been performed in children extensively but might well be of benefit in increasing joint motion and reducing injury to tendons.

Hand

Examination of the hand should begin by shaking hands with the patient to ascertain strength and tenderness. Radial or ulnar deviation of the metacarpal joints or proximal interphalangeal joints should be observed. Erythema of the metacarpal and proximal interphalangeal joint dorsal surfaces occurs at times. Swelling of the metacarpal joints is best detected by a loss of bony prominence, but in the two- to three-year-old child with chubby fingers this manifestation is difficult to evaluate when swelling is minimal. Comparison of sulci between metacarpal joints with the fist clenched is most helpful in this situation. Swelling of the metacarpophalangeal joints is most often periarticular with accompanying synovial thickening. Significant effusion does occur but not frequently. Tenderness to direct pressure, and at the end of the range of motion, is common.

Atrophy of the interosseus, thenar, and hypothenar muscle groups usually accompanies significant involvement of the hand in juvenile rheumatoid arthritis. The ensuing muscular weakness is often pronounced and grip strength is grossly deficient. The apparent weakness is caused by a combination of muscular atrophy and limitation of joint motion due to functional contracture and pain on motion.

The normal range of motion for the metacarpal joint is up to 90 degrees from the neutral position in flexion, 25 degrees from the neutral position in extension, and 30 degrees from the neutral position in abduction. The proximal interphalangeal joint flexes up to 120 degrees from the neutral position normally, and does not extend beyond the neutral position. The distal interphalangeal joints of the fingers flex to about 80 degrees from the neutral position with no extension beyond the neutral position. Flexion of the metacarpal interphalangeal joint of the thumb is up to 60 degrees from the neutral position, 55 degrees in radial abduction, and 45 degrees in palmar abduction.

Range of motion is best evaluated quickly by having the patient make a fist and then extend the fingers and thumb to the maximum degree. Limitation of motion of the metacarpal joint more frequently occurs in flexion. The proximal interphalangeal joints usually have a fusiform type of swelling, with flexion contracture of 20 to 45 degrees occurring later in the course of the disease. Swelling is either lateral, with minimal tenderness, or dorsal, with significant tenderness. The dorsal swelling may be more frequently associated with the tendon sheath. Limitation of flexion of the distal interphalangeal joints, with or without swelling, occurred in 17 of our patients.

Extensor tendon sheath involvement and bursal swelling are frequent findings accompanying metacarpal joint involvement. Bursal swelling of the metacarpal joint of the thumb on the palmar surface can be particularly painful to the patient, although pain is not a usual symptom in this particular group of joints.

Cervical Spine

One of the more prominent findings in juvenile rheumatoid arthritis is early limitation of motion in the cervical spine. Cervical spine involvement is often best observed by having the child turn from one direction to another. If there is significant involvement of the cervical spine, the child tends to move his head, neck, and shoulders as a unit rather than simply turning his head from side to side. Examination of all directions of motion is important. Extension is evaluated by having the child tilt his head backward, and flexion by having the child place his chin on his chest. Rotation to the left and right is best ascertained by having the child touch his chin to his shoulder, and deviation by having him touch his ear to his shoulder. Exact degrees of measurement are difficult but limitation can be readily observed, and tenderness at the end of motions is quckly ascertained.

Many observers place significant importance on involvement of the cervical spine in juvenile rheumatoid arthritis in contrast to some of the other arthritides. In other joints, swelling or limitation of motion with pain or tenderness may be recognized as symptoms of the disease. In the cervical spine, limitation of motion is recognized as a symptom of the disease after excluding local muscular pain and spasm due to such things as cervical adenitis or myositis.

Local tenderness along the spine is a usual finding. Weakness of the paraspinal musculature in the cervical spine area, accompanied by muscle spasm of the upper trapezius muscle group, contributes to limitation of motion.

Ziff believes that cervical spine fusion, with evidence of involvement of the apophyseal joints in the adult, is evidence of juvenile rheumatoid arthritis in the past (Ziff, 1966). Late changes include fusion of the cervical spine (Fig. 1-19). Subluxation of the first and second cervical vertebrae can create signs of spinal cord compression and, on occasion, necessitate surgical intervention with fusion. One patient has been observed who had bony fusion of the cervical spine in the flexed position with the chin 1 cm. off the sternoclavicular notch. This deformity was caused by subluxation of the first and second cervical vertebrae with a forward tilting of the foramen magnum anteriorly. Changes may be caused by ligamentous relaxation and rupture.

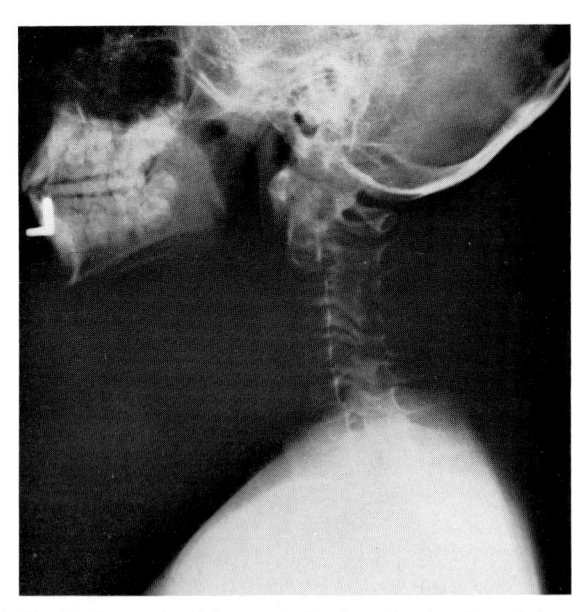

Figure 1-19 Radiograph of the cervical spine, showing loss of the normal lordotic curve with fusion of the articulating facets of the upper cervical vertebrae and marked reduction of the articulating joints in the lower cervical area. There is also partial loss of the intervertebral spaces between C3 and C4.

Vertebral bodies may become irregular in outline with reduction of height and narrowing of joint space. Overgrowth may also occur.

Thoracic and Lumbar Spines

Involvement of the thoracic and lumbar spines has been observed but is certainly unusual. In general, rheumatoid arthritis in children mainly involves the cervical spine and only rarely the dorsal and lumbar spine.

Hip

Hip involvement occurred in 39 per cent of 100 patients at Texas Children's Hospital. Detection of hip involvement is first observed while the patient is walking. The patient will often favor the affected extremity by leaning and giving way to the afflicted side. Pain present in the area of the hip may be referred to the thigh and knee. Clinical swelling of the hip joint in a child is almost impossible to ascertain. Localized tenderness, evident by direct palpation or, indirectly by having the patient move the joint into extremes of all ranges of motion, is a usual clue to hip disease. Atrophy of the muscles about the hip, including the gluteal muscle and the muscles of the thigh, occurs frequently.

Limitation of motion secondary to muscular spasm, or limitation due to fibrous ankylosis, often is the first indication of arthritis of the hip. Normal hip motion from neutral position ranges up to 125 degrees flexion, 10 degrees extension, 40 degrees adduction, 45 degrees abduction, and 45 degrees internal and external rotation.

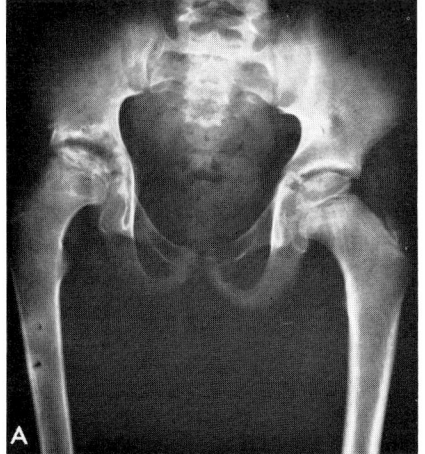

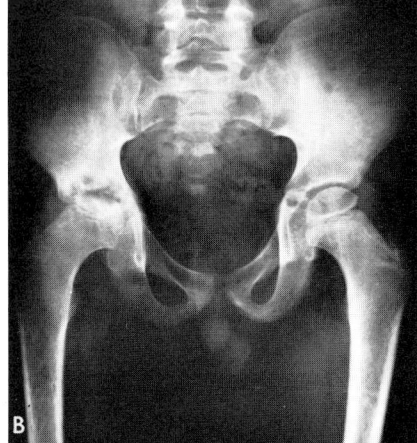

Figure 1-20 *A*, Reduction of the hip joint spaces is evident with extensive erosive changes affecting the articular structures, especially on the right. Flattening and increased density of the right capital femoral epiphysis are present. *B*, Repeat studies one year later show some regression of the disease in the joint space of the right hip and an increase in the destructive changes of the left hip.

Limitation of motion of the hip occurs in all ranges of motion, flexion contracture being the most important problem. An x-ray of the hip can reveal capsular swelling with an increase in joint space (Fig. 1-20 *A* and *B*).

A later manifestation of the disease is restriction of motion due to fibrous ankylosis. Osteoporosis accompanied by narrowing of the joint space, and actual destructive changes in the cortex of the head of the femur, along with destructive changes in the acetabulum, have been observed in five of our patients.

Overgrowth or undergrowth of the femoral head is also observed. At times, the limitation of motion is a result of thickening of the capsule, with marked synovial thickening. One of our patients exhibited this manifestation with almost complete functional loss of motion. The cortex of the acetabulum and the femoral head were not seriously involved.

Aseptic necrosis of the hip in conjunction with definite juvenile rheumatoid arthritis is well documented; it occurred in one of our patients.

Sacroiliac Joint

The sacroiliac joint was involved clinically in six of our patients. This involvement was evident by local tenderness over the area. By roentgenogram, the earliest change seen was subchondral sclerosis, primarily on the iliac portion of the joint. Localized areas of destruction sometimes appear, with progressive narrowing of the joint space and eventual fusion (Grokoest et al., 1962).

Temporomandibular Joint

In severely involved children, striking limitation of jaw movement can occur. Localized tenderness over the joint confirms local involvement. Swelling is not clinically detectable. A late change associated with involvement of the temporomandibular joint is hypoplasia of the entire mandible resulting in micrognathia. The face assumes an angular pinched expression with the mouth rounded and the lips held open. Overbite of the upper teeth is prominent. Hypoplasia of the mandible without involvement of the temporomandibular joint sometimes occurs.

Shoulder

Examination of the shoulder begins with observation of the patient walking. A shoulder drop, dislocation, or altered carrying angle becomes apparent, and atrophy of the deltoid muscle is often striking.

Normal shoulder motion ranges from neutral position are up to 180 degrees abduction, 40 degrees adduction, 180 degrees flexion, and 45 degrees extension. Abduction of the arm from the side to 90 degrees is the function of the central deltoid muscular group; continued abduction above the head involves the flexor and rotator muscle

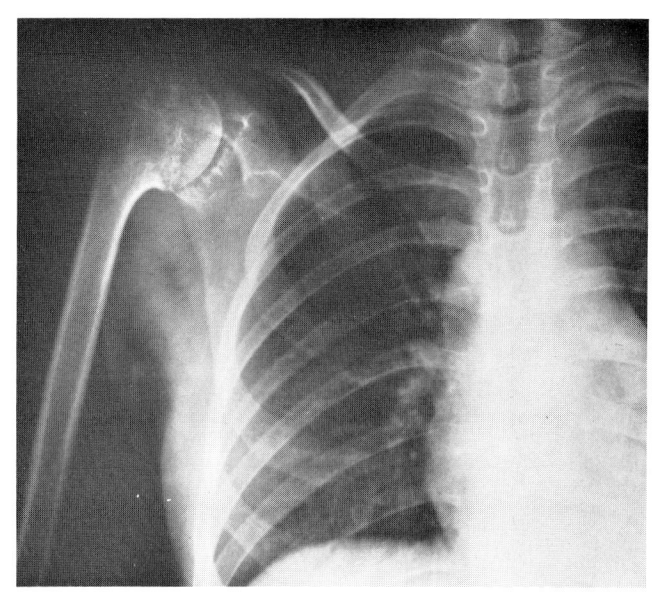

Figure 1-21 In this patient the joint space of the right shoulder is reduced and there is deformity of the surgical neck of the humerus with an associated lack of normal molding of the proximal humeral metaphysis. Erosive changes of the glenoid fossa are moderately advanced.

groups also. Abduction is often the first indication of a serious shoulder involvement, which may progress rapidly because of the rapid atrophy of the deltoid group and can lead to subluxation. Flexion and extension limitations of motion are not as prominent as limitation of abduction. Local pain is strikingly minimal or absent in this joint despite severe involvement. Swelling is difficult to detect. Tenderness is best elicited by palpation directly over the margins of the glenoid fossa. Bursitis in this area is not a usual finding but does occur.

Later changes that involve serious limitation of motion, restricting abduction to 40 degrees or less, are common. By x-ray examination, a narrowing of the joint space and cortical destruction of the head of the humerus with or without anterior subluxation can be detected (Fig. 1-21). Destruction of the glenoid fossa can also occur, as with the acetabulum of the hip. Such changes are common.

Elbow

Children with arthritis of the elbow usually develop functional limitation of motion and flexion rather quickly. Supination and pronation are also restricted. The normal range of motion for the elbow from the neutral position is up to 145 degrees flexion, and up to 90 degrees for supination and pronation of the forearm. Swelling about the elbow joint is usually periarticular, with synovial thickening and

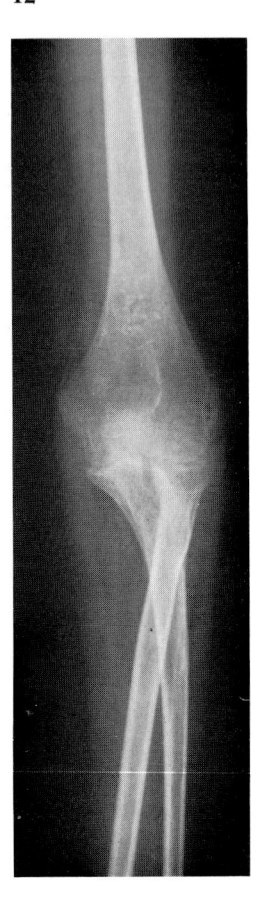

Figure 1-22 This anteroposterior radiograph of the elbow shows juxta-articular demineralization as well as reduction of joint spaces between the distal humerus and the radius and ulna. There is associated atrophy of the muscles.

minimal effusion. Swelling is best detected on the extensor surface, lateral and medial to the olecranon. Erythema is unusual but local tenderness is common when the elbow is involved. Pain on motion is frequent, but atrophy of the muscles around the joint is not as prominent as with the quadriceps about the knee area. Late manifestations include ankylosis (Fig. 1-22).

Metastatic Calcification of Soft Tissues

An unusual finding in rheumatoid arthritis is metastatic calcification in soft tissues. Two of our patients had soft tissue calcification about the ankle (Fig. 1-23). Grokoest reported patients with metastatic calcification of soft tissues on the lateral aspects of the wrist adjacent to the olecranon process of the ulna, the retroacetabular structures of the hip, the anterior aspects of the knee distal to the patella, and lateral to the first lumbar vertebra (Grokoest et al., 1962). Caffey reported ligamentous calcification of the coracoclavicular joint in juvenile rheumatoid arthritis (Caffey, 1961).

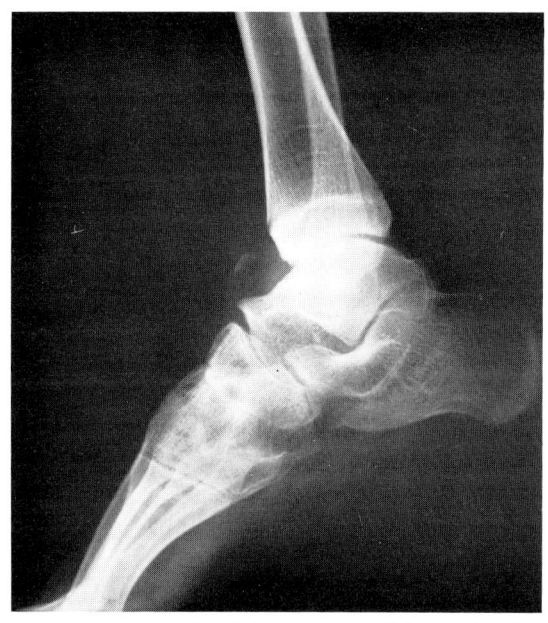

Figure 1-23 Mild rheumatoid arthritic changes of the ankle joint are seen as well as soft tissue calcification changes anterior to the talotibial articulation.

PROGNOSIS

Rheumatoid arthritis in children is rarely a fatal disease. The mortality rate from the disease alone is probably about 4 or 5 per cent. Mortality figures in the series reported in Table 1-6 have varied from 4 to 9 per cent, but most of the figures greater than 4 to 5 per cent probably result from therapeutic complications.

Valid, unbiased data with regard to the disease as it occurs in the general population have been impossible to obtain. Most series reported suffer from limitations of the institution or isolation from metropolitan areas; restriction of the type of patient admitted to the hospital; limitation of patients to hospital or clinic alone; or delay in patient referral beyond one year of disease. Some institutions, because of isolation or admission restriction requirements, never have the opportunity to see patients with mild cases of polyarthritis fulfilling the criteria of juvenile rheumatoid arthritis. The cases are of such short duration that referral is not accomplished. These patients recover uneventfully, with no residual disease or complications. In the United States, many such patients with mild polyarthritis are seen by other specialists such as orthopedic surgeons, and are never evaluated medically, even in the same institution. The duration of disease activity differs, therefore, in series based on data collected from patients seen at the onset of illness from series in which patients are seen one or two years after the onset of disease. This difference exists perhaps because the milder cases have been eliminated by duration. Another obstacle in

Table 1-6 Functional Effects of Rheumatoid Arthritis

	Number of Patients Followed	Complete Functional Recovery (%)	Minimal or Moderate Crippling (%)	Severe Crippling (%)	Deaths (%)
Laaksonen (1966)	544	30.1	40.2	29.7	4
Pickard (1947)	35	40	25.7	25.7	8.6
Laurin and Fauvreau (1963)	31	50	25	25	—
Barkin (1952)	51	41	—	39	20
Norcross, Lockie, and MacLeod (1958)	62	77.4	17.8	—	4.8
Lindbjerg (1964)	75	36	35	22	7
Brewer (1966)	100	33	51	11	5
Sury (1957)	151	39	32	29	—
Calabro (1965)	50	74	10	14	2

ascertaining the usual duration of disease is the length of time required to follow patients before truly knowing that recurrences will not develop.

One approach to evaluating prognosis has been to measure functional effects after several years of disease activity. Table 1-6 reveals that virtually all of the living patients had little or no restriction of functional capacity and were able to carry on useful lives.

These same results were obtained at five years from onset in Ansell and Bywaters' group (Ansell and Bywaters, 1959). Other groups have revealed a larger percentage of patients with significant crippling but, in general, the majority of patients recover without significant limitation of activity. Significant crippling of particular joints does occur in a considerable percentage.

Another prognostic evaluation method is estimation of the duration of total disease activity and determination of those manifestations of disease that have prognostic significance. Bywaters found that nearly one-half (95 of 216 patients) became inactive during observation of disease, with a range of one to 12 years and an average duration of 3.1 years. Over one-third of this group were in remission less than one year after onset. With an average follow-up of 10.4 years, 20 per cent of the 216 patients had recurrent disease activity. With an average follow-up of 6.2 years, 30 per cent of the group had continued activity of rheumatoid arthritis (Ansell and Bywaters, 1959). From these data it would appear that about one half of the patients can expect disease activity for an average of three years. The remaining group have an unknown and unpredictable duration.

Monarticular arthritis lasting longer than three months occurred in 12 of the initial 100 Texas Children's Hospital patients. The average age at onset was 5.9 years with a median of 3.5 years. The average duration of disease activity for the total group was 4.8 years with a median of 4 years, and an average follow-up of 3.5 years with a range of 1 month to 11.3 years. Six of 12 patients were inactive; five had disease activity of less than 3 years; one patient had disease activity of 10.3 years' duration. The remaining six have had their disease from 1.5 to 9.75 years, with all except one having greater than 5 years' duration. All had excellent functional capacity with good range of motion except for one patient who had atrophy, internal rotation of the hip, and a noticeable limp.

Patients with monarticular arthritis who have clinical remission with less than three years' activity probably have the best chance to avoid recurrence. When the disease lasts longer than three years, the chances of remission in less than ten years are remote.

Patients who develop subcutaneous nodules have continued activity but a more prolonged disease (Ansell and Bywaters, 1959). A positive rheumatoid factor test is also associated with more severe disease.

The prognosis of rheumatoid arthritis in children depends in large measure upon the severity of the disease. Mortality is rare and morbidity is basically related to joint deformity and limitation of motion. Those patients with mild polyarthritis who do not progress to erosive joint disease in the first few years of involvement have an excellent prognosis. The extent of permanent crippling can undoubtedly be minimized by proper physical therapy and other therapeutic modalities.

The disease is rarely fatal, with significant crippling developing in less than 25 per cent. The duration of the disease process is based on the severity of the polyarthritis and on whether or not progressive erosive arthritis occurs.

REFERENCES

Addair, J., and Snyder, L. H.: Evidence for an autosomal recessive gene for susceptibility to paralytic poliomyelitis. J. Hered., *33*:306, 1942.

Ansell, B. M., and Bywaters, E. G. L.: Growth in Still's disease. Ann. Rheum. Dis. *15*:295, 1956.

Ansell, B. M., and Bywaters, E. G. L.: Prognosis in Still's disease. Bull. Rheum. Dis., *9*:189, 1959.

Ansell, B. M., and Bywaters, E. G. L.: Rheumatoid arthritis (Still's disease). Pediat. Clin. N. Amer., *10*:921, 1963.

Ansell, B. M., Bywaters, E. G. L., and Lawrence, J. S.: A family study in Still's disease. Ann. Rheum. Dis., *21*:243, 1962.

Barkin, R. E.: The clinical course of juvenile rheumatoid arthritis. Bull. Rheum. Dis., *3*:1, 1952.

Baum, J., and Fink, C. W.: Juvenile rheumatoid arthritis in monozygotic twins: A case report and review of the literature. Arthritis Rheum., *11*:33, 1968.

Blegvad, O.: Iridocyclitis and disease of the joints in children. The Ophthalmic Department of the Finsen Institute and Radium Station, 1941.

Bunim, J., Burch, T. A., and O'Brien, W.: Influence of genetic and environmental factors on the occurrence of rheumatoid arthritis and rheumatoid factor in American Indians. Bull. Rheum. Dis., *15*:349, 1964.

Burch, T. A., O'Brien, W., and Bunim, J.: Family and genetic studies of rheumatoid arthritis and rheumatoid factor in Blackfeet Indians. Amer. J. Public Health, 54, *8*:118, 1964.

Bywaters, E. G. L., Glynn, L. E., and Zeldis, A.: Subcutaneous nodules of Still's disease. Ann. Rheum. Dis., *17*:278, 1958.
Caffey, J.: Pediatric X-ray Diagnosis. Chicago, Year Book Medical Publishers Inc., 1961.
Calabro, J. J., and Marchesano, J. M.: Juvenile rheumatoid arthritis: Observations on fever. New Eng. J. Med., *276*:11, 1967.
Coss, J., and Boots, R. H.: Juvenile rheumatoid arthritis. J. Pediat., *29*:143, 1946.
Edström, G. (1948). Discussed in Hill, D. F.: Climate and arthritis. In Hollander, J. L.: Arthritis and Allied Conditions, Ed. 7. Philadelphia, Lea & Febiger, 1966, p. 588.
Edström, G.: Rheumatoid arthritis and Still's disease in children. A survey of 161 cases. Arthritis Rheum., *1*:497, 1958.
Franceschetti, A., Blum, J. D., and Bamatter, F.: Diagnostic value of ocular symptoms in juvenile chronic polyarthritis (Still's disease). Trans. Ophthalmol. Soc. U.K., 1951.
Griffin, P. P., Tachdjian, M. O., and Green, W. T.: Pauciarticular arthritis in children, J.A.M.A., *184*:145, 1963.
Grokoest, A. W., Snyder, A. I., and Schlaeger, R.: Juvenile Rheumatoid Arthritis. Boston, Little, Brown & Co., 1962.
Grossman, B. J., Ozoa, N. F., and Arya, S. C.: Problems in juvenile rheumatoid arthritis. Med Clin. N. Amer., *49*:33, 1965.
Harris, H. A. (1933). Discussed in Ansell, B. M., and Bywaters, E. G. L.: Growth in Still's disease. Ann. Rheum. Dis., *15*:315, 1956.
Hatherley, E.: Uveitis and band-shaped keratitis in a case of Still's disease. Proceedings Royal Soc. Med., 1951, p. 978.
Herndon, C. N., and Jennings, R. G.: A twin study of susceptibility to poliomyelitis, Amer. J. Hum. Genet., *3*:17, 1951.
Hewitt, D., Westropp, C. K., and Acheson, R. M. (1955). Discussed in Ansell, B. M., and Bywaters, E. G. L.: Growth in Still's disease. Ann. Rheum. Dis., *15*:315, 1956.
Hill, L. (1939). Discussed in Hill, D. F.: Climate and arthritis. *In* Hollander, J. L.: Arthritis and Allied Conditions, Ed. 7. Philadelphia, Lea & Febiger, 1966, p. 588.
Hollander, J. L. (1961). Discussed in Hill, D. F.: Climate and arthritis. *In* Hollander, J. L.: Arthritis and Allied Conditions, Ed. 7. Philadelphia, Lea & Febiger, 1966, p. 588.
Isdale, I. C., and Bywaters, E. G. L.: The rash of rheumatoid arthritis and Still's disease. Quart. J. Med., New Series XXV, *99*:377, 1956.
Johnson, N., and Dodd, K.: Juvenile rheumatoid arthritis. Med. Clin. N. Amer., *39*:459, 1955.
Kelley, V. C.: Rheumatoid disease in childhood. Pediat. Clin. N. Amer., *7*:435, 1960.
Kuhns, J. G., and Swaim, L. T.: Disturbances of growth in chronic arthritis in children. Amer. J. Dis. Child., *43*:1118, 1932.
Lawrence, J. S. (1963). Discussed in Hollander, J. L.: Arthritis and Allied Conditions, Ed. 7. Philadelphia, Lea & Febiger, 1966, p. 594.
Masi, A. T., and Shulman, L. E.: Familial aggregation and rheumatoid disease. Arthritis Rheum., *8*:418, 1965.
Mendez-Bryan, R., Roger, N. L., and Gonzalez-Alcover, R. (1963): Abstract discussed in Hollander, J. L.: Arthritis and Allied Conditions, Ed. 7. Philadelphia, Lea & Febiger, 1966, p. 594.
Meyerowitz, S., Jacox, R. F., and Hess, D. W.: Monozygotic twins discordant for rheumatoid arthritis: A genetic, clinical and psychological study of 8 sets. Arthritis Rheum., *11*:1, 1968.
Mikkelsen, W. M.: The epidemiology of rheumatic disease. *In* Hollander, J. L.: Arthritis and Allied Conditions, Ed. 7. Philadelphia, Lea & Febiger, 1966, p. 551.
Moesmann, G.: Factors precipitating and predisposing to rheumatoid arthritis as illustrated by studies on monozygotic twins. Acta Rheum. Scan., *291*:303, 1959.
Norcross, B. M., Lockie, L. M., and MacLeod, C. C.: Juvenile rheumatoid arthritis. *In* Talbot, J. H., and Lockie, L. M. (eds.): Progress in Arthritis. New York, Grune & Stratton, 1958.
Pickard, N. S.: Rheumatoid arthritis in children. Arch. Int. Med., *80*:771, 1947.
Ragan, C., and Farrington, E. (1962). Discussed in Ragan, C.: The clinical picture of rheumatoid arthritis. *In* Hollander, J. L.: Arthritis and Allied Conditions, Ed. 7. Philadelphia, Lea & Febiger, 1966.
Rawson, A. J., Abelson, N. M., and Hollander, J. L.: Studies on the pathogenesis of rheumatoid joint inflammation. II. Intracytoplasmic particulate complexes in rheumatoid synovial fluids. Ann. Int. Med., *62*:281, 1965.

Schlesinger, B. E., et al.: Observations on the clinical course and treatment of one hundred cases of Still's disease. Arch. Dis. Child., *36*:65, 1961.

Short, C. L., Bauer, W., and Reynolds, W. E.: Rheumatoid Arthritis. Cambridge, Harvard University Press, 1957.

Smiley, W. K., May, E., and Bywaters, E. G. L.: Ocular presentations of Still's disease and their treatment—iridocyclitis in Still's disease: Its complications and treatment. Ann. Rheum. Dis., *16*:371, 1957.

Sokoloff, L.: The pathology of rheumatoid arthritis and allied disorders. *In* Hollander, J. L.: Arthritis and Allied Conditions. Ed. 7. Philadelphia, Lea & Febiger, 1966.

Still, F. G.: On a form of chronic joint disease in children. Med.-chir. Trans., *80*:47, 1897.

Vaughan, J. H.: Infectious and immunological considerations in rheumatic diseases. *In* Hollander, J. L.: Arthritis and Allied Conditions, Ed. 7. Philadelphia, Lea & Febiger, 1966.

Vesterdal, E., and Sury, B.: Iridocyclitis and band-shaped corneal opacity in juvenile rheumatoid arthritis. Acta Ophthalmol., *28*:321, 1950.

Ziff, M., and Baum, J.: Laboratory findings in rheumatoid arthritis. *In* Hollander, J. L.: Arthritis and Allied Conditions, Ed. 7. Philadelphia, Lea & Febiger, 1966.

Chapter Two

CARDITIS WITH RHEUMATOID ARTHRITIS

Dan G. McNamara, M.D.*
and Earl J. Brewer, Jr. M.D.

Despite the usual benign nature and rarity of carditis with rheumatoid arthritis, serious, potentially lethal cardiac sequelae occasionally do occur. Intent on preventing the dreaded joint deformities and relieving the persistent high fever, the clinician treating Still's disease may not be particularly concerned about the rare chance of significant heart involvement.

In fact, once acute arthritis in a child proves to be rheumatoid arthritis rather than rheumatic fever, the small chance of permanent cardiac damage to some extent consoles both family and physician despite other problems of the disease.

Comparison of Rheumatoid and Rheumatic Carditis

Characteristically, the carditis of rheumatoid arthritis is well known to be unlike that of rheumatic fever, though in a few cases valvulitis or a combination of valvulitis and myocarditis in rheumatoid arthritis resembles that of rheumatic fever. However, isolated pericarditis, characteristic of rheumatoid arthritis, probably does not occur in the acute rheumatic fever patient. Carditis in the two types of arthritis is compared in Table 2-1.

TYPES OF CARDITIS

Pericarditis

Pericarditis has been clinically identified in about 10 per cent of patients with rheumatoid arthritis. At post mortem examination the

---

*Associate Professor, Department of Pediatrics, Baylor College of Medicine; Director of Pediatric Cardiology, Texas Children's Hospital, Houston, Texas

Table 2-1 Carditis in Rheumatoid Arthritis and in Rheumatic Fever

	Rheumatoid Arthritis	*Rheumatic Fever*
Incidence	5 to 10%	50 to 65%
Pericarditis	Most frequent form of carditis. Occurs as an isolated clinical manifestation of carditis.	Least frequent form of carditis (1.5%). Rarely an isolated manifestation of carditis in rheumatic fever; usually a part of generalized pericarditis.
	Not an indication of severe or permanent cardiac sequelae.	Presence suggests severe permanent cardiac disease with poor prognosis.
Myocarditis	Isolated granulomatous myocarditis in adults but not in children.	Rarely an isolated manifestation of rheumatic heart disease. Occurs as part of severe pancarditis.
Valvulitis	Rarely occurs clinically. Adult or adolescent patients more likely to have valve involvement than children.	Occurrence common (50 to 60%). Incidence of mitral or aortic valvulitis more frequent in children than adults. The younger the child, the more severe the carditis.
	Clinical features of mitral or aortic valve involvement are similar for both diseases.	
Electrocardiogram	T wave or S-T segment shift, or both, usually present.	Increase in QRS voltage may occur with cardiac enlargement. S-T and T wave changes less frequent.

arthritis incidence is higher—as much as 45 per cent. Pericarditis was reported by Still in his first description of the disease.

Mild Pericarditis. Rheumatoid carditis usually presents as isolated pericarditis, so mild as to be difficult to identify clinically. It subsides spontaneously, produces few or no symptoms and only subtle and fleeting physical signs, causes inconstant and nonspecific electrocardiographic changes, and seldom leaves sequelae or recurs. Signs and symptoms that do appear last only a few days. Although the physician relies on the pericardial friction rub for diagnosis by physical examination, the rub is a difficult sound to learn to hear at all, and disappears entirely after a few days. The rub has a low intensity (Grade I–II/VI) and may occupy only a brief part of systole or diastole. It may be necessary to place the patient in different positions and listen carefully in quiet surroundings using the diaphragm rather than the bell of the stethoscope while the patient holds deep expiration for a moment.

Electrocardiographic changes last longer than the friction rub but are less specific. Contrary to general opinion, the most commonly identifiable electrocardiographic change in pericarditis with rheumatoid arthritis is in the T wave rather than in the S-T segment (V. I.).

Moderately Severe Pericarditis. The disability from the less common, moderately severe type of pericarditis is primarily pain. Such pain is left precordial, in the shoulder, or in the neck, and is aggravated on assuming the supine position and by deep inspiration, the latter suggesting pleurisy. In more severe cases one is likelier to hear a friction rub and both signs and symptoms last longer—10 to 14 days. Clinical recovery may be quite as complete as in milder cases but the acute symptoms are nevertheless more alarming and may require a brief course of steroid therapy for prompt relief.

Severe Pericarditis. The rare severe form can cause, in addition to precordial pain, an unpleasant shortness of breath, even at rest, and rarely accumulation of enough fluid to interfere with ventricular filling. Thus, heart failure may develop in what appears to be an abrupt manner. The friction rub is likely to disappear at this point. The patient who has an increase in cardiac silhouette radiographically, orthopnea, and electrocardiographic changes should be considered for pericardiocentesis whether there is a friction rub or not. The enlarged cardiac silhouette, of course, may prove to represent ventricular dilatation due to myocarditis rather than fluid accumulation (see Figure 2-1, A and B).

Constrictive Pericarditis. Rare as it may be, constrictive pericarditis must be mentioned as a possibility in reviewing the spectrum of pericarditis in rheumatoid arthritis. One case has been reported which required surgical treatment.

Myocarditis

Myocarditis may be responsible for heart failure and can be suspected when the radiographic increase in heart size proves, by peri-

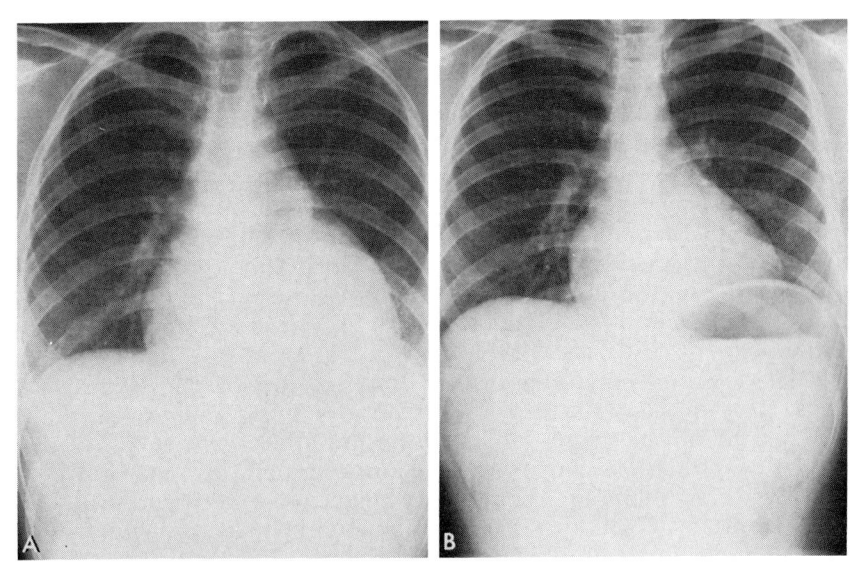

Figure 2-1   A, Pericardial effusion. Chest radiograph shows large cardiac silhouette. Clinical findings also signified pericardial effusion. B, Same patient, two months later; heart size is within normal limits.

cardial tap or other reliable means, to be unrelated to pericardial fluid. The electrocardiographic signs of myocarditis overlap too much with those of pericarditis to be of differential aid in this regard. Myocarditis that produces cardiac enlargement is an indication for corticosteroid therapy.

Valvulitis

Valvulitis, either aortic or mitral, is more common in the adult with rheumatoid arthritis and appears infrequently in children. In those few cases in which carditis precedes joint manifestations, clinical signs of mitral or aortic valvulitis would suggest rheumatic fever.

Medical management of valvulitis does not differ, however, whether the origin is rheumatoid or rheumatic, except for the administration of long-term penicillin prophylaxis for the rheumatic fever patient. Because of the murmur, valvulitis should be recognized by physical examination more readily than pericarditis or myocarditis. Unless a diagnosis of juvenile rheumatoid arthritis is without question, any patient with polyarthritis and valvulitis must be considered to have rheumatic fever.

Electrocardiograms in Carditis

T Wave. The most distinctive and the best known electrocardiographic change in pericarditis is S-T segment shift. However, primary change in the T wave alone without S-T segment shift occurs more often and, moreover, precedes S-T segment shift when this does occur.

Primary T wave change in the frontal plane implies that the mean frontal plane axis of the T wave varies by 60 degrees or more from the mean frontal plane axis of a normally oriented QRS complex. If, for example, the T axis were found to be minus 30 degrees on the frontal plane in the patient with rheumatoid arthritis and the mean QRS were plus 60 degrees, one would suspect pericarditis. If, however, in another patient the T wave were minus 30 degrees and the QRS axis 0 degrees as sometimes occurs in normal individuals, the QRS-T angle would be normal. In other words, the T wave change is important only in its relation to the QRS complex. The QRS complex remains normal in pericarditis that is uncomplicated by myocarditis, thus significant T wave changes usually are primary (Fig. 2-2, *A* and *B*).

Primary T wave change in the precordial leads is present when the maximal positive T wave lies three or more chest leads away from the lead with the tallest R wave. The T wave in left chest leads may thus be discordant with the R wave yet remain positive in these leads (as demonstrated in Figure 2-3, *A* and *B*), but an isoelectric or negative T wave in the left precordial leads (V4, V5, or V6) is more definitive evidence of epicardial injury, suggestive of pericarditis (Fig. 2-3, *A* and *B*).

S-T Segment. Because of the importance of S-T segment abnormality in the identification of pericarditis and the often misunderstood electrocardiographic manifestations of epicardial and subepicardial injury, a brief review of the origin of the S-T segment may be of value.

At the completion of ventricular activation (QRS complex) there is

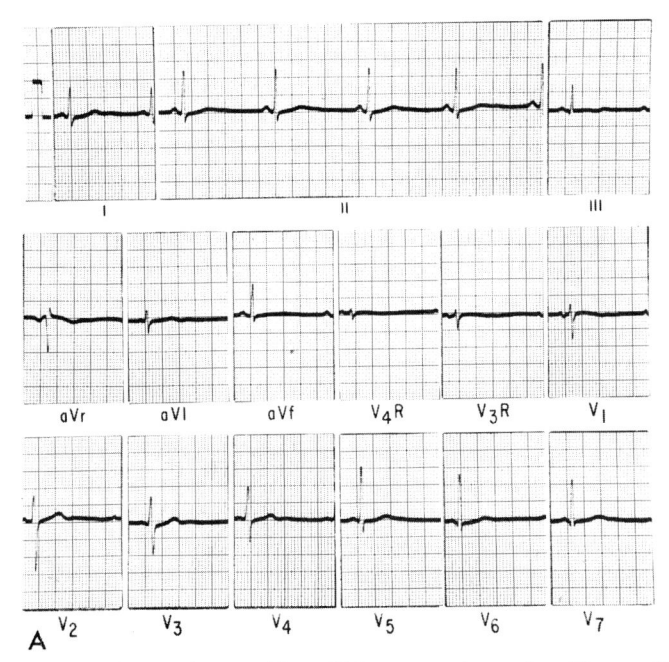

Figure 2-2, A T wave change without S-T segment change in a 17-year-old girl with pericarditis and rheumatoid arthritis. The mean frontal plane axis of the T wave is 0° whereas the mean frontal plane axis of QRS is normally oriented at +70°. The T waves in the left chest leads are positive, however; the most positive T wave is at V2, three chest lead positions away from lead V5 which has the greatest R wave.

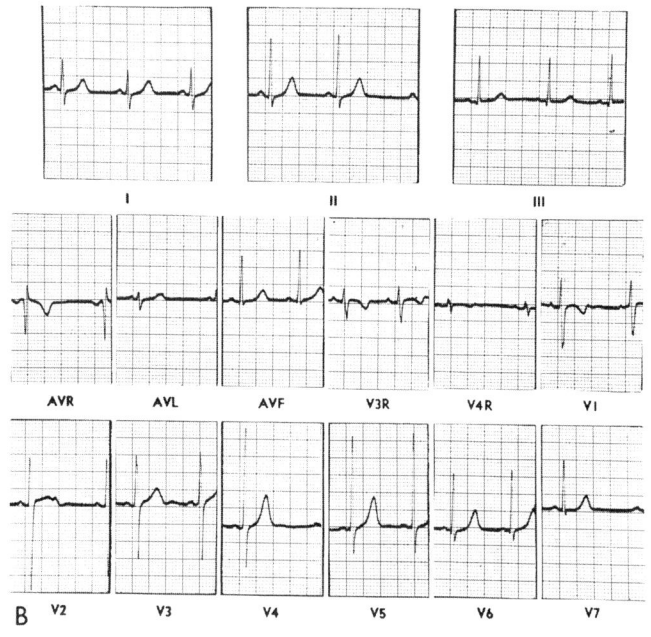

Figure 2-2, B Normal ECG from the same patient in Figure 2-2, *A*, prior to the development of pericarditis. There is a normal QRS-T angle on the frontal and horizontal planes. The frontal plane T wave axis is +45° and the QRS is +70°, giving a normal QRS-T angle of 25°. The greatest positive T wave in the chest leads is in V4, which also has the tallest R wave, giving a normal relationship of QRS and T.

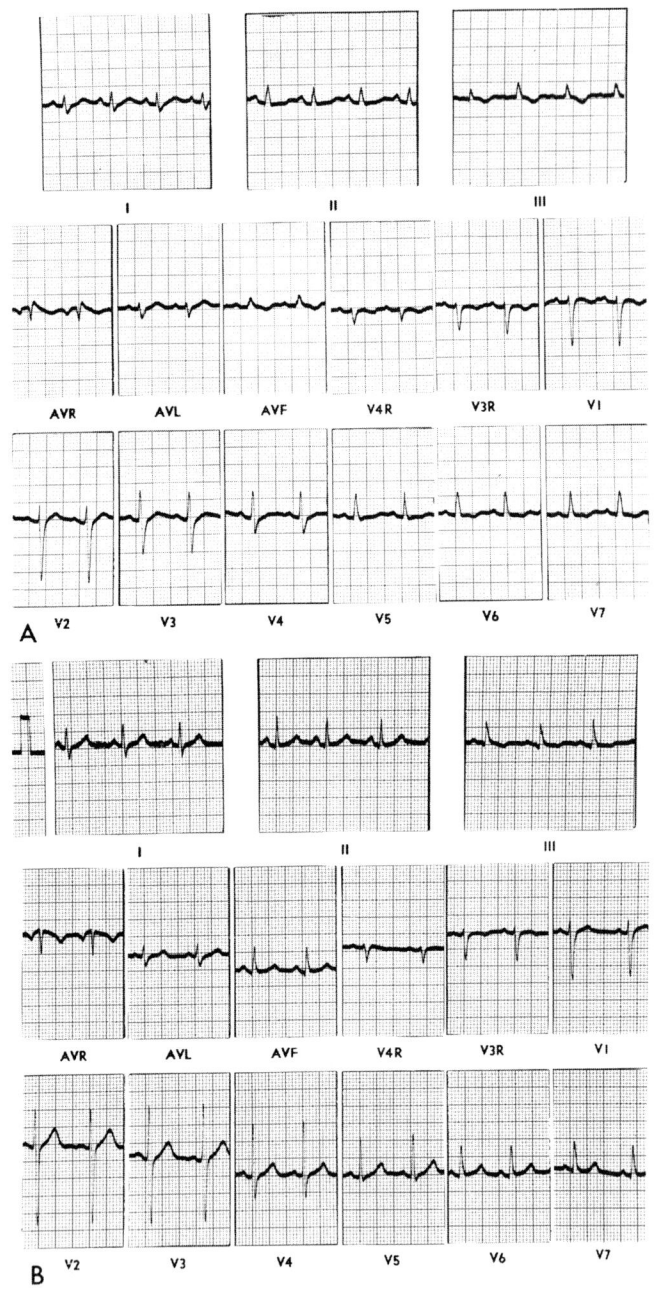

Figure 2-3, A ECG manifestation of subepicardial injury in an 11-year-old boy with pericarditis and rheumatoid arthritis. Note inverted T waves in left chest leads in the absence of definite S-T segment changes.

Figure 2-3, B Same patient in Figure 2-3, *A*, after recovery from pericarditis. The T waves appear normal. Compare with Figure 2-3, *A*.

CARDITIS WITH RHEUMATOID ARTHRITIS

a short period of electrical inactivity (S-T segment) prior to electrical reactivation of the ventricles (T wave). In pericarditis the ventricular myocardium subjacent to the involved pericardium is evidently altered, at least electrically, to the extent that depolarization of this portion of the muscle persists for a longer period than in the uninvolved myocardium. This electrical activity continues into the period that is usually electrically inactive (the S-T segment), thus the continued electrical activity causes displacement of the baseline toward the direction of the maximal activation and away from the area of least activation.

To the frustration of electrocardiographers, it is often stated that "elevation" of the S-T segment indicates pericarditis. This loose jargon implies that the mean S-T segment vector in the patient with pericarditis often is positive to *most* of the standard leads, such as leads I, II, AVL, and AVF (Fig. 2-4). To search for S-T segment elevation, as opposed to depression, as the criterion for pericarditis is to ignore the fact that the shifted S-T segment is "elevated" (positive) in only one half of the chest and is "depressed" (negative) in the other half. In the example given, the mean S-T segment vector on the frontal plane lies at about plus 30 degrees. However, in other instances of pericarditis the S-T segment vector may be "elevated" (positive) to lead AVR and lead III and "depressed" (negative) in other leads (Fig. 2-5).

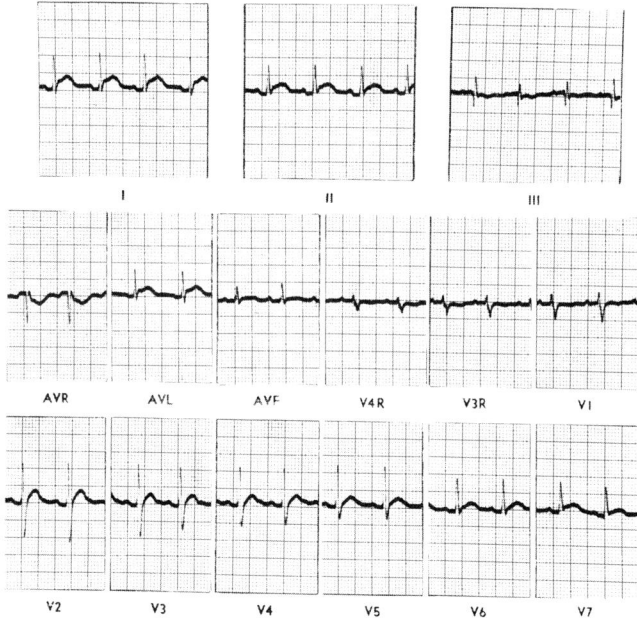

Figure 2-4 Scalar ECG in a 7-year-old boy with rheumatoid arthritis and pericarditis. The S-T segment is elevated (positive) to standard leads I, II, AVL, and AVF. The S-T segment is "normal" (isoelectric) to lead III and is depressed (negative) in lead AVR. Thus the mean frontal plane vector of the displaced S-T segment is +30°. On the horizontal plane, the S-T segment is positive "elevated" in leads V2 through V7. It is perpendicular to right chest leads V4R through V1 and thus no displacement of S-T segment is seen in these leads.

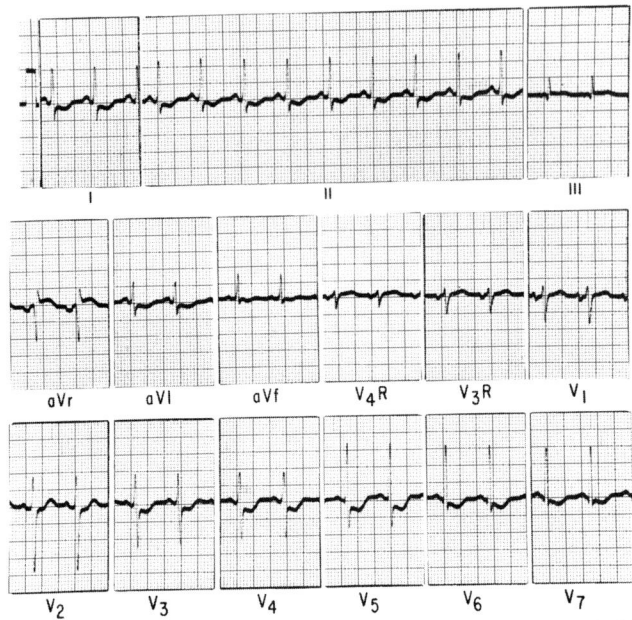

Figure 2-5 Scalar ECG in a 17-year-old girl with rheumatoid arthritis and pericarditis, unusual because the displaced S-T segment vector is toward 180° and thus is negative or "depressed" in most of the standard limb leads. The S-T segment is, in fact, "elevated" (or positive) but only in lead AVR. On the horizontal plane, the S-T segment is only slightly elevated in lead V4R, isoelectric in V3R and V1, but is "depressed" in leads V2 through V7. This tracing is from the same patient whose ECG obtained at an earlier stage of illness is seen in Figure 2-2, *A*.

In the example given in Figure 2-5, the S-T segment has a mean vector on the frontal plane of about 180 degrees. In this tracing most of the frontal plane leads will have a "depressed" S-T segment, as in leads I, III, and AVL. An S-T segment cannot be *only* elevated. If the S-T segment is nonisoelectric only half the torso has an elevated (positive) S-T segment; the other half is depressed (negative).

An electrical force traveling toward one lead (positive to that lead) travels away from the opposite lead (negative to that lead). The same holds true for the precordial leads.

The altered S-T segment may be positive to the left chest leads and thus elevated in leads V2 through V7, but the S-T vector may be positive to the right chest leads V4R, V3R, and V1, and show a negative deflection in the left chest leads (Figs. 2-4, 2-5).

There is no single explanation for this difference in direction of the S-T segment vector in different cases of pericarditis. It may be related to age of the child, location of the pericarditis, or other reasons, but there is no clear prognostic implication from these differences.

Relationship of S-T Segment Vector to T Wave Vector. The abnormally shifted S-T vector and the T vector usually vary together so that if the S-T vector is positive in the left chest leads the T wave vector will be positive also. Since the T wave is normally positive in the left chest leads, "isolated" S-T segment change without an obvious T wave change can be seen in the example in Figure 2-4.

If the S-T vector is positive (elevated) to the right chest leads, and negative (depressed) to the left chest leads, then the T vector is likewise positive in the right chest leads (upright) and negative (inverted) to the left chest leads, which is the abnormal direction for T waves (Fig. 2-5). Attention and concern over this additional abnormality are not justified. This phenomenon explains why some patients with pericarditis have only S-T segment change and others have both S-T and T wave changes.

The problems in electrocardiographic interpretation in pericarditis may account in part for some of the difficulty in diagnosis. Other reasons may be the difficulty in hearing the friction rub and the short duration of the pericarditis.

Course of Disease

Lietman and Bywaters (1963) reported the duration of clinical manifestations to be one to 15 weeks with a mean duration of seven weeks. In five of 12 patients recurrent episodes of pericarditis were present. Effusion duration was from three days to 14 weeks with an average length of seven weeks. Effusion was present intermittently in one patient. Death occurred in 10 per cent of Bywaters' series, representing about 1 per cent of the total group. This would indicate that about a fourth of all deaths in juvenile rheumatoid arthritis are related to cardiac disease.

Therapy

Patients who are significantly ill with pericarditis with some risk of failure or tamponade, in the opinion of the authors, should be treated with corticosteroid medication. Morbidity is certainly reduced significantly and patients improve promptly after 24 to 48 hours on appropriate corticosteroid medication. Patients who are not clinically ill with pericarditis probably require no corticosteroid therapy.

The corticosteroid ordinarily used is hydrocortisone parenterally, initially at a dosage of 240 mg./m^2 per day for several days. The dosage is then reduced according to clinical response and changed to oral prednisone in a dosage of 10 to 20 mg. daily for as short a time as possible, as determined by clinical judgment—usually a matter of a few weeks. Bywaters feels that salicylates and corticosteroids should not be given together to patients with clinical pericarditis. He has observed deterioration of the patient's condition when both medications were given. The reason for this is obscure but it is worth noting.

Prognosis

Almost all juvenile rheumatoid arthritis patients with pericarditis recover completely after several months. Exceptions are those few patients who have had intermittent recurrences of disease over a period of a year or two. In Bywaters' series only one patient was totally disabled and three patients had considerable limitation of physical activity.

In the authors' experience no children have sustained limitation of physical activity secondary to pericarditis. The mortality rate, as previously stated, is about 10 per cent.

REFERENCE

Lietman, P. S., and Bywaters, E. G. L.: Pericarditis in juvenile rheumatoid arthritis. Pediatrics, *32:* 856, 1963.

Chapter Three

RADIOGRAPHIC DIAGNOSIS OF RHEUMATOID ARTHRITIS IN THE PEDIATRIC PATIENT

Edward B. Singleton, M.D.*

Although the pathogenesis and pathologic findings of rheumatoid arthritis in the juvenile patient are basically the same as in the adult, the clinical features and systemic complications are frequently different. The radiographic changes may also vary from the usual adult manifestations, both in distribution and severity. A number of articles have appeared describing the clinical and radiographic findings of rheumatoid arthritis in the pediatric age group (Grokoest et al., 1962; Martel et al., 1962).

The early radiographic changes are frequently nonspecific, but as progression of the disease develops, the x-ray changes become more specific. Although careful correlation of the clinical and radiographic changes is important during all phases of the disease, serial radiographic studies are, in typical cases, virtually diagnostic. Radiographic examination of all joints should be obtained when the patient is first suspected of having rheumatoid arthritis, in order to have a base-line study for future comparisons.

The radiographic manifestations may be divided into soft tissue abnormalities, demineralization of the osseous structure (particularly the juxta-articular regions), and alterations of the joint spaces and articular surfaces.

Soft Tissues

The earliest manifestation of both juvenile and adult rheumatoid arthritis consists of soft tissue swelling at the sites of joint involvement.

---

*Associate Professor of Radiology, Baylor College of Medicine; Director of Radiology, St. Luke's and Texas Children's Hospitals, Houston, Texas

This swelling can be identified on radiographs of the involved areas, whether the involvement is monarticular or polyarticular, and can be seen to best advantage in the interphalangeal areas, manifested by an increase in the soft tissue densities surrounding the interphalangeal joints (Fig. 3-1).

Similar soft tissue involvement may be seen about the knees and ankles, but its identification is less reliable than in similar changes involving the hands. Soft tissue involvement of the shoulders, elbows, carpal and tarsal areas, hips, and spine is frequently difficult to recognize.

The identification of early joint effusion is also difficult. An increase in the joint space is rarely appreciated but obliteration or displacement of the pericapsular fat lines may provide presumptive evidence of effusion. In early knee effusions, an increase in the soft tissues of the suprapatellar area with obliteration of the fat of the suprapatellar bursae is commonly seen. These changes are much more difficult to appreciate in the infant.

Focal soft tissue calcifications adjacent to involved joints have been reported (Martel et al., 1962). In some instances these have been of linear configuration suggesting ligamentous calcification. Digital arterial calcification has also been reported but is a rare finding (Martel et al., 1962).

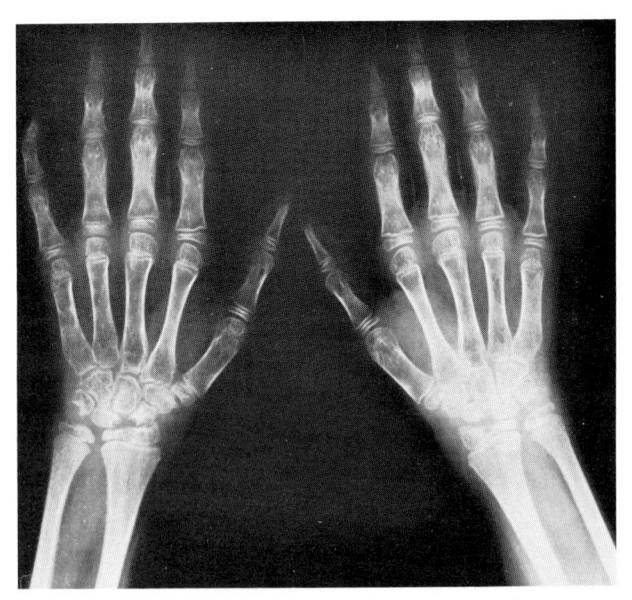

Figure 3-1 Generalized osteoporosis is present, especially pronounced at the juxta-articular areas. Soft tissue swelling about the interphalangeal joints is evident as well as reduction in the metacarpophalangeal and interphalangeal joints. The carpal bones show bone erosion with associated reduction in the intercarpal spaces. Small cysts are present in the carpal bones as well as in the distal left radial epiphysis.

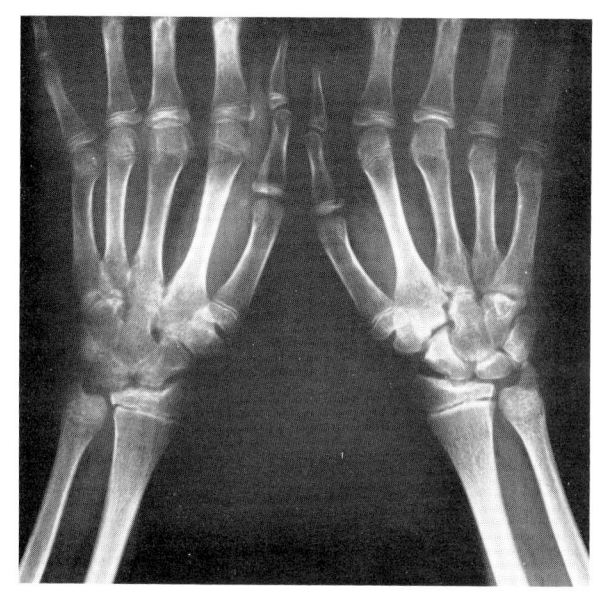

Figure 3-2 Marked reduction in the intercarpal joint spaces is evident with fusion of most of the carpal bones on the left. The radiocarpal joint spaces are reduced with considerable bone erosion involving the distal radial epiphysis. Ulnar deviation of the phalanges is present with associated reduction in the metacarpophalangeal joints.

Demineralization

Juxta-articular demineralization frequently accompanies the soft tissue swelling (Fig. 3-2). This is probably a response to the hyperemia associated with the inflammatory process and is an early finding in the course of the disease. The degree of juxta-articular osteoporosis is apparently related to the severity of the acute process. Later in the course of the disease, as the involved areas become less mobile, disuse osteoporosis undoubtedly plays a part. Naturally, in those cases in which steroids are used therapeutically, the osteoporosis is more generalized. This is especially apparent in radiographs of the spine. Band-like zones of metaphyseal rarefaction, similar to those seen in leukemia and other chronic debilitating diseases, may be seen in the metaphyseal areas of the long bones. These are nonspecific findings and simply reflect a generalized disturbance in bone growth. Associated growth arrest lines frequently accompany these radiolucent bands. Later in the disease, if more advanced changes occur, the juxta-articular osteoporosis is less noticeable, possibly because of a more generalized osteoporotic process or perhaps because there is less acute hyperemia of the joint area.

Destruction of Joint Cartilage

Alterations in the joint space are usually late manifestations of rheumatoid arthritis, and invariably there is accompanying osteoporosis and soft tissue swelling. It is important to realize that the cartilaginous surfaces of the joints are not visible on ordinary radiographs, and consequently destruction of the cartilage must occur before changes develop in the bone and become radiographically demonstrable. The radiographic findings reflect the gross pathology of the disease. The granulation pannus progresses over the articular surfaces and is associated with destruction of the cartilage and the underlying bone. Consequently several radiographic changes may occur: alteration in the height of the affected joint space, bone erosion, pseudocyst formation, ankylosis, and skeletal deformities. Reduction in the height of the joint space is best seen in radiographs of the wrists, but a similar decrease in joint space may be identified in any of the joints, depending on the degree of involvement (Fig. 3-3).

Narrowing of the interosseous joint space is often very pronounced in the carpal area and is at times more severe here than in the metacarpal, phalangeal, or interphalangeal areas. In adults the reverse is usually the case, with carpal involvement occurring relatively late as compared to interphalangeal involvement. Bony erosions tend to occur at the joint margins where the articular cartilage and the synovial reflection begins, and also where the collateral ligaments attach. Although these notch-like defects are common in the metacarpophalangeal and interphalangeal joints in adults, in children they are best seen in the carpal areas. In neglected or unsuccessfully treated

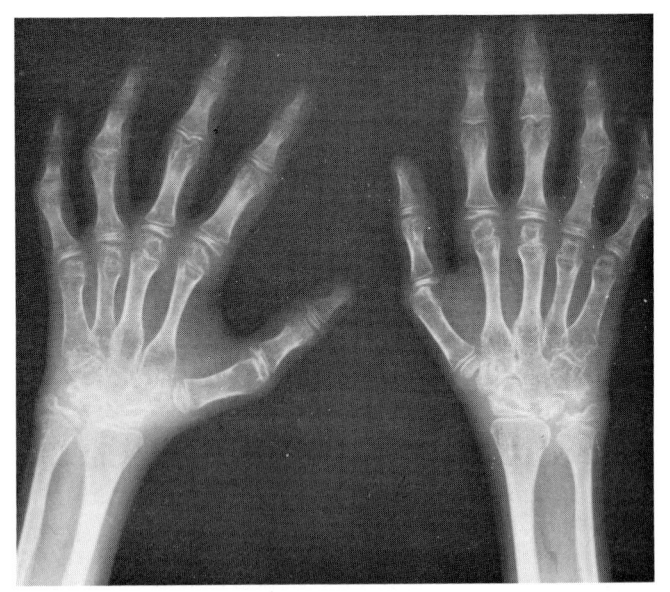

Figure 3-3 Juxta-articular osteoporosis is present as well as marked reduction in the interphalangeal joint spaces. Erosion and fusion of the carpal bones have occurred to a marked degree with similar changes involving the distal radial and ulnar epiphyses. There is also deformity of the proximal interphalangeal joint spaces, especially the fourth and fifth fingers bilaterally. Mild subluxation of the proximal metacarpophalangeal joints of the thumbs is evident.

patients, the joint spaces disappear completely, being obliterated by the solid bony ankylosis that develops (Fig. 3-4, *A* and *B*).

Erosive changes involving the proximal ends of the metacarpals may be seen later in the course of the disease, with a sharpening of the ends of these structures. Notch-like erosions at the distal radioulnar joint may also develop, but this is less common in children than in adults. Similar erosive changes of the ulnar styloid may be seen late in the course of the disease. Small pseudocysts accompany the diminution of the joint space and the erosive changes of the articulating surfaces. The development of pseudocysts, which are apparently areas of synovial proliferation, is less commonly seen in children than in adults.

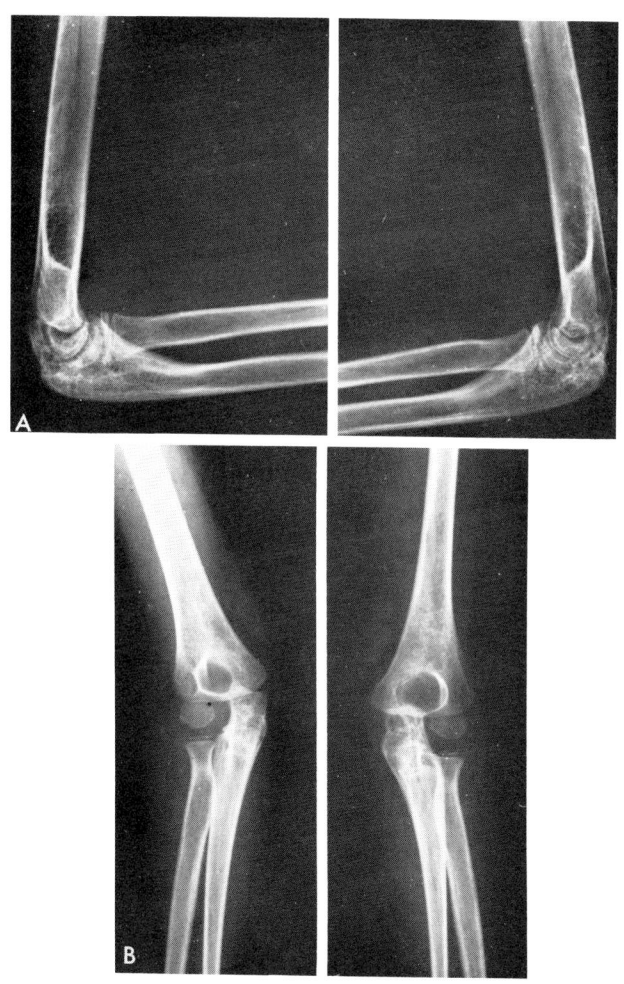

Figure 3-4, A and *B* Mild juxta-articular osteoporosis is present and a coarsening of the trabecular pattern of the proximal ulna has occurred, with reduction in the articulating space of the humeroulnar joint. Associated joint erosion is also evident in this area.

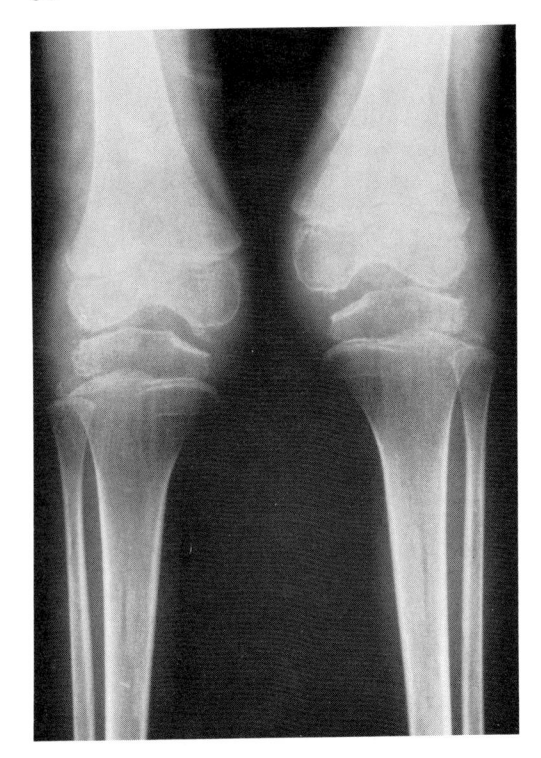

Figure 3-5 Soft tissue swelling is present about the knee joints and also reduction of the knee joint space, especially the lateral aspects of the knee joints. Erosion of the medial aspect of the proximal tibial epiphyses has occurred, with associated osteoporosis of the articulating structures.

Periosteal New Bone Formation

Periosteal new bone formation may occasionally occur, particularly in the phalanges and metatarsals adjacent to the affected joints. This is not necessarily a late finding, but may be seen early in the disease at a time when the soft tissue involvement is the predominant feature (Fig. 3-5). Associated chronic hyperemia may be responsible for these changes. The prevalence of periosteal new bone formation in children and its rarity in adults probably reflect the relative increase in vascularity of subperiosteal tissues in children.

Overgrowth and Undergrowth

Overgrowth of involved areas may occur, perhaps as a result of hyperemia. In addition, there may be an increase in the number of osseous maturation centers or "increased bone age," possibly as a result of the increased vascularity associated with the inflammatory process (Fig. 3-6, *A, B* and *C*). Undergrowth of a severely affected extremity may also occur, probably as a reflection of disease and muscle atrophy.

Spine

The spinal column may be involved early or late in the course of the disease. The condition involves primarily the articulating facets,

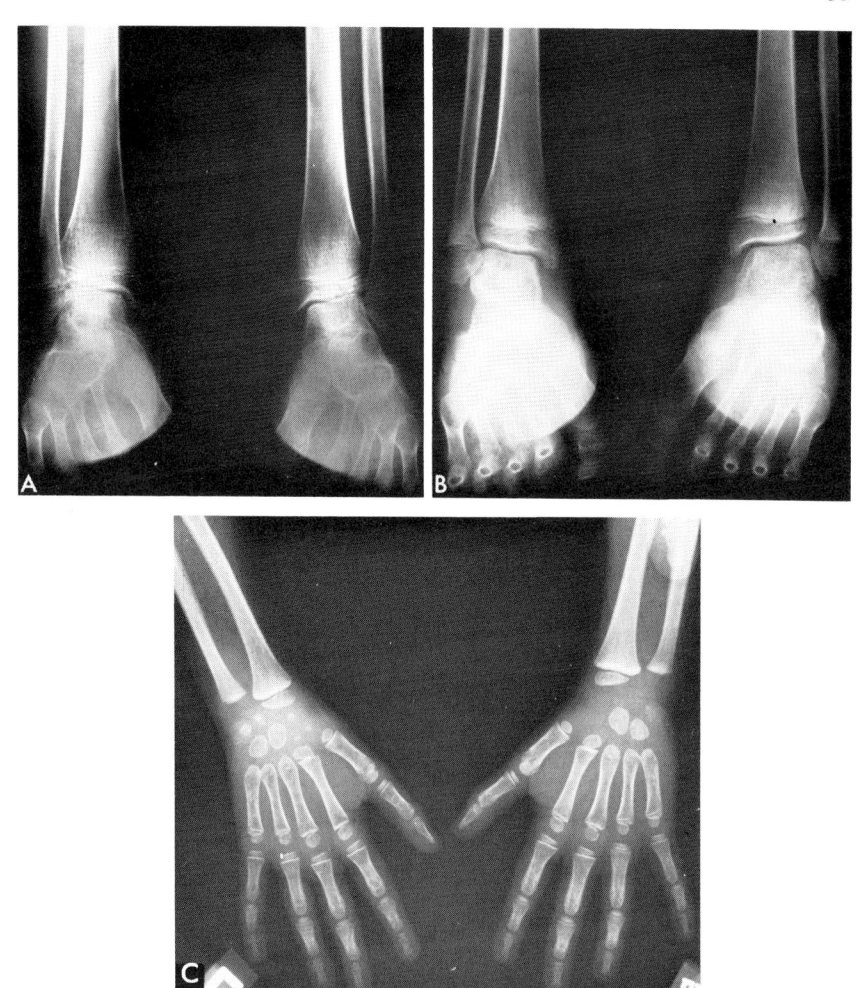

Figure 3-6 A, Soft tissue swelling is present by the ankle joints with reduction of the ankle joint spaces. B, Repeat studies four years later show an increase in the erosive changes and further reduction of the joint spaces. Cystic areas of bone destruction are seen in the distal tibial epiphysis. C, Advanced bone age, right wrist, in a 3-year-old child with rheumatoid arthritis. Seven ossification centers are identified on the right compared with three in the normal left wrist.

and consequently the radiographic features described in the other joints also apply to this portion of the osseous system. Further, demineralization of the articulating structures occurs, followed by a decrease in the articulating joints, and eventually ankylosis (Fig. 3-7).

Involvement of the cervical spine is common in juvenile rheumatoid arthritis, but involvement of the dorsal and lumbar spine areas is uncommon. The early involvement of the cervical spine is accompanied by a loss of the normal lordotic curvature, and once destruction of the articulating cartilage has occurred, the spine is maintained in a fixed, straight, and immobile position.

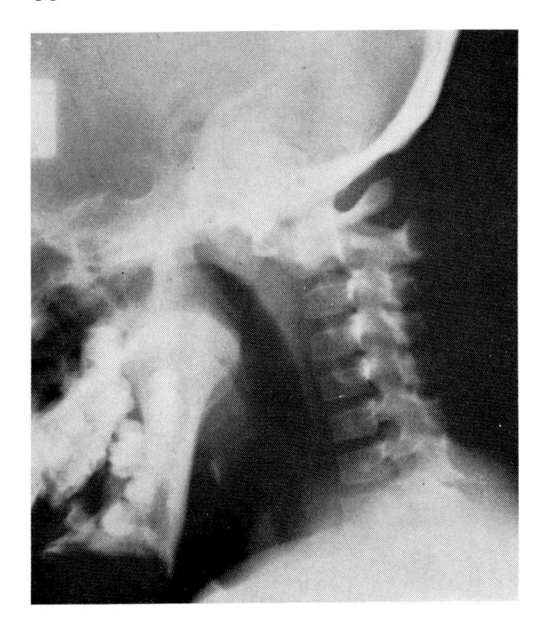

Figure 3-7 Obliteration of the apophyseal joint spaces is evident with associated marked straightening of the vertebral curve. Subluxation of the axis posterior to the anterior portion of the atlas is present. The intervertebral disc spaces are unaffected.

Differential Diagnosis

Such conditions as gout, degenerative arthritis, psoriatic arthritis, and villonodular synovitis, which must be considered in the adult patient, are naturally less common in the juvenile patient. The major conditions that must be differentiated from juvenile rheumatoid arthritis are tuberculosis, infectious arthritis, the inflammatory joint conditions that may complicate many of the collagen diseases, and osteochondrosis. Although monarticular arthritis is not uncommon in children, it is not usually associated with the degree of joint destruction seen in the polyarthritic type. Infectious arthritis, particularly staphylococcal arthritis, may produce monarticular joint swelling and rapid destruction of articulating cartilage. The rapidity of the process and the clinical manifestations serve to differentiate this condition from rheumatoid arthritis.

Single and multiple joint involvement may occur in tuberculosis, and the chronicity of the clinical features may suggest rheumatoid arthritis. Tuberculin testing and biopsy are important in the differential diagnosis. Arthritis complicating dermatomyositis, as well as some of the other collagen diseases, may mimic exactly the radiographic features of rheumatoid arthritis. Differentiation in these cases is made by recognizing the basic underlying disease.

Although many forms of osteochondrosis have been reported, there are only a few types for which radiographs showing necrosis are clinically important and which may possibly lead to a mistaken diagnosis of rheumatoid arthritis. The most common of these is Perthes' disease or aseptic necrosis of the capital femoral epiphysis. The early changes in this disease of subarticular demineralization of the femoral

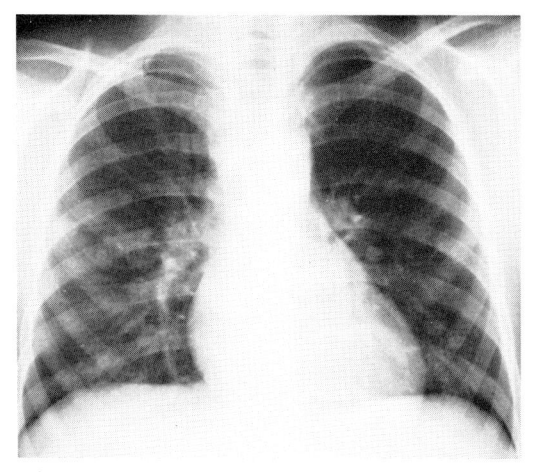

Figure 3-8 Chest radiograph shows multiple small nodules in both lungs. A few of the nodules have extravasated, leaving small cavities.

head with associated demineralization along the growth plate without diminution in the joint space serve to separate it from rheumatoid arthritis. Progressive destruction of the femoral head with associated flattening and sclerosis, followed by secondary changes in the femoral neck, is characteristic of Perthes' disease and should not be confused radiographically with rheumatoid arthritis. Osteochondritis can occur as a complication of rheumatoid arthritis. Multiple epiphyseal dysplasia, a congenital abnormality of epiphyseal development, although associated with some degree of joint immobility should not be mistaken radiographically or clinically for rheumatoid arthritis. Scheuermann's aseptic necrosis of the secondary ossification centers of the spine may be mistaken for spondylitis clinically, but the radiographic details, which show erosive changes of the vertebral bodies without abnormality of the synovial joints of the spine, are differentiating features.

Nodular Pneumonia

Nodular pneumonia occurs rarely in juvenile rheumatoid arthritis. The lesions are almost always asymptomatic and over a period of years can progress to cavitation. In Texas Children's Hospital study a 14-year-old patient had asymptomatic nodular pneumonia (Fig. 3-8). Serological tests for fungal diseases and skin tests for tuberculosis were negative.

REFERENCES

Grokoest, A. W., Snyder, A. I., and Schlaeger, R.: Juvenile Rheumatoid Arthritis. Boston, Little, Brown & Co., 1962.
Martel, W., Holt, J. F., and Cassidy, J. T.: Roentgenologic manifestations of juvenile rheumatoid arthritis. Am. J. Roentgen., *88*:400, 1962.

Chapter Four

LABORATORY DATA

HEMATOLOGICAL TESTS

Anemia

Anemia (less than 10 gm. per 100 ml. of hemoglobin or less than 34 per cent hematocrit) was present in 39 per cent (hemoglobin) and in 56 per cent (hematocrit) of the first 100 patients studied at the Texas Children's Hospital. The anemia is not characteristically persistent and occurs usually at some point during the disease process and lasts for varying periods of time (a few months to several years). The causes of anemia in juvenile rheumatoid arthritis are varied and can be related to the disease itself, to nutritional deficiencies, and to blood lost through stool from salicylate or steroid medication. Often a combination of these factors contribute to a significant anemia. The anemia of juvenile

Table 4-1 Hemoglobin (gm.%)

	Highest	Average	Lowest
Number of patients.. 100			
Number of determinations... 1544			
Patients with <10 gm.% Hgb some time during disease...... 39			
Range*...	19.6 to 9.9	–	17.5 to 5.2
Average**.......................................	–	11.9	–
Median***.......................................	13.5	–	10.4
Mean...	13.5	–	10.3
Standard deviation	1.4	–	2.0
Highest single determination...................	19.6	–	–
Lowest single determination....................	–	–	5.2
Number of determinations per patient..	136†	15.4	1
Duration of follow-up (in months per patient)..	136	41.6	1

*Range of each patient's highest and lowest values.
**The totaled average of each patient's average determination.
***Median and mean of all patients' highest values and lowest values.
†Prolonged, severely bleeding peptic ulcer requiring many hemograms.

Table 4-2 Hematocrit (%)

Number of patients...		100	
Number of determinations..		1637	
Patients with <34% Hct at some time during disease.........		56	
	Highest	*Average*	*Lowest*
Range*	59 to 30	—	52 to 18
Average**	—	36.3	—
Median***	41.1	—	33
Mean	41.0	—	32.6
Standard deviation	3.8	—	5.4
Highest single determination..................	59	—	—
Lowest single determination...................	—	—	18
Number of determinations per patient.......	132†	16.3	1
Duration of follow-up (in months per patient)...........	136	41.6	1

*Range of each patient's highest and lowest values.
**The totaled average of each patient's average determination.
***Median and mean of all patients' highest values and lowest values.
†Prolonged, severely bleeding peptic ulcer requiring many hemograms.

rheumatoid arthritis has not been well studied in pure form because medication and nutritional disturbances are important variables that are difficult to control.

Studies of adult rheumatoid arthritis patients have revealed a mild hemolytic process that is insufficient to explain the degree of anemia usually found (Lewis and Porter, 1960; Richmond et al., 1961; Roberts et al., 1963). The bone marrow in children with rheumatoid arthritis is usually hyperplastic, and the erythroid elements are increased. The serum iron is usually decreased. Iron absorption is thought to be normal (Roy et al., 1955; Weinstein, 1959). Freireich et al. (1957) have postulated that release of iron from reticuloendothelial tissues is impaired. Thus, an iron deficiency anemia could be present despite normal iron absorption. Adults with rheumatoid arthritis do not usually respond well to iron medication and the anemia present may be related to the chronic inflammatory process.

Children with rheumatoid arthritis often do not respond well to oral iron medication, but a significant number of children do have a nutritional deficiency of iron which is corrected with iron medication administered properly between meals, with no milk to diminish absorption. Failure to respond to iron medication often results from improper administration as well as from refractoriness of the anemia due to disease.

Significant bleeding does occur in patients receiving long-term salicylate therapy. Blood loss is reported to vary from five to 90 ml. per day (Holt, 1960), and may be even greater in patients actively bleeding. Occult blood loss has been reported in the stool in as many as 78 per cent of patients (Holt, 1960; Stubbe, 1958; Pierson et al., 1961; Muir and Cossar, 1959).

Table 4-3 White Blood Count (cells per cu. mm.)

Number of patients..		100	
Number of determinations...		1380	
	Highest	*Average*	*Lowest*
Range*...	86.0 to 4.2	–	12.7 to 1.1
Average**.....................................	–	9.28	–
Median***....................................	12.0	–	5.2
Mean..	15.7	–	5.6
Standard deviation	11.9	–	1.7
Highest single determination..................	86.0	–	–
Lowest single determination...................	–	–	1.1
Number of determinations per patient...	86	13.8	1
Duration of follow-up (in months per patient)...	136	41.6	1
Patients with > 12,000 WBC at some time during disease............................			50
Patients with < 5,000 WBC at some time during disease............................			40

*Range of each patient's highest and lowest values.
**The totaled average of each patient's average determination.
***Median and mean of all patients' highest values and lowest values.

Leukocytosis

Leukocytosis greater than 12,000 leukocytes per cu. mm. occurred at some time during the course of the disease in about half the patients. The highest cell count recorded in this group was 86,000 cells per cu. mm. There is marked variability in the leukocyte count, and as might be suspected, variation in the count is related to the severity of acute exacerbations as well as to the presence of other inflammatory diseases. Various respiratory diseases elevate the leukocytes significantly. Twelve children had leukocyte counts in excess of 25,000 at some time during the disease. Leukocytosis of this magnitude is not constant, and is always related to a serious exacerbation.

The polymorphonuclear leukocytes are characteristically increased in juvenile rheumatoid arthritis. The increase, however, as with the total leukocyte count, is related to the severity and exacerbation of the disease and considerable fluctuation occurs.

Occasionally patients will have definite leukopenia which may or may not be associated with splenomegaly. Felty's syndrome includes splenomegaly, leukopenia, and arthritis. Several patients have developed leukopenia secondary to medication; one patient developed a significant leukopenia secondary to gold administration.

The leukocyte count would seem, therefore, to be a nonspecific reflection of inflammatory disease, but a large percentage of patients with active rheumatoid arthritis at no time had an elevation of the leukocyte count or an increase of polymorphonuclear leukocytes. In addition, leukocytosis can obviously occur with any acute infectious disease, and must be considered, therefore, completely nonspecific either for diagnosis or prognosis.

Table 4-4 Polymorphonuclear Leukocytes (%)

Number of patients		100	
Number of determinations		1284	
	Highest	Average	Lowest
Range*	92 to 25	—	71 to 1
Average**	—	54.5	—
Median***	72	—	39
Mean	70.1	—	38.9
Standard deviation	15.0	—	13.5
Highest single determination	92	—	—
Lowest single determination	—	—	1
Number of determinations per patient	87	12.8	1
Duration of follow-up (in months per patient)	136	41.6	1

*Range of each patient's highest and lowest values.
**The totaled average of each patient's average determination.
***Median and mean of all patients' highest values and lowest values.

An interesting observation has been the intermittent presence of eosinophilia greater than 5 per cent that occurred in 55 of 100 patients during the course of the disease. At times eosinophilia can be related to medication, but no correlation has been made in these patients. Parasites are particularly common in the southern part of the United States and certainly some of the eosinophilia observed resulted from the presence of parasites. Stool examination, however, has not revealed parasites in any significant numbers.

Table 4-5 Eosinophiles (%)

Number of patients		98	
Number of determinations		943	
Number of patients with > 5% eosin at some time during disease		55	
	Highest	Average	Lowest
Range*	40 to 1	—	13 to 1
Average**	—	3.4	—
Median***	6	—	1
Mean	7.6	—	1.5
Standard deviation	2.0	—	2.3
Highest single determination	40	—	—
Lowest single determination	—	—	1
Number of determinations per patient	41	9.6	1
Duration of follow-up (in months per patient)	136	41.6	1

*Range of each patient's highest and lowest values.
**The totaled average of each patient's average determination.
***Median and mean of all patients' highest values and lowest values.

Erythrocyte Sedimentation Rate

The erythrocyte sedimentation rate is the most valuable single laboratory test in following the course of activity in juvenile rheumatoid arthritis. The ESR is a nonspecific test that measures the rate at which erythrocytes settle by gravity in a standardized tube in a given period of time. The rate is entirely nonspecific, and is governed by rouleaux formation of erythrocytes with aggregation, fibrinogen levels, alpha and gamma globulin levels, surface tension at the top of the column, red cell volume, friction of resistance, plasma viscosity, heparin anticoagulant, prolonged storage of blood, alteration of temperature, and length of blood column. These variables produce a normal rate of fall; in the presence of inflammatory disease an increase greater than normal occurs for reasons not fully understood. The Wintrobe method of determination is used in most children's hospitals in the United States because less than one milliliter of blood is necessary for determination. The amount of fall is measured in millimeters during a one hour period. The normal, uncorrected Wintrobe erythrocyte sedimentation rate is 15 millimeters or less per hour in children (Wintrobe, 1961). Prior to 1961 a correction was made for anemia based on a normal adult female hematocrit of 42 per cent and a normal male hematocrit of 47 per cent. Such correction should be discontinued because the normal hematocrit is usually lower in children, and also differs in various altitudes (Wintrobe, 1961). In Houston, for example, the normal hematocrit for children is 34 to 38 per cent, and a correction of the erythrocyte sedimentation rate to 42 or 47 per cent produces a spuriously low sedimentation rate.

The Westergren method of measuring the sedimentation rate is

Table 4-6 Erythrocyte Sedimentation Rate
(mm./hr., uncorrected) (Wintrobe)

Number of patients		98	
Number of determinations		631	
Patients with rate of 15 mm./hr. at some time during disease		79	
	Highest	*Average*	*Lowest*
Range*	78 to 1	—	53 to 1
Average**	—	25.9	—
Median***	40.0	—	10.1
Mean	36.8	—	15.3
Highest single determination	78	—	—
Lowest single determination	—	—	1
Number of determinations per patient	29	6.4	1
Duration of follow-up (in months per patient)	136	41.6	1

*Range of each patient's highest and lowest values.
**The totaled average of each patient's average determination.
***Median and mean of all patients' highest values and lowest values.

undoubtedly more accurate than the Wintrobe method because a larger volume of blood is used and 20 per cent dilution with sodium citrate reduces the influence of red cell volume on the erythrocyte sedimentation rate. The normal value is 10 millimeters or less per hour in children. In the adult the normal rate varies from 7 to 13 millimeters per hour, depending on age in the male, and from 10 to 20 millimeters per hour in the female, also depending on age.

In the Texas Children's Hospital group of 100 patients the Wintrobe ESR ranged from 78 to 1.0 millimeters and was elevated in all but 19 patients at some point during the course of the disease. The sedimentation rate varies considerably during the course of the disease, but does not change rapidly in a few days or weeks. Sedimentation rate characteristically is elevated for many months or years, with some fluctuation, and is often still elevated after clinical manifestations of disease are no longer present. In those few patients who had no elevation of sedimentation rate during the course of juvenile rheumatoid arthritis, the disease was usually milder.

Other Acute Phase Reactants

The C-reactive protein test consists of incubation of an antiserum to C-reactive protein with the patient's serum in a capillary tube. The C-reactive protein is precipitated by reaction with the C-polysaccharide of the pneumococcus. C-reactive protein was positive in 31.3 per cent of children with juvenile rheumatoid arthritis. The C-reactive protein elevation parallels the erythrocyte sedimentation rate closely, with little depression by salicylates or corticosteroids (Ziff and Baum, 1966). False-positive serological tests for syphilis are not usually present in children with active rheumatoid arthritis. In the adult, false-positive serological tests for syphilis have been reported in 6 to 11 per cent of patients (Kievits et al., 1956; Waldenstrom, 1958).

Serum Uric Acid

Serum uric acid levels were determined in 64 patients, usually early in the course of disease. Values slightly greater than 6.5 mg. per 100 ml. were found in two patients. The serum uric acid, at least in this group of children, was not significantly elevated, and in the two children who did have minimal elevation no attempt was made to establish a familial pattern. Serum uric acid, therefore, in children with juvenile rheumatoid arthritis, rarely exceeds 6.5 mg. per 100 ml. (phosphotungstic acid test with p-semidene as a reducing agent).

Serum Proteins

The study of the serum proteins in patients with juvenile rheumatoid arthritis is extremely helpful in establishing the presence of inflammation. The serum proteins are altered nonspecifically, presumably secondary to inflammatory response, in a significant number

Table 4-7. Juvenile Rheumatoid Arthritis—Laboratory Manifestations*

	Hemoglobin	Hematocrit	White Blood Cells	Polymorpho-nuclear	Eosinophiles	Total Serum Protein	ESR	Uric Acid	Antistrepto-lysin O Titer	LE cells	Latex	Sheep Cell
Patients tested	100	100	100	100	98	81	98	64	72	79	75	86
Total number of determinations	1544	1637	1380	1284	943	147	631	80	115	90	75	264
Highest single determination	19.6	59	86.0	92	40	10.5	78	6.7	2500			1792
Lowest single determination	5.2	18	1.1	1	1	3.6	1	1.2	7			
Average determination (total of all averages)	11.9	36.3	9.3	54.5	3.4		25.9	3.3	179			
Average number of determinations per patient	15.4	16.3	13.8	12.8	9.6	1.8	6.4	1.2	1.6			
Number patients with any abnormal low report	39	56	40									
Number patients with any abnormal high report			50		55		79		16			
Number patients with positive titer or test										2	30	18
Tests repeated remaining positive												7
Patients with negative latex and positive sheep cell titer												8

*Texas Children's Hospital, study of 100 patients. Longest duration of follow-up: 136 months; Shortest duration of follow-up: 1 month; Average duration of follow-up: 41.6 months.

of pediatric patients. The total serum protein, as measured by paper strip electrophoresis, is rarely low. Only three children of 80 patients tested revealed a total serum protein of less than 6.0 gm. per 100 ml. The selective constituents of the electrophoretic pattern, however, were significantly altered.

Albumin

Sixteen patients of 80 tested had a serum albumin of less than 3.5 gm. per 100 ml. In addition, six had a reversal of the albumin-globulin ratio. Thus, nearly 30 per cent of the patients tested revealed a significant decrease in serum albumin. This observation has been noted previously in adult rheumatoid arthritis patients (Ogryzlo et al., 1959; Sunderman, 1964; Sydnes, 1963; Wilkinson and Jones, 1962). In all 16 patients who had a serum albumin of less than 3.5 gm. per 100 ml. at some point during the disease process, the disease was severe. Only one of the three patients who expired in this series had serum albumin less than 3 gm. per 100 ml. Serum albumin of 3.3 gm. per 100 ml. was present in the second patient who expired; no measurement was obtained on the third patient.

Jeremy (1966) has shown that destruction of albumin increases in proportion to the degree of inflammation in rheumatoid arthritis. Radioactive I^{131} labeled albumin was used in his study.

Alpha-1 and Beta Globulins

Alpha-1 globulins in 80 patients tested were not elevated. This is consistent with other studies in adult patients (Ogryzlo et al., 1959; Sunderman, 1964; Sydnes, 1963; Wilkinson and Jones, 1962).

Five patients had beta globulins in excess of 1.3 gm. per 100 ml. Only a few, therefore, exhibited an increase in the beta globulin fraction. The cause, as with the increase in other globulins, is unknown. The increase is nonspecific and not generally associated with rheumatoid arthritis. No increase in beta globulins has been found in adults (Ogryzlo et al., 1959; Sunderman, 1964; Sydnes, 1963; Wilkinson and Jones, 1962).

Alpha-2

Alpha-2 globulins were elevated in six children of 80 tested. The cause of the alpha-2 elevation is unknown. The elevation is nonspecific, but does seem to be frequently related to rheumatoid arthritis.

Gamma Globulin

Serum gamma globulin, as measured by paper-strip electrophoresis, is of particular interest in juvenile rheumatoid arthritis. Forty-one patients of 80 tested (approximately 50 per cent) had elevations greater than 1.2 gm. per 100 ml.

Marked elevation of the serum gamma globulin (greater than 2 gm. per 100 ml.) occurred in 12 patients and was always associated with prominent systemic disease. Only two patients have since continued a course of mild disease or remission, and of these two patients, one has had only periodic mild exacerbations of disease in nine years' follow-up. The other patient has serious aseptic necrosis of the right hip, but has been in remission now for several years. Another patient, with serious peripheral rheumatoid arthritis, had persistent hepatitis, indistinguishable from so-called plasma-cell hepatitis.

The measurement of the serum proteins is an important laboratory aid in evaluation of the patient with juvenile rheumatoid arthritis, and an index of the degree of inflammation.

Antistreptolysin O Titer

Sixteen of 72 patients tested for antistreptolysin O titers (22 per cent of those tested) had titers greater than 250 Todd units. These patients were not hyperreactive to other antigens, such as afebrile agglutination reactions (typhoid, paratyphoid, Brucella, Proteus OX-19). As stated previously, about 45 per cent of the patients had respiratory infections preceding the onset of disease, and it is not surprising that a significant number of these infections were due to beta hemolytic streptococcus. The chief observation here of importance to the clinician is that Group A beta hemolytic streptococcal respiratory infections can and sometimes do precede the onset of juvenile rheumatoid arthritis, and streptococcal infection in itself need not indicate rheumatic fever.

Rheumatoid Factor

Rheumatoid factor is a 19 S macrogammaglobulin demonstrated by coating an inert particle with some form of gammaglobulin and mixing with the patient's serum, resulting in an agglutination reaction. The test is positive in 60 to 70 per cent of adult patients with rheumatoid arthritis, but is significantly elevated in only a small number of patients with juvenile rheumatoid arthritis. Probably about 15 per cent of patients with juvenile rheumatoid arthritis have rheumatoid factor present (Hanson et al., 1969). The reason for the reduced incidence is unknown and there has been some speculation that epidemiologic studies of seronegative juvenile rheumatoid arthritis patients have shown a greater incidence of spondylitis in relatives. Ankylosing spondylitis is, of course, associated with seronegative rheumatoid factor also (Ansell and Bywaters, 1962).

The most commonly used tests for rheumatoid factor are the latex, sensitized sheep cell agglutination, and bentonite particle tests. Barnett has suggested that a positive titer rheumatoid factor should be a titer greater than is found in 95 per cent of normal individuals of the same age group, as performed in a qualified laboratory. A positive test, therefore, must be correlated with the normal of the laboratory concerned in all instances. An attempt is being made to achieve world-wide standardization of rheumatoid factor tests but no specific recommendations are present at this time. The author has not been favorably im-

LABORATORY DATA

Table 4-8 Tests for Detecting Rheumatoid Factors†

Test	Form of coating gamma globulin	Type of particle	Manner of attachment of gamma globulin to cell or particle
Bacterial Agglutination	Unaggregated Human 7 S (?)	Bacterial Cell	Antibody bond
Sens. Sheep Cell Agglutination	Unaggregated Rabbit 7 S	Sheep Cell	Antibody bond
F II tanned Cell Agglutination	Aggregated Human 7 S	Tanned Sheep Cell	Adsorption
Sens. Human Cell Agglutination	Unaggregated Human 7 S	Human Rh+ Cell	Antibody bond
Latex Flocculation	Aggregated* Human 7 S	Latex	Adsorption
Bentonite Flocculation	Aggregated Human 7 S	Bentonite	Adsorption

*The use of aggregated gamma globulin increases the sensitivity of the test, but unaggregated gamma globulin is satisfactory for agglutinations by many sera.

†From Vaughan, J. H.: The rheumatoid factors, in Hollander, J. L., Arthritis and Allied Conditions, Ed. 7. Lea & Febiger, Philadelphia, 1966, p. 88.

pressed with the qualitative slide agglutination latex particle test since a wide variety of nonrheumatoid arthritis conditions have a positive test, leukemia in particular.

A significant number of children with arthritis will have borderline sensitized sheep cell agglutination titers of 1:14 or 1:28, but only about 10 to 15 per cent will have persistently elevated titers greater than 1:28. The percentage of positive tests seems to increase with age (Hanson et al, 1969), and patients with sensitized sheep cell agglutination titers greater than 1:112 (SCAT) seem to have persistently elevated tests. In general, these patients have more severe rheumatoid arthritis.

LE Cell Phenomenon

The phenomenon of the LE cell occurs in about 3 to 5 per cent of children with rheumatoid arthritis at some time during the course of disease (Table 4-7). The finding is usually transient and does not persist. A patient with such minimal disease as monarticular rheumatoid arthritis occasionally will have transiently positive LE preparations (See Differential Diagnosis, Chapter 5).

Hanson et al. (1966) have reported the presence of antinuclear factor in about 60 per cent of juvenile rheumatoid arthritis patients. Fink and Ziff have been able to detect antinuclear factor rarely, if at all, in juvenile rheumatoid arthritis patients. The discrepancy between two excellent laboratories makes abundantly clear the poor standardization of this procedure. The test must be considered only a research tool for the foreseeable future.

REFERENCES

Ansell, B. M., Bywaters, E. G. L., and Lawrence, J. S.: A family study in Still's disease. Ann. Rheum. Dis., *21*:243, 1962.

Freireich, E. J., Ross, J. F., Bayles, T., Emerson, C. P., and Finch, S. C.: Radioactive iron metabolism and erythrocyte survival studies of the mechanism of the anemia associated with rheumatoid arthritis. J. Clin. Invest. *36*:1043, 1957.

Hanson, V., Drexler, E., and Kornreich, H.: The relationship factor to age of onset in juvenile rheumatoid arthritis. Arthritis Rheum., *12*:82, 1969.

Hanson, V., Kornreich, H., and Drexler, E.: Rheumatoid factor in children with lupus erythematosus. Amer. J. Dis. Child. *112*:28, 1966.

Holt, P. R.: Measurement of gastrointestinal blood loss in subjects taking aspirin. J. Lab. Clin. Med., *56*:717, 1960.

Jeremy, R., Schaller, J., Wedgwood, R. J., and Healey, L. A.: Juvenile rheumatoid arthritis persisting into adulthood. Arthritis Rheum., *9*:515, 1966 (Abstracts).

Kievits, J. H., Goslings, J., Schuit, R. E., and Humans, W.: Rheumatoid arthritis and the positive LE cell phenomenon. Ann. Rheum. Dis., *15*:211, 1956.

Lewis, S. M., and Porter, I. H.: Erythrocyte survival in rheumatoid arthritis. Ann. Rheum. Dis., *19*:54, 1960.

Muir, A., and Cossar, I. A.: Aspirin and gastric hemorrhage. Lancet, *1*:539, 1959.

Ogryzlo, M. A., Maclachan, M., Dauphinee, J. A., and Fletcher, A. A.: The serum proteins in health and disease; filter paper electrophoresis. Amer. J. Med., *27*:596, 1959.

Pierson, R. N., Jr., Holt, P. R., Watson, R. M., and Keating, R. P.: Aspirin and gastrointestinal bleeding. Amer. J. Med., *31*:259, 1961.

Richmond, J., Alexander, W. R. M., Potter, J. L., and Duthie, J. J. R.: The nature of anemia in rheumatoid arthritis. V. Red cell survival measured by radioactive chromium. Ann. Rheum. Dis., 20:133, 1961.

Roberts, F. D., Hagedorn, A. B., Slocumb, C. H., and Owen, C. A.: Evaluation of the anemia of rheumatoid arthritis. Blood, 21:470, 1963.

Roy, L. M. H., Alexander, W. R. M., and Duthie, J. J. R.: Nature of anemia in rheumatoid arthritis. I. Metabolism of iron. Ann. Rheum. Dis., 14:63, 1955.

Stubbe, L.: Occult blood in feces after administration of aspirin. Brit. Med. J., Nov. 1, 1958.

Sunderman, F. W., Jr.: Studies on the serum proteins. VI. Recent advances in clinical interpretation of electrophoretic fractionations. Amer. J. Clin. Path., 42:1, 1964.

Sydnes, O. A.: On the electrophoretic estimated serum proteins in relation to the latex test and Waaler's test in rheumatoid arthritis. Acta Rheum. Scand., 9:237, 1963.

Vaughan, J. H.: The rheumatoid factors. In Hollander, J. L.: Arthritis and Allied Conditions, Ed. 7. Philadelphia, Lea & Febiger, 1966, p. 88.

Waldenstrom, J., and Winblad, S.: Some observations on the relationship of certain serological reactions in various diseases with hypergammaglobulinemia. Acta Rheum. Scand., 4:3, 1958.

Weinstein, I. M.: A correlative study of the erythrokinetics and disturbances in iron metabolism associated with the anemia of rheumatoid arthritis. Blood 14:950, 1959.

Wilkinson, M., and Jones, B. S.: Serum and synovial fluid proteins in arthritis. Ann. Rheum. Dis., 21:51, 1962.

Wintrobe, M.: Clinical Hematology, Ed. 5. Philadelphia, Lea & Febiger, 1961, p. 331.

Ziff, M., and Baum, J.: Laboratory findings in rheumatoid arthritis. In Hollander, J. L.: Arthritis and Allied Conditions, Ed. 7. Philadelphia, Lea & Febiger, 1966, p. 236.

Chapter Five

DIFFERENTIAL DIAGNOSIS

CRITERIA FOR DIAGNOSIS

Children who have polyarthritis with swelling, pain, and limitation of motion over a period of several months usually present few problems in a definitive diagnosis of rheumatoid arthritis. Patients with polyarthritis who suffer from pericarditis almost always have rheumatoid arthritis. The rash of rheumatoid arthritis, accompanied by polyarthritis, aids in disease classification. The problem of diagnosis occurs in those patients whose early manifestations are vague and resemble several other conditions. A group of 17 clinics* across the United States, Canada, and England is currently evaluating patients with juvenile rheumatoid arthritis in order to help delineate these diagnoses. Following are portions of the tentative criteria being used.

Any diagnosis listed under Major Conditions to be Excluded (p. 82) eliminates juvenile rheumatoid arthritis from consideration.

  I. Polyarthritis (two joints or more involved) or monarticular arthritis lasting longer than three months is sufficient for diagnosis if other diagnoses are ruled out. Swelling of a joint must be present to fulfill criteria, or two of the following three modalities must be present: heat; pain and tenderness; limitation of motion. Carpals with wrist, tarsals with ankle, and all cervical spines are considered one joint for tabulation purposes.
  II. Polyarthritis (as just defined in I) present more than six weeks requires one of the following manifestations for diagnosis:
   A. *Rash of Rheumatoid Arthritis.* Rheumatoid rash is an evanescent salmon-pink, usually circumscribed macular rash varying in size from 2 to 6 mm. in greatest diameter for individual lesions. The larger lesions may have a pale center with extreme paleness of the skin immediately to the periphery of the outer border of the rash. The rash tends to become confluent. It is found predominantly on the chest, axilla, thighs, upper arms, and, less commonly, on the face. It may appear at any time during the course of the disease. It occurs most frequently in patients with high fever, splenomegaly, lymphadenopathy, and leukocytosis. The rash may occasionally precede the onset of arthritis.
   B. *Rheumatoid Factor.* Latex fixation and sensitized sheep cell agglutination tests are positive in a small percentage (± 15 per cent) of patients with juvenile rheumatoid arthritis. Seropositivity increases with age. Positive reactions may also occur in other illnesses.
   A positive test as defined by the American Rheumatism Association Serology Standardization Committee is acceptable for purposes of this criterion.
   C. *Iridocyclitis.* Anterior, nongranulomatous uveitis is found in as high as 20 per cent of patients with juvenile rheumatoid arthritis. The eye

---

*See page 112 for listing.

involvement may be unilateral or bilateral, and may be followed by nonspecific band keratopathy. The onset is characteristically insidious, and physical findings may be initially minimal except for pupil irregularity. The earliest findings on slit-lamp examination are cells in the anterior chamber and precipitates on the posterior surface of the cornea. Band keratopathy is characterized by an opaque, gray band with fenestrations, which extends across the midplane of the cornea. Sequelae to these lesions are posterior synechiae with secondary cataracts, secondary glaucoma, or phthisis bulbi. Uveitis should be considered a serious complication of rheumatoid arthritis and may lead to blindness. Repeated ophthalmologic examinations should be performed on all children to detect the lesions in the earliest stages.

D. *Cervical Spine Involvement* (two other joints must be involved). Limitation of range of motion in the cervical spine region indicates involvement of the cervical spine and occurs in about one third of the patients. Radiologic evidence of apophyseal joint disease may occur without limitation of range of motion.

E. *Pericarditis.* Clinical evidence of pericarditis occurs in about 10 per cent of children with rheumatoid arthritis, and this is the chief form of cardiac involvement in this age group. It may occur during or after the onset of arthritis, and on rare occasions may even precede joint involvement. It is usually associated with other systemic manifestations. Chest pain may herald this complication, but more often, patients have no symptoms referrable to the heart. The classic signs of pericarditis (friction rub, x-ray evidence of pericardial effusion, and electrocardiographic changes) are identical with the findings of pericarditis due to other causes. The clinical course is variable and recurrent bouts are not uncommon. Complications such as heart failure and cardiac tamponade may occur. Constrictive pericarditis rarely, if ever, occurs.

F. *Tenosynovitis.* Tenosynovitis occurs in many patients with juvenile rheumatoid arthritis. It involves chiefly the tendon sheaths near the wrist, hands, ankles, and feet.

G. *Intermittent Fever.* Various patterns of fever may be seen in juvenile rheumatoid arthritis. However, a persistent intermittent fever with diurnal variation to between 102 and 106° F. with return to normal is suggestive of rheumatoid arthritis only if other diseases such as sepsis and leukemia are excluded.

H. *Morning Stiffness.* Many children exhibit stiffness or difficulty of motion after sleep or inactivity. Such stiffness may last a few minutes to several hours. The stiffness or "jelling" often must be determined only from observation by the physician rather than from description by the child. This phenomenon of stiffness differs from pain alone.

General Discussion

I. There are patients who exhibit systemic manifestations before arthritis occurs. These patients may have such symptoms as fever, rheumatoid rash, pericarditis, splenomegaly, lymphadenopathy, weight loss, malaise, laboratory findings as listed previously in II, and minimal or no obvious joint manifestations.

II. Additional nonspecific laboratory findings include anemia, extreme leukocytosis, and increased acute phase reactants.

III. *Subcutaneous Nodules.* Subcutaneous nodules occur in juvenile rheumatoid arthritis, rheumatic fever, systemic lupus erythematosus and sometimes in children with no discernible disease. They occur most conspicuously in areas subject to pressure. Histologically, they appear to be a mixture of those features found in rheumatic fever and adult rheumatoid arthritis and are, therefore, not specific for diagnosis.

IV. *Joint Fluid Changes.* The fluid is clear to turbid with increased opacity, and may spontaneously clot in many cases. The total cell count is increased, averaging 15,000 cells per cu. mm., with a range of 500 to

65,000 cells per cu. mm. Polymorphonuclear neutrophilic leukocytes predominate. Bacteria and characteristic crystals of monosodium urate or calcium pyrophosphate are not seen. Joint fluids should be routinely cultured on suitable media for microorganisms.

V. *Joint Biopsy.* Synovial biopsy in juvenile rheumatoid arthritis reveals a nonspecific chronic inflammatory reaction with synovial cell hyperplasia, and with infiltration of plasma cells and lymphocytes. The chief value of joint biopsy is to rule out tuberculosis, other infectious disease, and rare lesions such as pigmented villonodular synovitis. In general, biopsy is not necessary, but in cases of monarticular arthritis in which classification is uncertain, biopsy should be performed.

VI. *Joint Grouping.* For purposes of enumeration, the cervical spine is to be considered a single joint. The carpal and wrist joints, and the tarsal and ankle joints, in each extremity are considered as a single unit. All other joints are considered individually.

VII. *Early x-ray manifestations* usually consist of soft tissue swelling. Juxta-articular osteoporosis and juxta-articular periosteal new bone formation occur early. Altered epiphyseal growth, erosions, and ankylosis are later changes.

Major Conditions to be Excluded

A. Rheumatic fever
B. Connective tissue diseases
 1. Systemic lupus erythematosus
 2. Dermatomyositis
 3. Polyarteritis
 4. Scleroderma
C. Infectious diseases
 1. Pyogenic arthritis
 2. Sepsis
 3. Viral disease
 4. Tuberculosis
 5. Syphilis
 6. Fungal disease
D. Allergic reactions
E. Anaphylactoid purpura
F. Ulcerative colitis and regional ileitis
G. Hematologic diseases
 1. Leukemia
 2. Sickle cell anemia
 3. Hemophilia
 4. Thalassemia
H. Trauma
I. Miscellaneous diseases
 1. Plasma cell hepatitis
 2. Reiter's disease
 3. Sarcoidosis
 4. Agammaglobulinemia
 5. Hypertrophic osteoarthropathy
 6. Ankylosing spondylitis
 7. Villonodular synovitis
 8. Gaucher's disease
 9. Mucopolysaccharidoses and bone dysplasia

PERPLEXING PRESENTING PROBLEMS

Fever of Undetermined Origin

In the daily practice of pediatrics the physician sees many children who have fever of poorly explained origin. Most of these children are not seriously ill and prompt remission of fever usually occurs without therapy; these patients are sometimes said to have "viral infection." Occasionally a patient has a low grade fever of undetermined origin lasting for several weeks, while still others have intermittent daily pyrexia exceeding 102° F. Obscure localized abscesses, such as perinephric abscess, may occur and these can be difficult to determine.

Neoplastic diseases such as lymphoma and leukemia may occur with no clinical manifestations other than fever. Hemograms and platelet count may be completely normal. In such instances as many as five or six bone marrow determinations, and even liver biopsies, have been necessary over a period of six to 12 months before a definitive diagnosis could be established. Such patients can have joint pain and even arthritis before manifestations of leukemia become apparent in the peripheral blood smear. Hodgkin's disease can also be present in this manner. Lymph node biopsies, or percutaneous needle liver biopsies when indicated, usually are the only way to demonstrate the characteristic Sternberg-Reed cells. Sepsis is also an important consideration in patients with fever of undetermined origin.

It is essential and important to remember that most hospital laboratories usually retain blood cultures for about ten days only and therefore the laboratory must be directed to preserve blood cultures for as long as six weeks in cases of this nature. Organisms such as partially anaerobic gamma streptococci may require six weeks for growth and identification. Other organisms, such as unusual neisseria species, may require 15 to 20 days for growth. For this reason, multiple cultures should be taken to avoid the confusion of possible contamination.

Pyelonephritis does occur in the absence of pyuria, and at times is demonstrable only by carefully performed urinary tract cultures. Partially treated bacterial meningitis must always be ruled out, particularly in infants.

Allergic reactions, particularly to various medications, can cause prolonged, significant, intermittent daily fever for a period of weeks or months. Antibiotics especially are known to produce this effect. Many patients with fever of undetermined origin have been "cured" by discontinuing all medication. A rash or other manifestations do not always occur with fever in cases of allergic reaction.

Fever preceding the onset of polyarthritis is known to occur. In Calabro's series, 18 of 50 patients had significant fever antedating the onset of articular manifestations, with a median duration of three and one-half months (Calabro and Marchesano, 1967). In our experience at Texas Children's Hospital, patients almost always have signs of minimal arthritis within a few weeks of the onset of fever. Patients in this category must, by necessity, wait for other manifestations of rheumatoid arthritis before a definitive diagnosis can be seriously considered. Response to salicylates has been thought by many observers to be helpful in differentiating rheumatoid arthritis from other conditions such as rheumatic fever. Some children with rheumatoid arthritis do, however, respond dramatically to salicylates from the first dose, and a few patients with rheumatic fever will require salicylate therapy for several days before remission of fever occurs.

Hepatosplenomegaly, Lymphadenopathy, and Fever

When these symptoms occur the same infectious diseases discussed previously must be considered as well as parasitic diseases such as amebiasis. Subacute bacterial endocarditis and neoplastic diseases must be definitely ruled out. Children with plasma cell hepatitis, in addition to hepatosplenomegaly, lymphadenopathy, and fever, will have greater than 3 gm. per 100 ml. gamma globulin as measured by protein paper strip electrophoresis. Ascites is a prominent finding in these patients.

Patients with early rheumatoid arthritis may have hepatosplenomegaly, lymphadenopathy, and fever, but polyarthritis may be minimal or absent early in the course of disease. These patients, more often than not, must await the test of time and the exclusion of other prominent possibilities.

Peripheral Articular Joint Swelling with no Systemic Manifestations

Children who have swelling in multiple joints lasting more than six weeks, with no findings by x-ray other than soft tissue swelling, more often than not will later be diagnosed as having juvenile rheumatoid arthritis. Allergic reactions, however, can produce the same manifestations, along with systemic lupus erythematosus, rheumatic fever, agammaglobulinemia, Reiter's disease, sarcoidosis, psoriatic arthritis, and even ulcerative colitis and regional ileitis. Even though extremely rare, gout also sometimes occurs in older children.

Characteristically, during the first six weeks of juvenile rheumatoid arthritis, few, if any, destructive changes occur that are evident by x-ray.

Rash of Rheumatoid Arthritis

Juvenile rheumatoid arthritis patients have a wide variety of rashes including hives, erythema multiforme, and rarely erythema marginatum or rheumatic papules. One particular rash, termed the rash of rheumatoid arthritis, is probably diagnostic of the disease. This rash, as described in Chapter One, usually occurs in conjunction with more serious manifestations of disease such as fever, nodules, and lymphadenopathy, but can occur with fever alone and no obvious joint manifestations; it may even precede articular manifestations by several weeks. When the definite rash of rheumatoid arthritis is present with fever, a presumptive diagnosis can probably be made, but a definitive diagnosis must wait for the development of articular manifestations always.

Uveitis

Iridocyclitis, not a common ophthalmologic abnormality in the pediatric age group, is to be considered serious because of its chronicity and failure to respond to therapy (see Chapter One). Band keratopathy, cataract, secondary glaucoma, and even choroiditis are known to occur as sequelae. The possibility of blindness as a complication demands careful attention to the manifestation when present.

Rheumatoid arthritis is the disease most frequently associated with uveitis. Occasionally viral disease such as mumps and measles can cause acute uveitis, which ordinarily subsides with the disease process. Focal infection is frequently stated to be a cause of uveitis but then often no focal infection is ever found.

Iridocyclitis is known to occur many years prior to or following remission of rheumatoid arthritis; however, well documented cases of iridocyclitis have also occurred when no rheumatic disease has become apparent at any time.

Subcutaneous Nodules in Polyarthritis

Subcutaneous nodules occur in juvenile rheumatoid arthritis, rheumatic fever, systemic lupus erythematosus, and in children with no discernible disease. Subcutaneous nodules are not of diagnostic value in differentiating between the three diseases, but they help in differentiating the three conditions from other diseases.

The natural history of the histologic findings is not known with regard to subcutaneous nodules. As an example, the rheumatic fever nodule may well present its characteristic picture because of earlier development while the rheumatoid arthritis nodule may present its characteristic appearance because of the duration of its existence. Further work in this area will be necessary before it is known whether subcutaneous nodules can differentiate the two diseases.

Monarticular Arthritis

Monarticular arthritis is the presenting articular symptom in approximately one-fourth of children with rheumatoid arthritis; however, only about 10 per cent persist with monarticular arthritis more than three months (Chapter One). The remainder develop significant polyarticular disease and the diagnosis becomes easier. The children who persist with essentially monarticular disease usually, at some point in the disease process, manifest slight swelling in one or two other joints. The initial joint involved, often the knee, remains the major involvement during the entire course of the disease.

Patients with monarticular disease rarely present with systemic manifestations such as high fever, lymphadenopathy, or hepatosplenomegaly, although an increase in sedimentation rate is usually present. The usual child with rheumatoid arthritis presents with an insidious swelling of the knee or ankle which is mainly periarticular; massive joint effusion is unusual. There is no erythema of the skin overlying the joint, but slight warmth can be present. Tenderness is usually not severe but the patient has a noticeable limp. Atrophy of the surrounding muscles is rapid and limitation of motion is often present.

At this point the clinician must decide whether to actively pursue diagnosis with the tools at his disposal or adopt a "watchful waiting" attitude for a period of several weeks or even months. It is the author's feeling that monarticular arthritis deserves and demands early diagnosis, and whatever tools are at the disposal of the physician to make a valid, accurate, and early diagnosis should be utilized. This course should be pursued to avoid overlooking a child with pyogenic arthritis due to microorganisms such as staphylococci or tubercle bacilli. If joint fluid is obtainable, the joint should be immediately aspirated, and a search made for microorganisms by stain and culture. A search should also be made by polarized light microscopy for calcium pyrophosphate and sodium monourate crystals. The author's personal opinion is that if joint fluid is not available percutaneous needle biopsy with a Parker-Pearson needle or open biopsy should be performed, principally to rule out tuberculosis or other bacterial infection. The synovial biopsy of rheumatoid arthritis reveals nonspecific chronic synovitis with hyperplasia of the villi and increased cellularity of mononuclear cells such as plasma cells and lymphocytes. The rare patient with villonodular synovitis or hemangioma is also diagnosed in this manner. Another very good reason for consideration of early biopsy in the monarticular patient is that often the disease process may last for many years. Before entering into a long-term program of therapy, a serious attempt at accurate diagnosis should be accomplished in any patient with long-term chronic disease.

Patients with systemic lupus erythematosus and rheumatic fever may at the start have monarticular arthritis. Usually the arthritis is not severe and is not erosive. Appropriate tests such as the LE preparations help with the diagnosis. Early in the course of the disease, a definitive diagnosis may not be possible. Patients with rheumatic fever who have essentially monarticular arthritis are rare. Such patients usually have systemic manifestations such as fever and carditis. The carditis may not become apparent for several weeks so patients who have monarticular arthritis and fever must be carefully observed.

The major cause of confusion in monarticular arthritis is trauma. Patients who subsequently develop rheumatoid arthritis may begin with an episode of trauma, and the clinician must decide at what point trauma ends and rheumatoid arthritis begins. Usually, the joint swelling of trauma, secondary to twisting injury of the knee, or a blow, will last only about one week. If, however, the patient uses the injured joint, repeated minor trauma can cause persistence of the joint swelling and joint effusion for many weeks. Joint effusion is a prominent feature in traumatic arthritis, and the fluid is usually serosanguineous or even the normal straw color. It is here that the mucin test is of great help because the viscosity of the fluid in traumatic arthritis is high, and in rheumatoid arthritis it is low. Measurement of the viscosity, either by spreading a drop between the thumb and forefinger and checking the viscosity visually, or by the use of the more elaborate viscometer or Ropes test, is very helpful. There are usually less than 2000 leukocytes per high power field in the fluid with a good mucin clot.

Monarticular arthritis must be carefully evaluated by the physician to establish a diagnosis. The author is not in favor of unselectively placing a cylinder cast on every child with nonspecific synovial effusion, to "see how they will do" over a period of several weeks, and then providing medical evaluation if the patient persists with arthritis.

Significance of Rheumatoid Factor Test

Rheumatoid factor is present at some time during the course of disease in about 15 per cent of children with rheumatoid arthritis. In children under five years of age the percentage of rheumatoid factor is greatly diminished. The Serology Standardization Committee of the American Rheumatism Association has not formulated a specific definition of positive and negative tests for rheumatoid factor in either adults or children. Barnett has suggested that a positive titer of rheumatoid factor should be a titer greater than that found in 95 per cent of "normals" of the same age group, as performed in a qualified laboratory (1968).

The definition, however, does specify a quantitative test, and not a qualitative test. There are commercial slide agglutination qualitative test kits on the market which, at the present time, do not fulfill the preceding criteria. These tests often are reported as mildly reactive or reactive; however, they are positive in a wide variety of nonspecific conditions. Patients with conditions such as sepsis and leukemia have been found to have positive slide agglutination latex particle tests, but the interpretation of such tests must be regarded with great doubt, and they must always be followed by a quantitative sheep cell agglutination test or quantitative latex particle agglutination test.

The Serology Standardization Committee of the American Rheumatism Association, at the present time, is attempting to prepare kits through the Ortho Research Foundation to eliminate the problems that have occurred with qualitative tests.

A child with a positive quantitative rheumatoid factor test and polyarthritis should be considered to have juvenile rheumatoid arthritis until proved otherwise. For patients with only a qualitatively reactive slide agglutination latex particle test, the same significance should not be attached.

Significance of LE Cells and Antinuclear Factor

A small percentage of children with rheumatoid arthritis will have a few LE cells present in the peripheral blood. In such instances the clinician is hard pressed to state definitely that the patient has rheumatoid arthritis, but until other manifestations occur the diagnosis should be juvenile rheumatoid arthritis with LE cell phenomenon, and these patients need not be considered in a separate category of observation. Condemi et al. found that 33 per cent of children with juvenile rheumatoid arthritis showed an antinuclear factor (1965). Fink and Ziff have been unable to confirm this observation. One probable explanation for the apparent discrepancy is that the status of antinuclear factor test standardization is, at best, uncertain. There is apparently little correlation at the present time among different laboratories using the same sera.

The Patient with Polyarthritis, Elevated Antistreptolysin Titer, and Absence of Carditis

Children whose presenting symptoms are polyarthritis with an elevation of the ASO titer, and no clinically apparent carditis in the first four or five weeks of illness, must be considered to have acute rheumatic fever until proved otherwise. However, not all of these patients will have rheumatic fever; a significant number of children with juvenile rheumatoid arthritis have elevation of ASO titer secondary to a preceding streptococcal infection. Unless there are other clinical manifestations that lead the clinician to suspect rheumatoid arthritis or other diseases more than rheumatic fever, a presumptive diagnosis of rheumatic fever must be entertained. Any polyarthritis lasting longer than four or five consecutive weeks is not caused by rheumatic fever. Markowitz has observed patients whose initial polyarthritis lasted longer than four weeks and who subsequently were proved not to have rheumatic fever.

Pericarditis with or without Polyarthritis

Pericarditis with polyarthritis, in the absence of myocarditis or clinically detectable valvular lesions, is almost always characteristic of rheumatoid arthritis. Isolated pericarditis is known to rarely precede the onset of articular disease (Lietman and Bywaters, 1963). In those patients with both polyarthritis and pericarditis, systemic lupus erythematosus must be considered and effectively excluded. Usually there are other multisystem indications of lupus erythematosus. These include renal involvement, polyserositis, positive LE cell preparation or positive antinuclear factor, malar flush, hemolytic anemia, thrombocytopenia, Raynaud's phenomenon, or leukopenia. Pericardial effusion sufficient to impair function and cause tamponade is rare in systemic lupus erythematosus (Shulman and Harvey, 1961).

The pericarditis of rheumatic fever is almost always found in conjunction with myocarditis or clinically apparent valvulitis. Isolated pericarditis in rheumatic fever is extremely rare.

Idiopathic or acute benign pericarditis occurs in the absence of polyarthritis. A very perplexing problem presenting to the clinician is the patient whose isolated pericarditis precedes onset of rheumatoid arthritis. Time alone and the appearance of articular manifestations can solve this problem.

Constrictive pericarditis as a late sequelae is almost always due to conditions other than juvenile rheumatoid arthritis. There was not a single case found in the literature reviewed of constrictive pericarditis following the pericarditis of juvenile rheumatoid arthritis.

DIFFERENTIAL DIAGNOSIS OF SPECIFIC DISEASES

Rheumatic Fever

The revised Jones criteria for guidance in the diagnosis of rheumatic fever is helpful for differentiation of juvenile rheumatoid arthritis from rheumatic fever.

Jones Criteria (Revised) for Guidance in the Diagnosis of Rheumatic Fever

MAJOR MANIFESTATIONS	MINOR MANIFESTATIONS
Carditis	*Clinical*
Polyarthritis	Fever
Chorea	Arthralgia
Erythema marginatum	Previous rheumatic fever or rheumatic
Subcutaneous nodules	heart disease
	Laboratory
	Acute phase reaction
	Erythrocyte sedimentation rate,
	C-reactive protein, leukocytosis,
	prolonged PR interval

DIFFERENTIAL DIAGNOSIS

PLUS

Supporting evidence of preceding streptococcal infection (increased ASO or other streptococcal antibodies; positive throat culture for Group A streptococcus; recent scarlet fever).

The presence of two major criteria, or of one major and two minor criteria, indicates a high probability of the presence of rheumatic fever if supported by evidence of a preceding streptococcal infection. The absence of the latter should make the diagnosis suspect, except in situations in which rheumatic fever is first discovered after a long latent period from the antecedent infection (e.g., Sydenham's chorea or low-grade carditis).

Children who present with carditis and polyarthritis must be considered to have acute rheumatic fever until proved otherwise. Children with chorea, in addition to other manifestations listed, must be considered to have rheumatic fever. Although erythema marginatum is known to occur in juvenile rheumatoid arthritis, its presence with polyarthritis must be interpreted to indicate rheumatic fever unless definite evidence is available for the diagnosis of rheumatoid arthritis. As previously discussed, subcutaneous nodules are not diagnostic of rheumatic fever, rheumatoid arthritis, or systemic lupus erythematosus; however, their presence is helpful in differentiating the three diseases from other conditions in patients who have polyarthritis.

A major cause of concern and confusion is the patient who has polyarthritis and fever, with no carditis, and perhaps an increase in the sedimentation rate. Early in the course of the disease, the diagnosis is not clear. The committee of the American Heart Association has now added the requirement that strong supporting evidence of preceding streptococcal infection (in the form of an increased ASO titer or other streptococcal antibodies; positive throat culture for Group A streptococcus; or recent scarlet fever) is necessary before making a diagnosis of rheumatic fever. Occasionally a patient will still appear who is developing early juvenile rheumatoid arthritis after having a preceding streptococcal respiratory infection. The diagnosis of these patients will become apparent only after a six-week to three-month interval, with persistence of arthritis making the diagnosis clear. Polyarthritis of rheumatic fever is usually extremely migratory, and involves essentially the same joints as rheumatoid arthritis. Joint involvement in rheumatoid arthritis tends to be more stable, however, and true migratory polyarthritis is unusual. The joints in acute rheumatic fever often are more painful than in rheumatoid arthritis; erosive arthritis is virtually nonexistent in rheumatic fever. Polyarthritis lasting longer than five weeks in acute rheumatic fever is extremely rare.

The carditis of rheumatic fever is customarily associated with a significant organic murmur. The types of murmur accepted as signs are a significant apical systolic murmur, apical mid-diastolic murmur, or basal diastolic murmur. A significant change in the quality of the murmur is considered important. Cardiomegaly, or increase in cardiac size, in a patient with a past history of rheumatic heart disease constitutes another indication of carditis. Pericarditis, evident by pericardial effusion with muffled heart sounds, clinically detectable friction rub, or elevation of the S-T segments over the precordium, and concomitant changes in the limb leads with inversion of the T-wave, usually does not occur as an isolated manifestation but is associated with carditis or valvulitis. Congestive heart failure, in the absence of congenital heart disease, constitutes evidence of carditis, especially when associated with a significant murmur.

Systemic Lupus Erythematosus

Systemic lupus erythematosus can be extremely difficult to differentiate from juvenile rheumatoid arthritis. In general, the disease is unusual under the age of five years and occurs more frequently in girls, with a ratio of 5:1. The malar flush or the rash that occurs in some children with systemic lupus erythematosus is extremely helpful in differential diagnosis. The rash of rheumatoid arthritis is not known to occur in systemic lupus erythematosus. A markedly positive LE cell preparation is almost, but not always, diagnostic of the disease when attempting to differentiate from rheumatoid arthritis. Other lupus-like conditions such as drug reactions may or may not be diseases different from lupus erythematosus. A mildly positive LE cell preparation that has only a few cells per slide can occur in about 5 per cent of patients with juvenile rheumatoid arthritis at some time during the disease process, but a markedly positive LE preparation is most unusual and almost excludes the diagnosis. Antinuclear factor has achieved some prominence in the last few years as a more specific index of antinuclear antibody. Unfortunately the procedure is so new that standardization of the test among laboratories is not yet complete. Duplication among various medical center laboratories thus far is not possible until a more standard procedure is available, and the LE cell preparation should not be abandoned in clinical medicine in favor of the antinuclear factor test. Some laboratories have reported that as many as 33 per cent of juvenile rheumatoid arthritis patients have positive antinuclear factor tests (Condemi et al., 1965) and an even higher percentage of children with lupus erythematosus. These data have not been confirmed.

A sheep cell agglutination test or quantitative latex agglutination test is positive in 10 to 15 per cent of patients with juvenile rheumatoid arthritis, but almost never in children with systemic lupus erythematosus. This is not true of the adult, however; 60 per cent or more of adults with rheumatoid arthritis have positive rheumatoid factor tests and only about one-fourth of patients with systemic lupus erythematosus have positive rheumatoid factor tests.

Significant renal involvement is extremely rare in juvenile rheumatoid arthritis and is usually limited to amyloid degeneration. Two types of significant renal involvement seem to occur in systemic lupus erythematosus: massive proteinuria with a nephrotic-like syndrome, and mild proteinuria accompanied by hematuria with a clinical picture of chronic nephritis.

Significant hemolytic anemia occurs in children with systemic lupus erythematosus but is almost never apparent in juvenile rheumatoid arthritis. Leukopenia is a common finding in systemic lupus erythematosus but also occurs in juvenile rheumatoid arthritis. Polyserositis is a more prominent feature of systemic lupus erythematosus, but is unusual in rheumatoid arthritis, with pericarditis occurring in about 10 per cent of children with rheumatoid arthritis. Ascites usually does not occur in rheumatoid arthritis.

The polyarthritis associated with systemic lupus erythematosus is usually milder. Erosive arthritis is extremely unusual in children with systemic lupus erythematosus. Its presence or absence is helpful in diagnosis but not definitive. Clinically, there is no significant difference between the polyarthritis of lupus erythematosus and that of juvenile rheumatoid arthritis other than the milder nature of involvement in lupus erythematosus.

Salicylates have been said to provide a means of differentiating rheumatic fever, rheumatoid arthritis, and systemic lupus erythematosus. The rheumatic fever patient is purported to respond rapidly to salicylates, with a relatively poor response from the patient with rheumatoid arthritis, and no response from the patient with lupus erythematosus. In clinical practice, however, there are patients with rheumatoid arthritis and patients with systemic lupus erythematosus who do respond well and rapidly to salicylates. A patient with rheumatic fever occasionally does not respond immediately and requires many days to achieve abatement of fever.

The accompanying table may be helpful in differential diagnosis (Table 5-1).

Table 5-1 Differential Diagnosis of Rheumatic Fever, Rheumatoid Arthritis, and Systemic Lupus Erythematosus

	Rheumatic Fever	*Rheumatoid Arthritis*	*Systemic Lupus Erythematosus*
Age Trend	> 5 years	< 5 years	> 5 years
Sex Ratio	Equal	Girls 1.5:1	Girls 5:1
Joint Findings			
Pain	Severe	Moderate	—
Swelling	Nonspecific	Nonspecific	Nonspecific
Tenderness	Severe	Moderate	—
Bony X-ray changes	None	Frequent	Occasional
Morning Stiffness	Yes	Yes	Yes
Rash	Erythema marginatum	Rheumatoid arthritis rash	Malar flush
Chorea	Yes	No	Rarely
Clinical Carditis	+	Rare	Late
Laboratory Tests			
WBC	Normal to high	Normal to high	Decreased to normal
Latex	—	+(10%)	+ occasionally
Sheep cell agglut.	—	+(10%)	—
L.E. cell prep.	—	+(5%)	+
Biopsy			
Skin rash	Nonspecific	Nonspecific	Diagnostic
Nodules	Nonspecific	Nonspecific	Nonspecific
Response to salicylates	Rapid	Slow, usually	Slow or none

Polymyositis and Dermatomyositis

Both polymyositis and its more serious variant, dermatomyositis, occur in childhood. Polymyositis may occur in the total absence of any cutaneous lesions, muscular pain, or constitutional symptoms. It may be present in either very acute, subacute, or chronic insidious forms, and there may be systemic involvement of organs and tissues other than the skeletal muscles usually affected (Pearson, 1966).

The cardinal triad of symptoms is composed of extreme muscular weakness, muscular pain, and typical skin rash. In children, the weakness is usually sudden in onset, then progresses rapidly to the point that the patient is unable to rise from the bathtub or climb from a sitting position on the floor to a standing position. The muscular weakness is symmetrical and involves the extremities, predominantly the proximal muscles of the upper and lower extremities such as the thigh and pelvic girdle muscles. The weakness can spread to involve the distal musculature of the limbs and the muscles of the trunk, neck, and face. Swallowing is at times impaired by muscular weakness. Although minor weakness can be present in juvenile rheumatoid arthritis, extreme degrees of weakness are so unusual in children with juvenile rheumatoid arthritis that the diagnosis in such patients is suspect. Muscular pain or tenderness occurs in more than three-fourths of patients with polymyositis, and can be quite acute and severe. A significant myalgia is observed in juvenile rheumatoid arthritis at times, in particular in teen-age girls, and occasionally boys, who tend to have an exaggerated affectation with illness.

The rash of dermatomyositis is reasonably specific and is characterized by a facial butterfly pattern, erythematous to violaceous in color, accompanied by periorbital edema (Figs. 5-1, 5-2). In addition

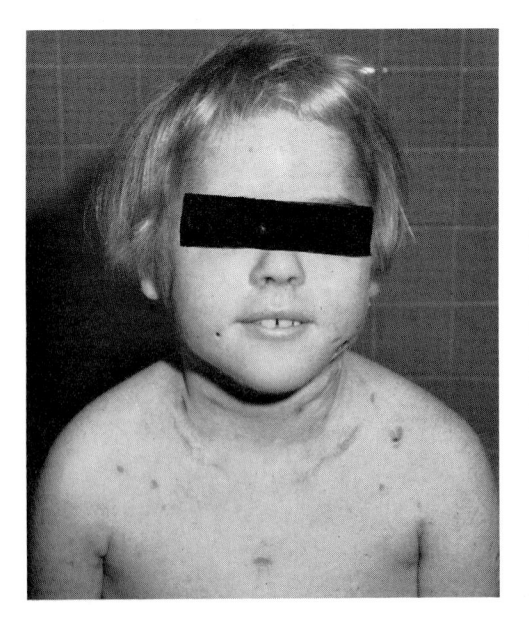

Figure 5-1 Dermatomyositis. Multiple scars represent previous areas of vasculitis and necrosis. On both cheeks are areas of pallor representing the first stage of vasculitis leading to necrosis of tissue with slough of skin, soft tissue, and even muscle. The lesions heal by secondary intention. A violaceous rash is present under the eyes.

DIFFERENTIAL DIAGNOSIS

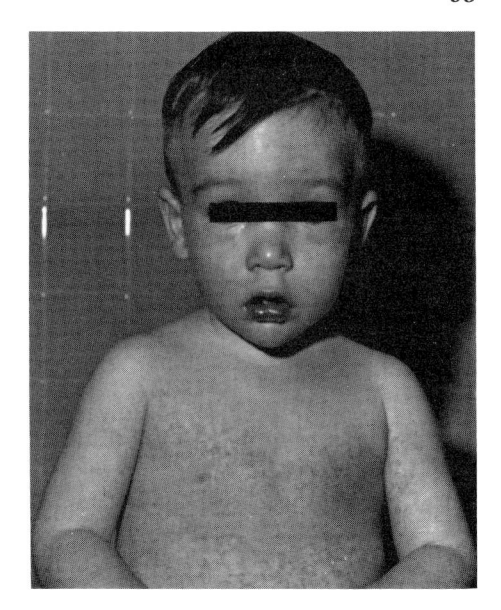

Figure 5-2 Dermatomyositis. Periorbital edema is apparent, along with a macular brownish confluent rash.

patients often exhibit an erythematous, shiny thickened rash over bony prominences such as the knees (Fig. 5-3). At times the extensor surfaces of the joints, especially the metacarpophalangeal, proximal phalangeal, and elbow joints, have scaling of the skin followed by depigmentation and ulceration. The lesions are almost always symmetrically distributed. Such a rash does not occur in juvenile rheumatoid arthritis.

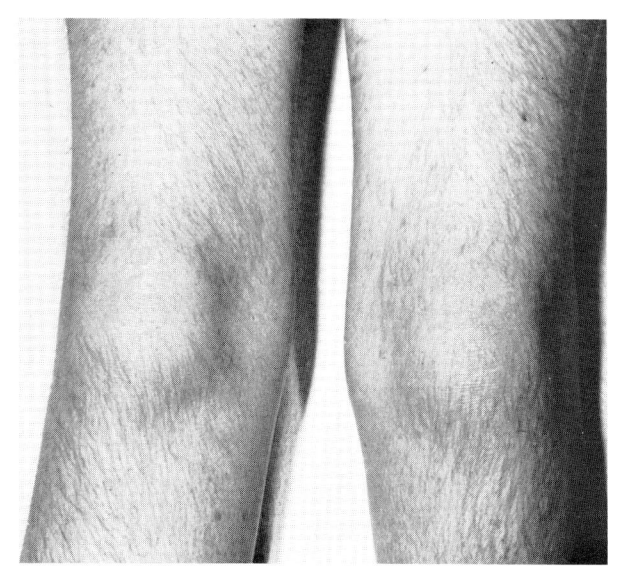

Figure 5-3 Lichenified shiny erythematosus rash of knees in patient with dermatomyositis.

Fever can be a prominent feature of this disease and can last over a period of many weeks; however, fever rarely precedes the onset of the disease by more than a week or two.

Transitory arthralgia or arthritis has been reported by Pearson in a third of all cases of polymyositis. Joint involvement is known to be accompanied by actual effusion, most frequently in the metacarpophalangeal joints and knees. Nonspecific synovitis with effusion is quite indistinguishable from juvenile rheumatoid arthritis (Pearson, 1966).

Fifteen per cent of patients with polymyositis and dermatomyositis have been reported to have splenomegaly, but hepatomegaly was not present in any of the patients. Pericarditis has not been reported as a complication for dermatomyositis. In children with rapid wasting of the voluntary musculature, calcification of the involved areas may become extreme. Calcium deposits are also known to occur occasionally in the soft tissues in rheumatoid arthritis.

Laboratory findings occasionally reveal mild, nonspecific anemia with a normal to slightly elevated leukocyte count. The sedimentation rate is usually elevated.

Specific helpful laboratory tests are lacking; the urinary excretion of creatine is increased, as one would expect with any disease producing marked atrophy of musculature. Creatine phosphokinase is reported by Pearson to be unpredictably elevated in polymyositis and thus cannot be relied upon as a measure of disease activity (Pearson, 1966). Values for serum glutamic oxaloacetic transaminase (SGOT) and for serum glutamic pyruvic transaminase (SGPT), as well as for aldolase, in our experience are often but not always elevated. These values are almost never elevated in rheumatoid arthritis. Electromyography, when performed by experienced and competent electromyographers, is extremely helpful in establishing a diagnosis. The findings include fibrillation and positive spike potentials, pseudomyotonic discharges occurring as short duration repetitive high frequency potentials which are seen at rest and activity, and the typical polyphasic wave appearing with voluntary activity; these potentials are greatly reduced in amplitude. The myogram is a valuable tool to locate inflammatory foci for biopsy.

Muscle biopsy is extremely helpful for a definitive diagnosis and differentiation from other connective tissue diseases. Rheumatoid arthritis is known to cause myositis, usually mild with nonspecific chronic inflammatory response present. In dermatomyositis, a local inflammatory focus usually contains significant necrosis, muscle fibers with phagocytosis, and evidence of regeneration.

The LE cell preparation is almost never positive in children with dermatomyositis and positive rheumatoid factor is not found in children with dermatomyositis.

Usually this variable and capricious connective tissue disease does not offer serious problems in differential diagnosis, except in those patients who have fever, polymyositis, and arthralgia or minimal arthritis. The extreme weakness usually present, and extreme muscular pain, offer the main aids to early differentiation of the two diseases. The rash is characteristic enough to be diagnostic of the disease.

Polyarteritis

Polyarteritis is a rare, necrotizing angiitis involving principally medium-sized arteries and, at times, veins. The disease affects males more than females in a ratio of 3:1. Initially described by Kussmaul and Maier (1866), the manifestations of the disease are protean and any organ can be involved. As observed by Arkin (1930), the kidneys are involved in 80 per cent of patients, the heart in 70 per cent, the liver in 65 per cent, the spleen, muscles, and nerves in 30 per cent, the gastrointestinal tract in 50 per cent, the lungs and pancreas in 25 per cent, and the central nervous system in 8 per cent. Most other organs have been reported involved, except the thyroid and pituitary glands. Hypertension is a prominent physical finding. Early in the course of the disease fever is often a prominent manifestation, and muscular aching with tenderness and joint pain can make early differential diagnosis difficult. Actual joint swelling occurs in about 10 per cent of patients (Shulman and Harvey, 1966).

Subcutaneous nodules of various sizes do occur in polyarteritis. They are usually painless, appear in clusters, and disappear after a short time. In addition, nodular swelling occurs along the course of blood vessels in some patients. Skin lesions are helpful in differentiating the disease from rheumatoid arthritis. Bizarre erythema multiforme type lesions often occur as well as angioneurotic edema, livedo testicularis, and purpuric lesions which lead to gangrene and sloughing of the part.

Laboratory findings reveal the presence of both anemia and leukocytosis in up to 80 per cent of the patients. Urinalysis reveals proteinuria accompanied by red cell casts, white cell casts, and fatty casts. The changes in urinalysis reflect the renal involvement present in up to 80 per cent of the patients. Sedimentation rate is elevated as it is in juvenile rheumatoid arthritis, and serum globulin fraction is also found.

The chief problem in differential diagnosis is to decide whether the disease is primary, is secondary to rheumatoid arthritis, or is a drug reaction resulting from dosage with steroids or some other chemotherapeutic agent. Patients being treated with steroids can develop the lesions of polyarteritis.

Diagnosis is made by skin-muscle biopsy. Other findings include edema and fibrinous exudate in the media of the blood vessels, followed by necrosis of the inner media and subendothelial tissues in the smaller vessels. Fibrinoid changes occur in the adventitia. The lesion may form an ellipse that parallels the axis of the vessel. The wall of the artery weakens and aneurysmal dilatation may occur. Another type of nodular lesion occurs which may be caused by the proliferation of granulomatous tissue or necrotic tissue about the wall of the vessel. Secondary pathologic changes may occur as a result of ischemia or rupture of an aneurysm. Healing is by fibrosis.

Muscle biopsy is not entirely diagnostic, for in as many as two of three cases later proved at autopsy, previously muscle biopsy may have shown no abnormality (Maxeiner et al., 1952).

Scleroderma

In childhood scleroderma is an extremely rare connective tissue disease. No cases have been recognized at the Children's Medical Center in Boston (Cook et al., 1963) and only one case has been recognized at the Texas Children's Hospital even though the disease has been reported as early as infancy (Talbott and Ferrandis, 1956).

The disease occurs most frequently in girls and is distinguished chiefly by involvement of the skin and subcutaneous tissue, characterized by stiffness, tightness and swelling, and brawny indurated swelling of the subcutaneous tissue, particularly of the fingers and face. The fingertips often become necrotic and hyperkeratotic, and palpable calcium deposits can be felt in the subcutaneous tissues of involved areas.

Arthritis does occur and at joints swelling, warmness, and even effusion are known. Joint stiffness usually seems to be secondary to periarticular soft tissue involvement.

Dysphagia, caused by involvement of the esophagus, is a prominent early finding as a result of hypomotility. One patient with lupus erythematosus, in Texas Children's Hospital, had changes in the small intestine compatible with scleroderma; hypomotility and edema of the bowel wall were prominent. Restriction in pulmonary function can be caused by fibrosis of the soft tissue of the chest wall as well as by interstitial fibrosis of the lungs. Comparable changes may occur in any other area of the body. X-ray examination often reveals unsuspected calcium deposition in the soft tissues. Resorption of bone is known, and osteoporosis and narrowing of the joint space have been seen in the joints.

Diagnosis is by biopsy of the skin and subcutaneous tissue, which reveals characteristic hyperplasia of connective tissue followed by fibrosis. Infiltration of mononuclear cells occurs later in the course of fibrosis with metastatic calcium deposition in the tissues.

Septic Arthritis

Acute septic arthritis is the single most important differential diagnostic consideration in any child with monarticular arthritis or polyarthritis. Definitive diagnosis and prompt therapy are essential in dealing with septic arthritis. Patients with monarticular arthritis especially must be carefully evaluated to rule out septic arthritis. Although the patient usually has fever and the joint is hot, red, and exquisitely tender with prominent effusion, mild cases also occur with few or none of these symptoms. Prompt examination of the joint fluid for microorganisms by a stained slide and adequate culture is essential. Patients who have been partially treated with antibiotics may reveal organisms on smear tests but cultures may show an inability to adequately grow such or-

Figure 5-4 Incidence of septic arthritis in childhood. (Redrawn from Borella, L., Goobar, J. E., Summitt, R. L., and Clark, G. M.: Septic arthritis in childhood. J. Pediat. 62:742, 1963.)

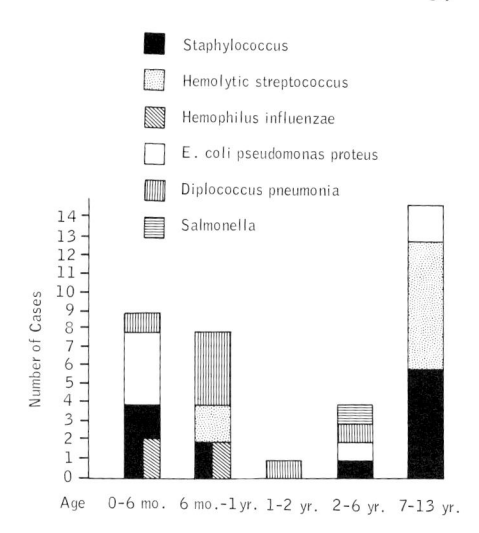

ganisms. These patients should be considered to have septic arthritis until proved otherwise. It is important to remember that patients with known juvenile rheumatoid arthritis may also have septic arthritis complicating their disease.

Examination of the synovial fluid of the patient with septic arthritis usually reveals turbid, purulent fluid, yellowish to sanguineous in color, with a poor mucin clot, low viscosity, and a leukocytic cell count of a few hundred to over 150,000 cells per cu. mm. The predominant cells are polymorphonuclear leukocytes.

Patients with septic arthritis may have a focus of primary infection. Septic arthritis can be caused by direct trauma to a joint or by contiguous spread from osteomyelitis. In some cases, the primary source of infection is never found. The age in incidence of septic arthritis is of some interest in differential diagnosis (Fig. 5-4) (Borella et al.). The peak incidence of septic arthritis differs significantly from that of juvenile rheumatoid arthritis.

The chief organisms involved in septic arthritis differ by age group as shown in Table 5-2 (Nelson and Koontz). Other specific bacterial organisms which can produce septic arthritis include meningococcus, brucella, and shigella.

Tuberculous Arthritis

Another difficult differential diagnostic problem in monarticular arthritis, and occasionally in polyarthritis, is tuberculous arthritis. The patient usually presents with a monarticular arthritis indistinguishable from other types of monarticular arthritis. The tuberculin skin test early in the disease, particularly in the first six weeks, is often negative, and only in about 50 per cent of the cases are associated visceral tuberculous lesions found (Henderson, 1936).

In the usual physical findings it is impossible to generalize about a single reliable feature consistently useful in differential diagnosis. Sys-

Table 5-2 Etiologic Agents and Ages of Patients†

Organism	Total	<2 yr.	2–5 yr.	6–10 yr.	11–15 yr.
Clostridium novyi	1	0	1	0	0
Staphylococcus, coagulase positive	30	5	11	9	5
Hemophilus influenzae, type b	28	26	2	0	0
Streptococci*	16	4	5	4	3
Neisseria gonorrhoeae	10	0	5	3	2
Staphylococcus, coagulase negative	6	2	3	0	1
Pseudomonas aeruginosa	7	3	2	2	0
Diplococcus pneumoniae	7	4	2	1	0
Aerobacter aerogenes	4	2	0	1	1
Neisseria meningitidis	3	1	1	1	0
Salmonella heidelberg	2	2	0	0	0
Bacteroides fundiliformis	1	0	0	0	1
Paracolon intermedium	1	0	0	1	0
Mycobacterium tuberculosis	1	0	1	0	0
Blastomyces dermatitidis	1	0	0	1	0
Staphylococcus, coag. pos., and Group A streptococcus	1	0	1	0	0
Klebsiella pneumoniae	1	1	0	0	0
Unknown	63	21	21	13	8
Total	183	71	55	36	21
Percentage	100	39	30	20	11

*Including 4 group A, 3 viridans, 2 not grouped, and 1 anaerobic.
†Modified from Nelson, J. D., and Koontz, W. C.: Septic arthritis in infants and children: A review of 117 cases. Pediatrics, *38*:966, 1966.

temic manifestations can be minimal. Roentgenographic examination early may reveal only soft tissue swelling and no evidence of destruction of joint or contiguous areas.

In this type of patient, the only satisfactory means of diagnosis is examination of the synovial fluid, and if tuberculous microorganisms are not demonstrated, synovial biopsy is essential. Tuberculous arthritis is rare, and omitting therapy until too late can be disastrous. For this reason patients with monarticular arthritis should have adequate diagnostic tests to rule out tuberculosis.

Gonococcal Arthritis

Gonococcal arthritis in children does indeed occur, and is particularly important because of the ease with which the diagnosis may be overlooked. Untreated cases of gonococcal arthritis can have a protracted course. Fink found the age in these patients ranged from two to twelve years (1965). The majority were girls with arthritis persisting for up to ten days after penicillin therapy was begun. The major joints affected seemed to be in the upper extremities, with the shoulder, wrist, and elbow most often involved. The knee was involved as the

Table 5-3. Clinical and Laboratory Data on Six Children with Gonococcal Arthritis**

Case No.	1	2	3	4	5	6
Age	2 yr., 3 mo.	4 yr., 10 mo.	3 yr., 5 mo.	7 yr.	12 yr., 11 mo.	11 yr., 2 mo.
Sex	F	F	F	M	F	F
Vaginal discharge	Present	Present	Present	—	Absent	Absent
Initial joint affected	Wrist	Knee*	Arm*	Ankle	Both ankles	Wrist
Subsequent joint affected (in order)	Arm, hip* and knee	Shoulder	Legs* and wrist	Hip, elbow and shoulder	Back, elbow and wrist	None
Major joint affected	Knee	Shoulder	Wrist	Shoulder	Elbow	Wrist
Maximum temperature	102 F.° (38.9 C)	102.8 F.° (39.4 C)	99 F.° (37.2 C)	101 F.° (38.4 C)	103 F.° (39.5 C)	102.2 F.° (39 C)
Days afebrile after penicillin therapy	1	2	Never febrile	1	1½	1½
Days joints symptomatic after penicillin therapy	10	2	3	7	10	9
Vaginal culture for N. gonorrhoeae	Negative	Positive	Positive	—	Positive	Negative
Vaginal smear†	Positive	Positive	Positive	—	Positive	Positive
Joint culture for N. gonorrhoeae	Positive	—	Negative	Positive	—	Negative
Fluorescent antibody test						
1:100‡	2+§	4+	3+	3+	2+	4+
1:200‡	1+	4+	—	2+	2+	2+
1:400‡	—	3+	—	1+	Absent	Absent

*Pain only.
†Gram negative intracellular diplococci resembling N. gonorrhoeae seen on smear.
‡Serum dilutions.
§Numbers refer to degree of fluorescence on a scale of 1+ to 4+.
**From Fink, C. W.: Gonococcal arthritis in children, J.A.M.A., 194:237, 1965.

major joint in only one patient. Differential diagnosis here is made by use of positive vaginal smears, cultures, or joint fluid culture. Fluorescent antibody tests were also helpful in these cases. (See Table 5-3.)

Meningococcal Arthritis

Meningococcal arthritis occurs in children with some frequency. Accurate data are not available regarding the incidence of arthritis in proved cases of meningococcemia or meningococcic meningitis. Four of the 11 patients reported by Pinals and Ropes were under sixteen years of age (1964). The joints involved were ankles, knees, hips, elbows, and metacarpophalangeal joints. The onset of swelling usually occurred within the first few days of illness and persisted up to two months. Usually the arthritis persisted a few weeks. No permanent x-ray changes were noted and one patient examined ten years later had no evidence of recurrence, residual disease, or rheumatoid arthritis.

Fever can occur with the polyarthritis and persist in conjunction with the polyarthritis long after the patient would have been expected to remain afebrile from chemotherapy of sepsis or meningitis.

The synovial fluid findings are the same as in other forms of bacterial arthritis. The diagnosis, more often than not is made from the accompanying disease rather than from local culture of the joint.

Viral Diseases

Definite polyarthritis, lasting from a few days to several weeks, can occur preceding, during, or following any number of viral diseases. The arthritis characteristically is transient and is not erosive. Among the diseases it may be associated with are rubella, rubeola, mumps, chickenpox, smallpox, infectious mononucleosis, viral influenza, and infectious hepatitis. The chief aid in diagnosis is associated proved disease, and the relatively short duration of time that the patient has polyarthritis. Early in the course of juvenile rheumatoid arthritis, a patient who has acute systemic manifestations such as fever, lymphadenopathy, and splenomegaly along with acute polyarthritis, may be impossible to adequately differentiate from one afflicted with a viral disease. Confirmation of a viral etiology can often be made after sera are examined for a rise in antibody titer.

Fungal Diseases

Mycotic disease such as coccidiomycosis, histoplasmosis, blastomycosis, actinomycosis, and cryptomycosis can produce arthritis. These diseases usually reveal involvement of bone with contiguous spread to joints thus allowing adequate differential diagnosis from juvenile rheumatoid arthritis. Skin tests, however, can often be negative in the first six weeks of involvement.

Allergic Reactions

Allergic reactions of a significant nature can cause polyarthritis, fever, and other manifestations found in juvenile rheumatoid arthritis.

The terminology used by many authors in discussing allergic reactions is confusing enough so that, for purposes of clinical discussion, all reactions can be practically included in one broad classification of allergic reactions, which implies the reaction of the host to the antigen. This would include serum sickness, atopy, hypersensitivity to infection, foreign protein reactions, contact dermatitis, and anaphylaxis. Children with significant host reactions can manifest disease with swelling of multiple joints lasting from a few days to several weeks. Joint swelling can be accompanied by periarticular swelling and joint effusion. A helpful hint is often the presence of angioneurotic edema involving a whole hand or a whole foot, or periorbital edema or edema of the lips. The joint swelling seldom lasts beyond a few weeks, and a careful history must be taken to establish relationship of the offending antigen, such as a food (e.g., egg), or a drug (e.g., penicillin).

Erosive arthritis does not occur in this type of disease. Any patient with juxta-articular osteoporosis or erosions would be eliminated from consideration. It is worthwhile noting that patients with rheumatoid arthritis do hyperreact to many drugs and other substances, and can have an allergic reaction superimposed on disease. Diphenylhydantoin (Dilantin) is particularly dangerous to use in children with arthritis (Rallison et al., 1961).

Fever may occur in allergic reactions and may be low-grade or an intermittent fever up to 104° or 105°. The fever may be present for a few days or several weeks. Mild lymphadenopathy may occur with some tenderness, but more often than not the lymphadenopathy is asymptomatic. An important manifestation that helps in differentiating the disease is the presence, in acute allergic reactions, of acute glomerular nephritis or diminished renal function. This may be manifest by oliguria, albuminuria, casts in the urine, or hematuria.

Rash in the form of urticaria accompanied by intense pruritis is common in allergic reactions, and may be helpful in differentiating rheumatoid arthritis from an allergic reaction. Urticaria, however, can also occur in rheumatoid arthritis, but is not as prominent as in acute allergic reactions. Nonspecific rashes such as erythema multiforme also occur in allergic conditions. These rashes are usually of reasonably short duration but may be intermittent and recurring, as in drug hypersensitivity, over a period of several months.

Laboratory findings are nonspecific. Patients with allergic reactions rarely have significant leukocytosis. Eosinophilia often is prominent. Sedimentation rate is usually normal in allergic reactions.

Examination of joint effusion reveals leukocytosis with an increase in polymorphonuclear cells and is no help in differential diagnosis. LE cell phenomenon is known to occur as a reaction to certain drugs such as hydralizine and isoniazid (Alarcon-Segovia et al., 1965).

Leukemia

Acute leukemia is second only to septic arthritis as the most significant differential diagnosis to be made in children presenting with polyarticular manifestations. Silverstein and Kelley reviewed children and adults with acute leukemia who had presenting symptoms primarily of bone and joint involvement (1965). Of 450 patients reported, including 173 children, more than 10 per cent of the children presented with a clinical course of bone and joint involvement. The percentage of boys affected was not significantly different from the percentage of girls. The predominant presenting symptom was pain of sudden onset lasting for several days to several months. The large weight-bearing joints were primarily involved but joints of the fingers were also involved. The joint involvement was often bilateral in the hands and knees. Migratory bone and joint pain were common. Nearly half of the patients had migratory swelling and painful and tender joints. Only three patients had associated erythema of the skin of the involved joint. Polyarthralgia occurred in 40 per cent of the patients, and monarticular arthritis in about 5 per cent.

Other clinical manifestations helpful in diagnosis were splenomegaly (in 50 per cent), hepatomegaly (in 37 per cent), lymphadenopathy (in 43 per cent), and purpura (in 20 per cent). Eleven patients had a completely normal physical examination, except for bone and joint manifestations.

A basic rule to remember in differentiating the arthritic manifestations of acute leukemia from other forms of arthritis is that the initial peripheral hemogram, including the hemoglobin, hematocrit, leukocyte, differential, and platelet counts, can be completely normal, initially and several months later. Initially the bone marrow may be normal and it may continue to be normal over a period of several months. A normal bone marrow and a normal hemogram do not eliminate leukemia from consideration. Several patients each year have been seen who have had the onset of articular and bone manifestations several weeks to several months prior to proof of leukemia.

The roentgenographic changes that are seen in leukemia are focal destructive cystic lesions, osteosclerosis, subperiosteal new bone formation, and transverse bands of diminished density at the growing ends of long bones. All of these changes are nonspecific (Holt et al., 1962). Cortical erosion is known to occur and Scott believes that there is no reason why erosion of articular cartilage should not follow involvement of underlying bones or synovium, although the relatively thicker cartilage at bone ends in children may have a protective influence (1965).

Lymphoma

In patients with lymphoma, biopsy of nodes or of liver is often necessary for definitive diagnosis. Hodgkin's disease in childhood is rare but does occur and the same manifestations may be apparent in this condition; diagnosis may be made only after appropriate biopsy of nodes, or of the liver or other involved organ.

Hemophilia

Hemophilia is a clinical syndrome caused by several distinct inborn errors of metabolism. The classic sex-linked hemophilia caused by a deficiency of antihemophiliac globulin (AHG) is one of several deficiencies that can produce similar problems with hemarthrosis. Hemarthrosis rarely presents difficulty in the differential diagnosis of juvenile rheumatoid arthritis or other arthritides other than trauma. Localized hemorrhage into the synovial space alone is common and may or may not be accompanied by purpura of the skin or other areas of hemorrhage.

Aspiration of the joint reveals frank hemorrhage, and early in the disease, other than synovial effusion, no changes are demonstrable by x-ray. Diagnosis is made by properly performed tests of bleeding time and clotting time. In addition, the thromboplastin consumption test, measuring the amount of prothrombin remaining in the serum after blood is clotted, is the most specific test for measuring AHG. Normally less than 25 per cent of the prothrombin originally present in the plasma should remain. Other deficiencies of coagulation factors such as PTC and PTA can, at times, result in significant hemorrhage into the joints.

Agammaglobulinemia and Hypogammaglobulinemia

Congenital agammaglobulinemia and acquired hypogammaglobulinemia are associated with polyarthritis but are distinguishable from rheumatoid arthritis. Five patients of 12 in Janeway's series (1956) and three patients of 11 in Good's series (1957) had polyarthritis indistinguishable clinically from that of juvenile rheumatoid arthritis. The reported incidence may not be valid, for milder cases now being recognized undoubtedly will reduce the incidence of arthritis found. The clinical course in the adult and child is indistinguishable from that of rheumatoid disease. Destructive changes as demonstrated by roentgenogram have been reported (Good et al., 1957). An interesting aspect of the condition is that in children the manifestation of polyarthritis seems to disappear with adequate gammaglobulin therapy.

Synovial Hemangioma

Neoplasms of the synovium in the adult or child are extremely rare. Hemangioma is an example of a neoplasm that does occur in the synovium. Although the disease is quite rare, in the differential diagnosis of monarticular arthritis care must be taken to rule out neoplasm. This can be done only by adequate biopsy.

Symptoms of hemangioma are recurrent episodes of swelling beginning early in childhood usually incident to mild trauma. The episodes may occur with varying frequency during the year, sometimes subsiding completely. There may be increasing synovial thickening, often over a period of years, before a diagnosis is made. Hemarthrosis is found upon joint aspiration and serial roentgenograms reveal progressive increases in soft tissue swelling of the synovial area. As stated previously, diagnosis is made by biopsy.

Juvenile Gout

Juvenile gout is an extremely rare disease in the pediatric age group. Decker reviewed 13 cases of juvenile gout with onset prior to age 17 (1962). Two of the patients discussed were under the age of seven years and were associated with the development of tophi. Articular pain was a later manifestation. Decker also reported an adolescent with gouty arthritis who developed crystalluria at six years of age followed by nephrectomy at 10½, and arthritis symptoms beginning at 13 years of age. Hyperuricemia was considered to be the cause of the renal calculi. Patients in the studies reviewed who began clinical onset of the disease after the age of 11 consisted of ten boys and one girl. Onset seemed to be associated with articular pain and excessively high serum uric acid levels.

Patients with articular pain who have serum uric acid levels in excess of 8 mg. per 100 ml. must be carefully considered for diagnosis of juvenile gout. Attempts should be made with each examination of the synovial fluid, under polarized light, to determine the presence of sodium monourate crystals or calcium pyrophosphate. Thus far, to the author's knowledge, no case of calcium pyrophosphate disease has been found in a pediatric patient, but undoubtedly this condition may occur.

Familial hyperuricemia is not necessarily associated with clinical gout (Popert and Hewitt, 1962). Patients who ingest a high purine diet, especially common in the upper income levels, have a higher than usual serum uric acid level, and levels between 6 and 8 mg. per 100 ml. are not unknown in otherwise normal individuals.

There is a familial disorder of uric acid metabolism and central nervous system dysfunction, reported originally by Lesch and Nyhan (1964). The cardinal features of the disorder were hyperuricemia related to hyperexcretion of uric acid and excessive formation of uric acid (up to 200 times normal). Other features of the disorder were mental retardation, cerebral palsy, choreo-athetosis, and self-destructive biting. These patients were not reported to have arthritis, a circumstance that may be related to the age of the individual.

Ankylosing Spondylitis

Ankylosing spondylitis, occurring as a disease separate from juvenile rheumatoid arthritis, is extremely rare. Although the majority of cases begin in the third decade of life, 10 to 15 per cent begin at around age 16. The onset in the majority of patients is insidious, with the first complaints referable to the lower back. The beginning of low back pain is often accompanied by periods of stiffness and transient arthralgia. In about 10 per cent of the patients the first symptom is sciatic pain (Boland and Present, 1945). When the onset is primarily in the sacroiliac or lumbar spine, with no peripheral arthritis, differential diagnosis is not difficult. However, in over 10 per cent of patients the lower back disability is preceded by involvement of the peripheral joints which is indistinguishable from rheumatoid arthritis (Boland and Present, 1945). The disease occurs predominantly in males at ratios of 4:1 to 8:1, depending on the reported series (Dunham and Kautz, 1941; Mikkelsen and Duff, 1961; Primer on the Rheumatic Diseases, 1964). Rheumatoid factor is rarely positive in ankylosing spondylitis.

Table 5-4 Principal Features that Differentiate Ankylosing Spondylitis from Rheumatoid Arthritis*

1. Greater prevalence in males (9:1).
2. Regular involvement of spine and other axial joints.
3. Infrequent involvement of small peripheral joints.
4. Early, constant, bilateral sacroiliitis on roentgenogram.
5. Stiffness more prominent than pain.
6. Absence of subcutaneous nodules.
7. Higher incidence of recurrent iritis.
8. Greater frequency of aortitis and conduction defects.
9. Negative serum rheumatoid factor.
10. More frequent spinal fluid protein elevation.
11. Lack of response to gold and antimalarials.
12. Selective response to local irradiation.

*From Calabro, J. J.: Management of ankylosing spondylitis. Bull. Rheum. Dis., 16:408, 1966.

About 30 per cent of patients are said to have an associated neuritis at some point in the disease.

This disease is to be differentiated from the cervical spine involvement present in juvenile rheumatoid arthritis. Ansell et al. found that the evidence of ankylosing spondylitis is greater in relatives of juvenile rheumatoid arthritis patients than in relatives of adult patients with rheumatoid arthritis (1962).

Sarcoidosis

Sarcoidosis is a chronic granulomatous systemic disease of unknown etiology that can resemble juvenile rheumatoid arthritis early in the course of the disease. A review of the 113 reported cases in the world literature, from the first description by Hutchison in 1875 until 1956, reveals that the onset of the disease most frequently occurred in late childhood, with almost 75 per cent of the patients between the age of nine and 15 years at onset. There was no difference in sex distribution. The youngest patient was a two-month old boy. Sarcoidosis is said to occur predominantly in the Negro, but of 87 reported patients in whom race was known, 63 were white. Heredity did not seem to be a factor in these patients (McGovern and Merritt, 1956).

The characteristic pathologic manifestations are epithelioid, noncaseating tuberculomas containing numerous multinuclear giant cells and doubly refractive bodies. The lesions have been found in almost every tissue and organ of the body, with the lymph nodes, lungs, skin, and eyes involved in more than half of 113 cases reported. Involvement of the bone occurred in about 30 per cent of the patients (McGovern and Merritt, 1956). (See Tables 5-5 and 5-6.)

When arthritis does occur in sarcoidosis, biopsy reveals a characteristic granuloma. The Kviem test involves intradermal antigen extract of sarcoid lymph node material. It is difficult to interpret and even more difficult to obtain. Arthritis is a rare manifestation.

Table 5-5 Organs Affected in 113 Cases of Sarcoidosis in Children*

	Reported Cases (104)	Authors' Cases (9)	Total Cases (%)
Lymph nodes (peripheral, thoracic)	66	10	76 67
Lungs (parenchyma, hilar nodes)	54	8	62 55
Skin	51	6	57 50
Eyes	51	4	55 49
Parotid gland	35	1	36 32
Bones	30	3	33 29
Spleen	24	1	25 22
Liver	13	3	16 14
Nervous system	11	1	12 11
Kidney	4	2	6 5.3

*From "Sarcoidosis in Childhood," by J. P. McGovern and D. H. Merritt, in *Advances in Pediatrics.* Copyright © 1956, Year Book Medical Publishers, Inc. Used by permission of Year Book Medical Publishers.

Table 5-6 Signs and Symptoms of Sarcoidosis in Children in Order of Frequency*

	Presenting		Occurring During Course of Disease	
	Reported Cases	Authors' Cases	Reported Cases	Authors' Cases
Fever	14	2	9	2
Weight loss	9	2	4	
Anorexia	8	2	1	
Dyspnea	7	1	5	1
Cough	6	2	3	1
Leg or foot pain	6		1	
Ocular pain	5		2	
Abdominal pain	5			
Eyelid disturbance	3		1	
Epistaxis	3		1	
Headache		3		1
Nausea	2			
Icterus	1		1	
Arthralgia	1	1		
Limitation of finger motion	1			
Back pain	1			

*From "Sarcoidosis in Childhood," by J. P. McGovern and D. H. Merritt, in *Advances in Pediatrics.* Copyright © 1956, Year Book Medical Publishers, Inc. Used by permission of Year Book Medical Publishers.

Traumatic Arthritis

Perhaps the most common cause of monarticular arthritis in children is trauma. The incidence of joint swelling secondary to sprains, strains, and twisting injuries is considerable. In most of these patients, juvenile rheumatoid arthritis is never seriously considered because of the self-limiting, short duration of swelling. In addition, a history of significant injury is usually known.

A disturbing problem in differential diagnosis, however, is that about 10 to 15 per cent of patients with juvenile rheumatoid arthritis have a history of significant trauma immediately preceding the onset of disease. One possibility in these patients is that the trauma brought attention to an already insidiously swollen joint. There are patients, however, who have significant trauma in the absence of previously noted disease, and then develop chronic monarticular arthritis or, indeed, polyarthritis. Therefore, in differential diagnosis one has to be ever mindful of the possibility that trauma may herald the onset of juvenile rheumatoid arthritis, or may be an incidental finding bringing attention to an already existing monarticular rheumatoid arthritis.

Reiter's Syndrome

Reiter's syndrome is a symptom complex characterized by polyarthritis, conjunctivitis, and urethritis (Reiter, 1916). First reported in children by Zewi (1947), the condition has been found in children as young as two years, but usually pediatric patients are between nine and 16 years of age. All recorded patients in childhood have been males. The syndrome has been closely associated for many years with epidemics of *Shigella flexneri*, a bacillary dysentery (Koster and Jansen, 1946). The typical patient with this condition develops polyarthritis five to 14 days after a bout of diarrhea, followed within a few days or weeks by urethritis and conjunctivitis.

The polyarthritis reported is indistinguishable from that of rheumatoid arthritis early in the disease, but the disease characteristically lasts only a few weeks to a few months with complete clinical recovery. The large weight-bearing joints of the lower extremity are the usual sites of occurrence, with the knee joint being involved in about half of the patients (Paronen, 1948). Considerable synovial effusion does occur, but erosive arthritis is virtually unknown. Roentgenograms are usually normal except for evidence of soft tissue swelling.

The most usual ophthalmologic manifestation is unilateral or bilateral conjunctivitis. However, involvement of the uveal tract and cornea have also been reported (Zewi, 1947).

The urethritis can be extremely mild, consisting only of dysuria, but albuminuria and pyuria are also known to occur. Other organ involvement has been reported, including lymphadenitis, skin lesions of the genitalia, pleural effusion, and cardiomegaly (Corner, 1950).

A condition known as keratosis blennorrhagica is manifested by urethritis, polyarthritis, and a peculiar skin lesion consisting of vesicular eruptions with crust formation and lichenification occurring on the trunk, extremities, and buccal mucous membranes. It has been reported associated with Reiter's syndrome, but is considered by some to be associated with sexual contact and gonorrhea (Corner, 1950).

Recently, Engelman et al. have isolated Bedsonia microorganisms from patients with Reiter's disease (1966), but antibody studies and isolation techniques are still not standardized or available for general use.

Hemoglobinopathies—Sickle Cell Anemia

The inherited hemolytic diseases involving alteration in hemoglobin, such as sickle cell disease and more rarely Christmas disease or hemoglobin C disease, can produce clinical manifestations that may mimic juvenile rheumatoid arthritis.

The most frequent age of onset of sickle cell disease, as with juvenile rheumatoid arthritis, is one to six years. Some cases are found earlier than one year of age. The most frequent clinical manifestations found by Porter and Thurman (1963) in sickle cell disease diagnosed in children under one year of age are shown in Table 5-7.

Of four recognizable clinical patterns outlined by Porter one includes patients who presented with painful, swollen hands or feet and significant anemia, and with no hepatosplenomegaly. The usual swelling of the hands and feet was without pitting, was particularly painful, and was not limited to a particular joint but involved the entire area. The cause was thought to be local thrombosis. The patient is usually irritable, and temperatures as high as 103° can occur.

In 20 cases of painful sickle cell crisis, among 173 cases of homozy-

Table 5-7 Signs and Symptoms of Sickle Cell Disease*

	No. of Cases	Per Cent
Hepatomegaly	47	73
Concurrent infection	45	70
Failure to thrive	45	63
Irritability and colic	40	63
Fever	37	58
Splenomegaly	32	50
Abdominal distention	27	42
Jaundice	23	36
Dactylitis	23	36
X-ray evidence of dactylitis	12	19
Pallor	21	33
Heart murmur	17	26
Nausea and vomiting	16	25
Cardiac enlargement (x-ray)	12	19
Facial edema	10	15
Cyanosis	8	5
Palpable mass in abdomen	2	3

*From Porter, F. S., and Thurman, W. G.: Studies of sickle cell disease. Amer. J. Dis. Child., 106:35, 1963.

gous S hemoglobin disease and 20 cases of hemoglobin S-C disease (Watson et al., 1963), radiographs were reviewed at the onset of painful swelling of feet and hands. No bony abnormalities were revealed but soft tissue swelling was prominent. The first bony changes were noted at seven to 14 days after onset, with the initial appearance of subperiosteal bone formation. Local radiolucency occurred, with destruction of the head of the metatarsal or metacarpal bones at times. The changes evident by x-ray in this particular syndrome are reversible and not permanent. The average duration is about one to two weeks.

Sickle cell anemia crises can mimic acute rheumatic fever or acute rheumatoid arthritis (Smith et al., 1953). Children have been reported with a hemolytic sickle cell crisis following scarlet fever, resulting in a sudden onset of anemia of less than 7 gm. per 100 ml., fever and extreme pain in the knees resulting in marked restriction of motion, a fixed position with the knees drawn to the chest, and marked aggravation by motion. Again, these upsets rarely last more than one to two weeks.

Another striking variation of sickle cell disease that may cause confusion with juvenile rheumatoid arthritis involves those patients with sickle cell anemia who develop pain in unusual bony areas such as the proximal radius or ulna near the elbow. These patients may have multifocal areas of pain in or near joints, and x-ray will reveal osteomyelitis. Local culture has revealed salmonella group organisms as the etiologic agent (de Torregrosa et al., 1960; Hughes and Carroll, 1957; Hendrickse and Collard, 1960). The bony changes of the hemolytic anemias, sickle cell anemia, and related conditions are probably related to hyperplasia of the bone marrow and local thrombosis, secondary to the disease. The changes reported (Rodnan, 1966) are widening of the medullary cavities, thinning of cortices, coarsening and irregularity of trabecular markings, and cupping of vertebral bodies. Osteoporosis, and even aseptic necrosis of bone, can occur secondary to thrombosis or local infarction.

Acute sickle cell crises rarely present problems in differential diagnosis of rheumatoid arthritis, but occasionally painful hydrarthroses do occur, and a diagnosis is usually made after sickle cell disease is considered.

Plasma-Cell Hepatitis

Various terms have been used for this disease, including lupoid hepatitis, Kunkel's disease, chronic active hepatitis with cirrhosis, and postnecrotic cirrhosis. Kunkel et al. (1951) and Bearn et al. (1956) published papers regarding teen-age girls who had hepatitis followed by cirrhosis, accompanied clinically by arthralgia or arthritis, skin rash, amenorrhea, obesity, and marked elevation in serum gammaglobulin concentration. Because an occasional patient with this syndrome has had a positive LE preparation, the term lupoid hepatitis has come into usage. Plasma-cell hepatitis is the term used here because of the preponderance of plasma cells that are found during acute phases of hepatitis associated with this disease (Page and Good, 1960).

In the author's opinion, this disease is not limited to the teen-age and adult group, but occurs in infants and children also. The usual onset is marked by significant jaundice, and skin lesions such as erythema multiforme, erythema nodosum, or various purpuric or necrotizing rashes. The patient is acutely ill with significant fever, and develops arthralgia and arthritis of the weight-bearing joints and hands. Effusion is usually minimal and pain is not extreme in the joints. There may be erythema over involved small joints such as the metacarpophalangeal joints of the hand. The patient develops significant and serious ascites with striae over the abdomen, accompanied by a massive enlargement of the liver and spleen. Pleural effusion and pericardial effusion can occur. The vast majority of patients are girls. In those past puberty, amenorrhea is a prominent finding, but disappears with remission of the disease spontaneously or by steroid therapy.

Table 5-8 reveals the diverse manifestations of a multisystem disease. The principal manifestation that differentiates this syndrome from rheumatoid arthritis is the marked hepatic involvement. Patients with plasma-cell hepatitis have been reported who have anicteric plasma-cell hepatitis with arthritis. Abnormal liver function tests and massive enlargement of the liver are virtually unknown in juvenile rheumatoid arthritis. The splenomegaly of rheumatoid arthritis is almost never as massive as in plasma-cell hepatitis. Lymphadenopathy is similar in both diseases.

The arthritis found in plasma-cell hepatitis is usually transient, and erosive arthritis has not occurred in the author's experience. The synovitis in plasma-cell hepatitis rapidly disappears—ordinarily when steroid therapy is begun. Characteristic joints involved are the same in rheumatoid arthritis as in plasma-cell hepatitis.

The skin manifestations in plasma-cell hepatitis have included erythema multiforme, necrotizing erythema of legs, severe acne, erythema nodosum, purpuric rash, necrotizing lesions of ankles, feet and hands, urticaria, and buccal mucosal ulcers (see Table 5-8). The characteristic rash of juvenile rheumatoid arthritis has not been reported to occur in plasma-cell hepatitis.

Laboratory data reveal leukocyte count of the peripheral blood to be normal or reduced (see Table 5-9). A few patients have positive LE cell preparations, and renal disease can occur with subsequent complications such as membranous nephritis or nephrotic syndrome (Maclachlan et al., 1965).

Liver function studies are markedly abnormal in plasma-cell hepatitis (see Table 5-10). The gammaglobulin determination reveals a marked hypergammaglobulinemia by the strip electrophoretic method. As patients begin remission the serum gammaglobulin decreases toward normal. Antinuclear factor was increased in 16 of 18 adults and teen-agers with plasma-cell hepatitis (Maclachlan et al., 1965). Rheumatoid factor was found in 11 of 19 patients, all of whom were adults. This syndrome is a distinct entity, in children and teen-agers at least, and can usually be differentiated from rheumatoid arthritis with ease.

Table 5-8 Clinical Manifestations of Patients with Plasma-Cell Hepatitis*

Patient	Sex	Age (Yr.)	Jaundice	Hepato-megaly	Spleno-megaly	Lymphad-enopathy	Skin Manifestations	Arthralgia	Arthritis
1	M	14	++	+++	++	++	Erythema multiforme, necrotizing erythema of legs, severe acne	++Shoulders +Hips	+Fingers +++Both knees ++Both elbows
2	F	13	+	+++	++	–	None	++Fingers ++Wrists +Ankles	+Wrists +Ankles +Toes
3	F	14	+++	++++	–	+++	Erythema nodosum, purpuric rash, necrotizing lesions on ankles, feet, and hands	+Shoulders +Hips	+Left ankle +Knees +++Fingers
4	F	13	++++	+++	?	++	None	None	None
5	F	12	++	++++	+++	+++	Erythema multiforme, purpuric erythema, giant urticaria	+Knees	+Toes ++Ankles ++Wrists ++Knees
6	M	19	+	++	++	–	Generalized maculopapular erythematous rash, recurrent buccal mucosal ulcers	None	None

*From Page, A. R., and Good, R. A.: Plasma-cell hepatitis, with special attention to steroid therapy. A.M.A. J. Dis. Child., 99:288, 1960.

Table 5-9 Routine Laboratory Studies on Patients With Plasma-cell Hepatitis*

Patient	Hgb.	WBC	PMN's	Lympho-cytes	Eosino-phils	ESR	Man-toux	Wasser-mann	Alb.	Urinalysis RBC	Urinalysis WBC	Casts	Platelets	LE
1	9.1	5100	2900	2040	0	132	Neg.	Neg.	1+	0	0	0	565,000	Pos.
2	12.6	4300	2580	1075	258	89	Neg.	Neg.	0	0	Occ.	0	Normal on smear	Neg.
3	11.1	9100	5800	1720	725	91	Neg.	Neg.	1+	Occ.	Occ.	Occ.	386,000	Pos.
4	12.0	5900	3120	2000	177	100	Neg.	Neg.	0	Occ.	Occ.	0	Normal on smear	Neg.
5	10.2	6650	2800	2950	1264	86	Neg.	Neg.	1+	0	Occ.	0	220,000	Pos.
6	12.9	4250	1910	2080	127	83	Neg.	Neg.	0	0	0	0	216,000	Neg.

*From Page A. R., and Good, R. A.: Plasma-cell hepatitis, with special attention to steroid therapy. A.M.A. J. Dis. Child., 99:288, 1960.

Clinics Evaluating Patients with Juvenile Rheumatoid Arthritis for Diagnostic Classification (see page 80)

1. University of Washington School of Medicine, Seattle, Washington
2. Canadian Arthritis and Rheumatism Society, Vancouver, B.C., Canada
3. Children's Hospital Medical Center, Boston, Mass.
4. University of Rochester Medical School, Rochester, N. Y.
5. Convalescent Hospital for Children, Cincinnati, Ohio
6. University Hospital, Ann Arbor, Mich.
7. University of Texas Southwestern Medical School, Dallas, Texas
8. The Children's Hospital, Columbus, Ohio
9. College of Physicians and Surgeons of Columbia University, New York, N. Y.
10. Robert Breck Brigham Hospital, Boston, Mass.
11. Sinai Hospital of Baltimore, Inc., Baltimore, Md.
12. Children's Hospital, Los Angeles, Calif.
13. Canadian Red Cross Memorial Hospital, Taplow, Berkshire, England
14. Texas Children's Hospital, Houston, Texas
15. Hospital for Special Surgery, New York, N. Y.
16. Stanford University School of Medicine, Palo Alto, Calif.
17. Veteran's Administration Center, West Los Angeles, Calif.

Table 5-10 Liver Function Studies on Patients with Plasma-cell Hepatitis*

Patient	Age (Yr.)	Sex	Serum Bilirubin, 1 Min., Mg. %	Serum Bilirubin, Total, Mg. %	Ceph. Chol. Flocc.	Thym. Turb. Units	Zinc Turb. Units	Alkaline Phosphatase K.A. Units
1	14	M	2.2	3.8	4+	31	75	38.2
2	13	F	1.4	2.6	4+	10	50	19.0
3	14	F	1.3	2.4	4+	34	64	15.6
4	13	F	18.5	26.7	4+	16	69	43.0
5	12	F	3.5	5.9	4+	27	51	9.5
6	19	M	2.0	3.2	4+	19	50	—

Patient	Sulfobromo-phthalein, % Retention 45 Min.	Prothrombin Time, Sec.	Total Serum Proteins, Gm. %	Serum Albumin, Gm. %	Serum Globulin, Gm. %	α-Globulin Gm. %	β-Globulin Gm. %	γ-Globulin Gm. %
1	0	—	15.3	0.8	14.5	1.7	2.9	9.9
2	28	—	11.2	2.7	8.5	1.2	0.9	6.4
3	24	Patient 17.2 / Control 13.0	13.0	2.2	10.8	1.4	1.1	8.3
4	18	Patient 20.5 / Control 12.4	11.6	2.1	9.5	—	—	7.1
5	15	Patient 16.4 / Control 13.3	12.0	2.3	9.7	1.5	2.3	5.9
6	27	—	11.1	2.4	8.7	0.8	1.0	6.9

*From Page, A. R., and Good, R. A.: Plasma-cell hepatitis, with special attention to steroid therapy. A.M.A. J. Dis. Child., 99:288, 1960.

REFERENCES

Alarcon-Segovia, D., Worthington, J. W., Ward, L. E., and Wakim, K. G.: Lupus diathesis and the hydralazine syndrome. New Eng. J. Med., *272*:462, 1965.
Ansell, B. M., Bywaters, E. G. L., and Lawrence, J. S.: A family study in Still's disease. Ann. Rheum. Dis., *21*:243, 1962.
Arkin, A. Discussed in symposium on periarteritis nodosa. Proc. Staff Meet. Mayo Cl., *24*:2, 19, 1949.
Barnett, E. V.: Personal communication, 1968.
Bearn, A. G., Kunkel, H. G., and Slater, R. J.: The problem of chronic liver disease in young women. Amer. J. Med., *21*:3, 1956.
Boland, E. W., and Present, A. J. Discussed by Boland, E. W.: Ankylosing spondylitis. *In* Hollander, J. L.: Arthritis and Allied Conditions, Ed. 7. Philadelphia, Lea & Febiger, 1966, p. 647.
Borella, L., Goobar, J. E., Summitt, R. L., and Clark, G. M.: Septic arthritis in childhood. J Pediat., *62*:742, 1963.
Calabro, J. J.: Management of ankylosing spondylitis. Bull. Rheum. Dis., *16*:408, 1966.
Calabro, J. J., and Marchesano, J. M.: Juvenile rheumatoid arthritis: Observations on fever. New Eng. J. Med., *276*:11, 1967.
Condemi, J. J., Barnett, E. V., Atwater, E. C., Jacox, R. F., Mongan, E. S., and Vaughan, J. H.: The significance of antinuclear factor in rheumatoid arthritis. Arthritis Rheum., *8*:1080, 1965.
Cook, C. D., Rosen, F. S., and Banker, B. Q.: Dermatomyositis and focal scleroderma. Pediat. Clin. N. Amer. *10*:1007, 1963.
Corner, B. D.: Reiter's syndrome in childhood. Arch. Dis. Child., *25*:398, 1950.
Decker, J. L., and Vandeman, P. R.: Renal calculi preceding gouty arthritis in a child. Amer. J. Med., *32*:805, 1962.
de Torregrosa, M. V., Dapena, R. B., Hernandez, H., and Ortiz, A. Discussed by Rodnan, G. P.: Arthritis associated with disorders of hemopoiesis and blood coagulation. *In* Hollander, J. L.: Arthritis and Allied Conditions, Ed. 7. Philadelphia, Lea & Febiger, 1966, p. 1095.
Dunham, C. L., and Kautz, F. G.: Discussed by Boland, E. W.: Ankylosing spondylitis. *In* Hollander, J. L.: Arthritis and Allied Conditions, Ed. 7. Philadelphia, Lea & Febiger, 1966, p. 636.
Engelman, E. P., Barnes, M. G., Jones, J. P., Jr., Schacter, J., and Meyer, K. F.: Arthritis associated with bedsonia infection (abstract). Arthritis Rheum., *9*:502, 1966.
Fink, C. W.: Gonococcal arthritis in children. J.A.M.A., *194*:237, 1965.
Fink & Ziff: Personal communication.
Good, R. A., Rötstein, J., and Mazzitello, W. F.: The simultaneous occurrence of rheumatoid arthritis and agammaglobulinemia. J. Lab. Clin. Med., *49*:343, 1957.
Henderson, M. S. Discussed by Balboni, V. G.: Tuberculous arthritis. *In* Hollander, J. L.: Arthritis and Allied Conditions, Ed. 7. Philadelphia, Lea & Febiger, 1966, p. 1018.
Hendrickse, R. G., and Collard, P. Discussed by Rodnan, G. P.: Arthritis associated with disorders of hemopoiesis and blood coagulation. *In* Hollander, J. L.: Arthritis and Allied Conditions, Ed. 7. Philadelphia, Lea & Febiger, 1966, p. 1095.
Holt, E. L., Jr., McIntosh, R., and Barnett, H. L.: Pediatrics, Ed. 13. New York, Appleton-Century-Crofts, Inc., 1962., p. 626.
Hughes, J. G., and Carroll, D. S. Discussed by Rodnan, G. P.: Arthritis associated with disorders of hemopoiesis and blood coagulation. *In* Hollander, J. L.: Arthritis and Allied Conditions, Ed. 7. Philadelphia, Lea & Febiger, 1966, p. 1095.
Janeway, C. A., Gitlin, D., Craig, J. M., and Grice, D. S.: "Collagen Disease" in patients with congenital agammaglobulinemia. Trans. Assoc. Am. Physicians, *69*:93, 1956.
Koster, M. S., and Jansen, M. Discussed by Corner, B. D.: Reiter's syndrome in childhood. Arch. Dis. Child., *25*:398, 1950
Kunkel, H. G., Ahrens, E. H., Jr., Eisenminger, W. J., Bongiovanni, A. M., and Slater, R. J.: Extreme hypergammaglobulinemia in young women with liver disease of unknown etiology (abstract). J. Clin. Invest., *30*:654, 1951.
Kussmaul, A., and Maier, R.: Periarteritis nodosa. Deutsches Arch. Klin. Med., *1*:484, 1866.

Lesch, M., and Nyhan, W. L. Discussed by Wyngaarden, J. B.: Etiology and pathogenesis of gout. *In* Hollander, J. L.: Arthritis and Allied Conditions, Ed. 7. Philadelphia, Lea & Febiger, 1966, p. 915.

Lietman, P. S., and Bywaters, E. G. L.: Pericarditis in juvenile rheumatoid arthritis. Pediatrics, *32*:855, 1963.

Maclachlan, M. J., Rodnan, G. P., Cooper, W. M., and Fennell, R. H., Jr.,: Chronic active ("lupoid") hepatitis. A clinical, serological, and pathological study of 20 patients. Ann. Int. Med., *62*:425, 1965.

Markowitz, M. A.: Personal communication, 1968.

Maxeiner, S. R., McDonald, J. R., and Kirklin, J. W. Discussed by Shulman, L. E., and Harvey, A. McG.: Polyarteritis, *In* Hollander, J. L.: Arthritis and Allied Conditions, Ed. 7. Philadelphia, Lea & Febiger, 1966, p. 802.

McGovern, J. P., and Merritt, D. H.: Sarcoidosis in childhood. Advances Pediat., *8*:97, 1956.

Mikkelsen, W. M., and Duff, I. F. Discussed by Boland, E. W.: Ankylosing spondylitis. *In* Hollander, J. L.: Arthritis and Allied Conditions, Ed. 7. Philadelphia, Lea & Febiger, 1966, p. 636.

Nelson, J. D., and Koontz, W. C.: Septic arthritis in infants and children: A review of 117 cases. Pediatrics, *38*:966, 1966.

Page, A. R., and Good, R. A.: Plasma-cell hepatitis with special attention to steroid therapy. A.M.A. J. Dis. Child., *99*:288, 1960.

Paronen, I. Discussed by Corner, B. D.: Reiter's syndrome in childhood. Arch. Dis. Child., *25*:398, 1950.

Pearson, C. M.: Polymyositis. Ann. Rev. Med., 1966.

Pinals, R. S., and Ropes, M. W.: Meningococcal arthritis. Arthritis Rheum., 7:241, 1964.

Popert, A. J., and Hewitt, J. V.: Gout and hyperuricemia in rural and urban populations. Ann. Rheum. Dis., *20*:154, 1962.

Porter, F. S., and Thurman, W. G.: Studies of sickle cell disease. Amer. J. Dis. Child., *106*:35, 1963.

Primer on the Rheumatic Diseases: Ankylosing spondylitis. J.A.M.A., Part II, *190*:425, 1964.

Rallison, M. L., Carlisle, J. W., Lee, R. E., Jr., Vernier, R. L., and Good, R. A.: Lupus erythematosus and Stevens-Johnson syndrome, occurrence as reactions to anticonvulsant medication. Amer. J. Dis. Child., *101*:725, 1961.

Reiter, H. Discussed by Corner, B. D.: Reiter's syndrome in childhood. Arch. Dis. Child., *25*:398, 1950.

Rodnan, G. P.: Arthritis associated with disorders of hemopoiesis and blood coagulation. *In* Hollander, J. L.: Arthritis and Allied Conditions, Ed. 7. Philadelphia, Lea & Febiger, 1966, p. 1095.

Scott, J. T.: Joint involvement in bone diseases. *In* Dixon, A. St. J. (ed.): Progress in Clinical Rheumatology. Boston, Little, Brown & Company, 1965, p. 305.

Shulman, L. E., and Harvey, A. McG.: Systemic lupus erythematosus. *In* Hollander, J. L.: Arthritis and Allied Conditions. Philadelphia, Lea & Febiger, 1961.

Shulman, L. E., and Harvey, A. McG.: Polyarteritis. *In* Hollander, J. L.: Arthritis and Allied Conditions, Ed. 7. Philadelphia, Lea & Febiger, 1966, p. 806.

Silverstein, M. N., and Kelly, P. J.: Bone and joint involvement in acute leukemia. Rheumatism, *21*:67, 1965.

Smith, E., Rosenblatt, P., and Bedo, A. V.: Sickle-cell anemia crisis. J. Pediat., *43*:655, 1953.

Talbott, J. H., and Ferrandis, R. M.: Collagen diseases. New York, Grune & Stratton, 1956.

Watson, R. J., Burko, H., Megas, H., and Robinson, M.: The hand-foot syndrome in sickle-cell disease in young children. Pediatrics, *31*:975, 1963.

Zewi, M. Discussed by Corner, B. D.: Reiter's syndrome in childhood. Arch. Dis. Child., *25*:398, 1950.

Chapter Six

PSYCHOLOGICAL ASPECTS OF JUVENILE RHEUMATOID ARTHRITIS

SIDNEY E. CLEVELAND, PH.D.*
AND EARL J. BREWER, JR., M.D.

Rheumatoid arthritis in children creates many personality problems that must be handled by the physician. Parent, child, and physician are all involved in emotional interplay that will last over the many years of disease activity. Rheumatoid arthritis is a disease of unknown etiology, which has a capricious and variable course, and no specific cure is available. The physician therefore is faced with the task of interpreting to the parent how it is possible to diagnose a condition with no known cause. He must plan a course of therapy with inadequate tools and must necessarily be vague concerning the ultimate outcome. In addition the services of several other specialties, such as orthopedics, cardiology, and ophthalmology, are necessary during the course of the disease along with the efforts of paramedical personnel such as physical therapists, laboratory technicians, and social workers. The physician treating the child must therefore assume the role of central figure in planning and executing the program.

REACTION TO DISEASE

Reaction of the Parent

Juvenile rheumatoid arthritis, in the minds of most parents, connotes a serious and dreadful disease leading to lifelong crippling. There is usually the immediate fear and anxiety by parents over the knowledge that their own child is afflicted with such a dreadful condi-

---

*Professor of Psychology, Department of Psychiatry, Baylor College of Medicine, Houston, Texas

tion. If the physician fails to establish careful rapport at this point, then several unfortunate effects can occur. Some parents look immediately for innumerable other physicians to confirm or deny the existence of arthritis in their child. This series of changes of physician is not based on the idea of further consultation but on the hope that somehow the disease will disappear. At this point parents are most susceptible to the camp followers of medicine with nostrums such as sea water, elaborate mechanical devices, or séances as instant answers to the problem.

One of the two main reactions of the mother to the diagnosis is an enormous feeling of guilt, a feeling that somehow she has failed the child, or that she has caused the condition in some unwitting way. Such feelings are particularly difficult to erase in view of medicine's lack of knowledge of etiology. The feeling of guilt can be overwhelming and usually persists in one form or another all during the course of the disease, and the physician must be constantly on guard to reduce or minimize this feeling.

The second common reaction of parents, particularly of mothers, is a total denial of the disease's existence. If this idea is allowed to take root and continue, the entire therapeutic program is doomed to failure. The mother can and does totally repress belief in the very existence of the disease or hopes that in some mysterious way it will disappear. This represents not only denial of the existence of the disease but repression of the parent's responsibility for it and can represent an inability or refusal to accept the reality of the situation.

Reaction of the Child

The severity of the emotional reaction to juvenile rheumatoid arthritis is in large measure dependent upon the severity of symptoms, limitation of activity, and age of the child. A patient with severe multiple joint swelling and significant pain presents a completely different problem from a patient who has one or two joints minimally involved with little or no pain and no restriction of motion. In children who have a significantly severe onset of the disease the usual reaction is the same as in any child with an acute serious illness, a reaction of irritability and concern over what has gone wrong. Mood depression and fear are usually transmitted directly from the mother, father, and physician. At this point of the disease the attitude of the physician is the key to later success or failure. If the physician approaches the patient and family as the voice of doom and offers little hope, a practical therapeutic program becomes difficult if not almost impossible for a later physician or consultant.

Studies performed at the Arthritis Clinical Research Center at Texas Children's Hospital have shown that there are no personality patterns specific to juvenile arthritis (Cleveland et al., 1965). Children react instead according to basic individual personality patterns, which are not unique for this disease. Some children were often described as being more active physically than other children prior to the onset of the disease but this impression may have been distorted by retrospective reminiscences on the part of the parents.

REACTION TO THE THERAPEUTIC PROGRAM

Reaction of the Parent

There are two chief reactions, particularly by the mother, that often occur and must be eliminated by the physician initially. First, there is a natural concern about the limitations of activity, with the mother tending to overprotect the patient. In a short term illness this can be desirable, but in a disease state that may well last for several years the concept has to be firmly established that discipline and training must be continued as near to the usual routine as possible. An overprotective attitude affects not only the patient but siblings as well. If undue attention is paid to the patient, or more attention than is necessary, the other children in the family feel the change in emphasis and excessive sibling rivalry develops.

The second serious reaction of the parent to the therapeutic program is a feeling of overt or covert hostility toward the effort necessary to help prevent serious crippling. In the study performed at Texas Children's Hospital a significant number of mothers felt that they were being "put upon" by the illness and the demands of therapy (Cleveland et al., 1965). This attitude led to a grudging acquiescence at best and at times to a complete rejection of the whole program.

Perhaps the most serious problem in therapeutic programs designed to prevent serious joint deformity is related to the boredom and inertia that develop from the routine of day to day medication, warm baths, and physical therapy over a period of years. The results of such programs are often difficult to ascertain because the maintenance of normal or near normal joint function is difficult to assess.

Reaction of the Child

Reaction to therapeutic programs is largely dependent upon the age of the subject as well as the severity of the disease. Patients under four years of age have difficulty in following a planned exercise program. More often than not the mother and physical therapist have to conduct the exercises desired, and other exercises must be designed to get the patient himself to use a range of motion to a maximum degree, in addition to the resistance exercises conducted by the parent. The reaction of this age group to moist heat is also predictable. Care must be taken to ensure pleasure, if possible, during the heat and exercises. Such efforts as gait training for patients with problems of abduction or adduction are difficult in this age group. Excessive depression and mood alteration, other than irritability when pain or fever occur, are unusual, but in this age group, as with other age groups, the patient does have good days and bad days, good periods of time and poor periods of time.

From about four years of age until adolescence patients are easier to handle and can be taught assistive and strengthening exercises and gait training with relative ease. The attention span of this age group, however, is still short and any therapeutic program must be measured in terms of the patient's attentive limits. Constant reassurance must be given during this time by the therapist and the parent. Discouragement comes easily and is probably the biggest problem. Patients in this age group do become depressed about illness, and they worry about the duration of symptoms as well as exacerbations even when doing the best job possible with exercise, heat, and medication.

Patients in the teen-age group present particular problems, as they have a greater concern about self image and body image. The arthritis unit at Texas Children's Hospital has the subjective impression that teen-agers, particularly girls, experience more subjective pain and exquisite tenderness than those in the younger age group. Teen-agers are usually easy to engage in participation in a therapeutic program but discouragement does come easily and constant reassurance is particularly necessary here, with definite goals established that are attainable.

Relationships Between Psyche and Soma—Theoretical Background

Body Image

A concept that has been found useful in understanding some of the relationships between personality and behavioral processes on the one hand and physiological and somatic functioning on the other hand is that of body image. Body image refers to the body as a psychological experience and involves the individual's feelings and attitudes toward his body. Body image is concerned with the individual's subjective experiences with his body and the manner in which he has organized these experiences. The assumption is that as each individual develops he has the difficult task of meaningfully organizing the sensations from his body—one of the most important and complex phenomena in his total perceptual field. It is a phenomenon relatively more complex and difficult to organize perceptually because of the individual's unique simultaneous role, as a participant in the perceptual process and also as the object of this same perceptual process. In other words the body as a perceptual object is unique in that it is simultaneously that which is perceived and also a part of the perceiver. Thus, when an individual touches himself, he concurrently has a sensation of touching and of being touched. No other perceptual object ever occupies such a dual position or participates so intimately in the perceptual process. Secondly, an unusually intense level of ego involvement is evoked by one's body as an object of perception. When the individual reacts to his own body, he is stirred and aroused in a manner that rarely occurs when he reacts to the non-self world. This is not simply a theoretical presumption but has been demonstrated in a variety of studies. For example, it has been shown that when individuals unknowingly respond to pictures of their own bodies they express more emotional response than they do when reacting to pictures of other people.

There are indications that the individual starts early to organize his body perceptions. He begins to highlight certain areas and to minimize others. Some body areas may be persistently in the forefront of awareness, and others may be denied to the point where they almost do not exist in a perceptual sense. Two psychologists, Kagan and Moss (1962), have demonstrated the continuity and consistency to be found in the development of body attitudes. They have shown that the degree of fearfulness about one's body in adulthood is significantly correlated with the level of such fearfulness in early childhood. Furthermore, they found that early body anxiety appears to have the consequence of encouraging certain long-term modes of behavior. For example, boys with high body anxiety were found to avoid athletic activities and to invest an increasing proportion of their time in intellectual tasks.

Those who have explored the body image concept, e. g., Schilder (1935), usually make the assumption that the manner in which the individual accomplishes the difficult task of organizing his body attitudes and perceptions becomes one of the primary dimensions in his overall system of standards for interpreting the world. A person's body image is literally an image of his own body that he has evolved through experience. The word image is possibly misleading because it might be interpreted as referring only to those attitudes that he has of which he is consciously aware. Actually the term body image is not limited by one's awareness of such attitudes and feelings. Indeed, the more we learn about body image the more apparent it becomes that some of the most important attributes of body image involve feelings of which the individual is totally unaware and incapable of reporting, either to himself or to others. Thus, body image is not synonymous with physical appearance. The concept of body image usually involves something more and something different from one's physical size, shape, or stature. Body image refers to a representation of attitudes and expectancy systems, conscious or unconscious, entertained by each individual. The resulting body image evolved is less influenced by the actual physical appearance of the individual than by the kinds of experience he has encountered with his body. We often see individuals who are perfectly formed, with bulging muscles or graceful curves, yet who entertain the most depreciatory and negative image of their body. Conversely, persons with even severe disability may retain a positive and constructive image of themselves.

Neurological and Psychiatric Contributions. It is among neurologists that one finds the earliest references to body image phenomena. Patients with various brain lesions often manifest a wide range of distorted ideas about their bodies. Henry Head, the famous British neurologist, made body image one of the most important constructs in his system of thinking about neurological problems. He has been followed by Gerstman, Critchley, and many others in reporting the fascinating body image distortions accompanying certain brain lesions. In the area of psychiatric study, Schilder, Fenichel, and Freud himself have described the often weird body delusions and ideas entertained by schizophrenics and depressed patients. But the body image attitudes of normal individuals and the body image distortions produced by conditions other than neurological or psychiatric illness have attracted relatively little explicit interest, probably because they are not as highly visible as those manifested by sick and disturbed patients.

The existence and importance of the boundary dimension is difficult for most people to grasp because in the normal course of events people do not experience any special concern about their body boundaries. They seem to know well enough where these boundaries end and where the outer world begins, but there are various pathological states in which the individual does grossly lose the ability to identify his body boundaries. In such instances the actual existence and functional value of the body boundary become apparent. It has already been noted that brain-damaged and also schizophrenic patients often have marked difficulty in deciding whether certain stimuli come from outside the body boundry or arise from the body itself. Although such gross variations do not normally occur, we have evidence that even among normal people there are many instances in which individuals perceive themselves as not clearly demarcated from what is "out there."

Research on Body Image. The experimental study of body image has been slowed because the concept is not a unitary trait, nor do body attitudes lend themselves easily to measurement and objective study. There are many facets to one's body image and it is by no means clear which dimensions are the more important and powerful determinants of behavior. Attitudes involving body size, smallness vs. large size, beauty vs. ugliness, strength vs. weakness, and masculinity vs. femininity are all obviously interesting and important psychological variables pertaining to the body. However, these are difficult dimensions to quantify and experimental study in this area has been slow.

A program of research conducted by Fisher and Cleveland (1958) has explored the dimension of body image involving the boundaries or periphery of the body. The tendency of individuals to establish definite and well articulated body image boundaries and the consequences for a wide variety of behaviors of well defined vs. poorly defined body boundaries have been examined in their studies.

The research by Fisher and Cleveland grew out of the view that it was important to have a means for investigating the correlation and consequences of variations in boundary definiteness. Beginning in 1951 a series of studies were conducted that established the concept of distinct individual differences in the definiteness or articulation that one ascribes to the boundary regions of one's body.

Although the investigations were later extended to normal, healthy subjects, this research and the concept of body boundary began with the examination of persons suffering from somatic illness. Originally chosen for study were groups with somatic symptoms having emotional involvement and overlay, syndromes usually recognized as falling within the group of illnesses referred to as the psychosomatic diseases, e.g., peptic ulcer and neurodermatitis, as well as rheumatoid arthritis.

Originally interest was focused only on adult arthritics because a ready supply of patients was available and they seemed to represent an interesting group to subject to clinical study. In addition, rheumatologists and physiatrists working with these arthritics were impressed by the emotional and personality factors at play among their patients and were interested in knowing something more about their psychological makeup.

Clinical evaluation of adult male patients with rheumatoid arthritis revealed certain seemingly unique personality patterns through the use of psychological tests and interviews in the later Fisher and Cleveland studies (1960). It was noted that arthritics, in response to the Rorschach or ink blot test, produced fantasies that suggested a link between the way they perceived their bodies and the nature of their psychosomatic symptomatology. Arthritics tended to give responses to the Rorschach test emphasizing the containing, protective, and enclosing properties of the periphery of things. Their fantasies reflected some of the rigidity and armor-like characteristics of their stiffened joints, limbs, and muscles. The kinds of Rorschach fantasies I am referring to included such responses as "a cave with rock walls," "a man in a suit of armor," "a post embedded in concrete," and "a hard-shelled crustacean."

A comparison group of patients with symptoms somewhat similar to those of the arthritics in terms of the pain, discomfort, and limitation of motion imposed—patients with low back pain—did not produce these unique fantasies. Moreover, psychosomatic groups with symptoms involving the interior of the body, patients with duodenal ulcer, not only did not produce these fantasies underlining the boundaries of objects but instead described objects whose periphery was weakened, vulnerable, and diffuse. Thus, ulcer patients would describe the Rorschach cards in such terms as "a body cut open," "a rotten log with holes in it," and "a bullet piercing flesh."

Body Image Scoring Indices. Two formal body image scoring indices were devised from these contrasting response series. One index, constructed of the responses involving boundary definiteness, was termed the barrier score. The barrier score represents the sum of those responses in an ink blot record depicting objects with sharply defined and clearly delineated boundaries, responses such as the ones just mentioned, "cave with rock walls," "man in armor," and "post in concrete." In all responses of this type the protective, containing, and enclosing properties of the periphery are highlighted. The second body image index, termed the penetration score, is derived from the ink blot fantasies highlighting the weakness and diffuseness of boundary properties. The penetration score represents the sum of ink blot responses characterizing the boundaries of objects as either poorly defined, vulnerable, or weak, e.g., "a body cut open," "an x-ray of the body," and similar responses.

These body image indices were next applied to normal groups, and it was found that persons with no demonstrable somatic or psychiatric illness placed themselves along a continuum on the barrier and penetration scores. A series of studies was carried out to determine the personality and behavioral characteristics associated with high or low scores on the barrier scale. These studies showed that an individual with definite and clearly defined body image boundaries (high barrier score) is likely to behave autonomously, to manifest high achievement motivation, to be the type of person who pushes his way through his environment and who is interested in employing his muscles in an active, assertive manner. He is likely to be a person with an unusual interest in physical exertion, competitive sports, and hard physical labor. By way of contrast, persons with diffuse body boundaries tended to be more passive, relied more on external cues for guidance of their behavior, and were generally less assertive and achieving.

Body Image Scores and Arthritic Patients. Returning now to arthritic patients, it was found that arthritic groups scored very high on the barrier scale. At the fantasy level they emphasized the containing and armoring qualities of their body image boundaries. The protective and enclosing attributes they assigned to the peripheries of Rorschach percepts were analogous to the characteristic symptomatic stiffening of their muscles and joints. From these findings a link was postulated between certain aspects of the individual's way of perceiving his body and the geography or site of his psychosomatic symptomatology. Noted further was the fact that psychosomatic symptomatology could be roughly conceptualized as falling along a continuum in terms of whether the exterior body layers, the skin and striped muscles, were involved at one extreme or the internal viscera, at the other extreme. The intriguing possibility then arose that there might be a relationship between the individual's manner of picturing his body boundaries and the site of his psychosomatic symptoms relative to the body's exterior-interior continuum. It should be noted that this exterior-interior dimension refers to the psychological domain of body exterior and interior and not to any formal physiological or neurological pattern. For example, rheumatoid arthritics think of their symptoms as involving primarily the exterior of their body, and their psychological investment is primarily centered on what they conceive of as the outer layer or shell of their body. However, ulcer patients, colitis patients, and others with symptoms involving stomach pains and vomiting without a demonstrable organic basis ignore the body's exterior and focus their psychological attention on the interior of the body. For these patients the defensive value of their body image boundary is minimal, and they conceive of their body periphery as vulnerable, diffuse, and ill-defined.

This depiction of contrasting views of the body boundary among pathological groups was arrived at by extensive comparison of separate groups of adult rheumatoid arthritics, an ulcer group, and a group with neurodermatitis, all equated for age, education, socioeconomic status, and other pertinent variables. Arthritis and dermatitis patients significantly exceed ulcer and colitis patients on the barrier scale, with the reverse being true for the penetration scale.

Whether these special fantasies elicited in response to an ink blot series are merely a reaction to and a reflection of the distress imposed by somatic symptoms or whether they represent a more basic personality element is, of course, a primary question. In an attempt to answer this question appropriate control groups were also studied when possible. As has been mentioned, patients with low back pain, usually involving a slipped disc syndrome, were employed as a control group for the arthritis study. Patients with unsightly scars produced by industrial burns and chemical reactions were used as a control group for the dermatitis cases. In these control groups the barrier score was not elevated and was significantly lower than for either the arthritis or the dermatitis groups.

Another analysis was made to determine whether duration of symptoms affected the body image scores produced in response to ink blots. Arthritis and dermatitis groups were divided at the median for duration of symptoms. Those with relatively recent, acute symptomatology did not differ significantly from chronic patients in their scores on the barrier scale. Symptom duration was not related to body image score.

It is recognized that some may find fault with the choice of these particular control or comparison groups. However, considering the realities of the available clinical population, the choice of patients with low back pain and those with industrial skin lesions as control groups appears to be a logical compromise between the ideal and the practical.

Perception and Body Image. A puzzling question that arises is why body feelings should find representation in ink blot percepts. Why should there be an almost isomorphic relationship between patterns of exterior-interior body sensations and the properties ascribed to the boundary regions of ink blot images? The possibility that immediately presents itself is that when an individual is asked to react to highly unstructured stimulus materials, the background of sensations represented by his own body in the total perceptual field may intrude with sufficient force to impose some patterning on his reactions. Thus, if his body persistently appears to him as an object whose periphery is emphasized and highlighted, he may be stimulated to see similar patterns with highlighted peripheries in perceptual targets that lack form or structure of their own. Actually this possibility was first implicitly suggested by Hermann Rorschach, who speculated that human movement responses elicited by ink blots represented projections of an individual's kinesthetic sensations. It is also very pertinent that investigators have discovered that when specific patterns of tonus are induced in an individual, either by the use of drugs or by mechanical stimuli such as heat or cold, they may affect his perception of ambiguous pictures and designs. There is the noteworthy possibility that a significant part of response to ink blots and similar stimuli is contributed by the background matrix of body experiences.

The relationship between the barrier score and the patterning of interior-exterior body perception may be derived from two sources:

First, there are indications that the person with clear-cut boundaries learns during his socialization to assign great significance in his body scheme to the boundary regions of his body, particularly the musculature, because these boundaries take on unusual import for him as a method of coping in an active and "voluntary" manner with the outside world. But the individual with vague boundaries, who is less actively oriented, ascribes less importance to his body's exterior and more to its interior. Presumably this difference could result in focusing differential attention upon the areas in question. Therefore, the high barrier subject whose boundary region is of relatively special significance to him would scan it with great attentiveness, and similarly the low barrier subject would be sensitive to sensations in his body's interior.

Secondly, evidence exists that the high barrier subject exceeds the low barrier subject in level of physiological arousal of exterior body areas (Fisher, 1963). However, the low barrier subject manifests higher arousal of interior regions than the high barrier subject. Early in the program of research described here, it was speculated that since persons were found to differ in their psychological investment in different body areas, there might be a concomitant difference in their physiological response in these same areas. In two separate studies, one carried out by Fisher and Cleveland (1960) and one by Williams and Krasnoff (1964), this was found to be true. Male arthritics and male ulcer patients were compared for physiological response under stress. Physiological recordings were made for galvanic skin response, muscle potential, and, in one of the studies, basal skin resistance. The measure of heart rate activity was also recorded. Stress was induced in one study by intense and unpleasant loud sound and in the second study by an exasperating intellectual task. Under these stressful conditions, arthritics were characterized by a significantly lower heart rate, a higher number of galvanic skin responses, and higher muscle potential than ulcer patients. In other words, arthritics under stress tended to respond maximally with increased muscle and skin arousal whereas ulcer patients gained in heart rate.

Probably this difference in physiological reactivity results in a differential density of sensations at the body sites in question. Therefore, at least partially the correlation of the barrier score with body sensation patterns may be a function of the contrast in actual arousal levels of the body's exterior and interior. Perhaps the differences in sensation between exterior and interior that are related to the physiological factors acquire in their persistence over time an influence of their own in reinforcing the psychological dominance of the exterior or interior in the body schema. It is likely that long-term richness of sensation from one body sector could in its own right make that sector a prominent body schema landmark.

A definitive study joining barrier score and bodily function would be a predictive study. If body image scores were obtained in late adolescence or early adulthood and if these scores predicted the development of physical symptoms in later life, conclusive support for a strong linkage between perceptual processes and body response would be at hand. Attempts have been made in this direction, but there are practical limitations to this type of study, mainly involving the relatively low order of frequency of occurrence of any single psychosomatic illness such as rheumatoid arthritis in a given population; thus enormous numbers of subjects are needed for evaluation in order to identify positive cases. Perhaps an even more limiting factor to a predictive longitudinal study is the long waiting period, measured in decades, before the emergence of somatic illness.

Personality and Rheumatoid Arthritis

To return to findings involving personality and emotional factors in rheumatoid arthritics, some of the more general research results are of interest in describing personality characteristics in arthritics. Fisher and Cleveland studied two separate groups of adult male rheumatoid arthritics, using clinical interviews and psychological tests including the Rorschach, TAT, and figure drawings. As has been mentioned, comparison groups similarly studied included in one case a low back pain group and in the second study male duodenal ulcer patients. One of the principal findings regarding personality and control of emotional expression in the arthritic groups concerned their inhibition and suppression of anger. Arthritics severely overcontrol hostile expression and appear as conforming, compliant, and docile individuals.

Interview results indicated that the arthritic appeared to be calm, composed, and optimistic, rarely, if ever, expressing or even consciously feeling anger. He boasted of never fighting or getting angry, although he admitted that a "smart alec or braggart" or a "loud mouth guy" could get him angry. The arthritics complained of social shyness and inadequacy, tended to shun the limelight, and desired to be "just average and not stand out at all." Maintaining composure and reflecting an unruffled manner were important for the arthritics. Indeed, the psychological function of their arthritic symptoms is seen as limiting and restricting aggressive action. Arthritics view their muscle and joint stiffness as a constraint on hostile expression.

Chronic inhibition of rage with a consequent overconforming and compliant manner has also been a characteristic of arthritic patients reported in other studies. For example, Moos and Solomon (1965) recently studied 16 female arthritics and their healthy siblings and were impressed with the difficulty arthritics experienced in expressing anger and rage. These investigators described their arthritic subjects as masochistic, self-sacrificing, inhibited in the expression of anger, compliant, and subservient. They speculated, as have other investigators, e.g., Gottschalk et al. (1950), that chronically repressed and inhibited rage may lead to higher muscle tension, increased joint pressure, pain, and joint damage. Chronic muscle tension is viewed as a predisposing or contributing factor in the development of arthritic symptoms. In the Fisher and Cleveland studies it has been shown that arthritics under stress respond maximally with increased muscle tension. A crucial test of the role played in arthritis by muscle tension would be the evaluation of the same subjects either prior to the onset of symptoms or during a period of complete remission, in order to assess the disruptive effect produced by the symptoms themselves.

Another finding emerging from the study of arthritic groups concerns the unusual interest and investment in physical activity, gross muscle utilization, and a generally energetic manner reported by arthritics as characterizing their life style prior to the onset of symptoms. Other reports are available attesting to the mobile life style of arthritics, for example, Ludwig (1952) and Johnson et al. (1947). If this description does not represent some sort of retrospective falsification on the part of the arthritic, that is, a longing for a return to a period when he was more mobile, there exists the possibility that at one point in their lives arthritics manifested a more aggressive, competitive, and active life style. The arthritic may be considered an individual who from an early period in his life habitually channeled excitation and physiological response via his muscles whenever he was under stress. In the psychological dimension the arthritic is the individual who has elaborated on the boundary or periphery of his body image. He is the sort of person who has gone to extraordinary lengths to establish a defensive and protective boundary about himself, so much so that in his unconscious fantasies he perceives these boundaries as a kind of armor plating or bulwark.

It is not contended that chronic inhibited rage, converted into chronic muscle tension, together with an unusual psychological investment in the periphery of the body, leads inevitably to the development of arthritic symptoms. Indeed, it is not possible to differentiate on the basis of body image formulation among a number of different disease groups, e.g., rheumatoid arthritis and neurodermatitis. Also, in normal adults the pattern of high muscle response under stress combined with a well-articulated body image is a common finding. The development of rheumatoid arthritis is obviously an enormously complex and multivariate process. A history of unusual participation in physical activity, utilization of striate muscles as a major stress response mechanism, and the creation of a body image characterized by rigid and well-articulated boundaries are not sufficient factors to explain the occurrence or nonoccurrence of arthritic symptoms. What is suggested is that these factors, so prominent in groups with active arthritic symptoms, may play a contributing role in the etiology and development of the disease.

Psychological Studies in Juvenile Rheumatoid Arthritis

The research reported thus far with adult arthritics has been extended to the study of children with rheumatoid arthritis. Cleveland et al. (1965) evaluated 30 arthritic children and their mothers, using psychological tests and interviews. A comparison group of 25 asthmatic children was similarly studied. Like their adult counterparts, arthritic children also score high on the barrier body image index, indicating unusually well-defined body image boundaries. Mothers of arthritic children rate them as much more physically active than the average child prior to the onset of symptoms. Moreover, arthritic children score higher on intellectual tasks emphasizing motor skills than they do on problems requiring purely verbal capacity. By contrast, asthmatic children do not differ in verbal or psychomotor performance. Motility and physical activity, together with the development of well-defined and heavily articulated body image boundaries, appear to characterize juvenile arthritics as well as their adult counterparts.

Needed Research in Rheumatoid Arthritis

This reported research represents only a beginning in the attempt to identify the possible role of psychological factors in rheumatoid arthritis. A few interesting leads have been identified, but much more extensive work remains. For example, the impact of the disabling arthritic symptoms on personality should be studied. Since arthritis, especially in its acute stage, is a capricious disease with symptoms appearing and disappearing spontaneously and suddenly, it should be an easy matter to study the psychological state of the same individual in remission and under acute symptom exacerbation. Yet such a study has not been made in a systematic way.

Identification of those psychological factors related to treatment response and rehabilitation outcome also require investigation. It is known from research with other disability groups, e.g., paraplegics, that pretraumatic personality factors, psychological attitude and morale, bear heavily on response to treatment. It is also possible that psychological variables are largely responsible for the sometimes almost magical remission of arthritic symptoms so often noted. Arthritics do not respond uniformly as a group to treatment. There are wide differences in individual response and we need to identify what personality factors, if any, are associated with good or poor treatment response.

There are puzzling methodological problems involved in attempting to isolate the responsible factors in disease development. The matter of proper control groups is an unresolved issue. Some studies have attempted to meet the problem by using other pathological groups, equating where possible the confounding effects of illness and hospitalization. Other investigators have approached this problem with a different solution. For example, Moos and Solomon (1965) have employed healthy siblings as controls for arthritic patients. But the use of healthy family members as controls introduces more problems. For one thing, one is then comparing healthy, nonhospitalized normal individuals with physically ill, hospitalized, or at least treated, patients, and the effect of ill health and medical treatment on behavior and personality is no longer constant for experimental and control groups. Even more important, in using family members as controls, too much may be eliminated; that is, control may be too stringent and the very factor one is looking for, perhaps a family trait, may be obscured. Unfortunately, the use of healthy siblings as controls in studying psychosomatic groups offers no solution to the problems of research in this area.

A recent survey of the literature by Moos (1964) reveals that some 70 scientific articles have appeared dealing with psychological and emotional aspects of rheumatoid arthritis. With only a few exceptions, this published research has reported on studies of adult arthritics; only a handful investigated psychological aspects of juvenile arthritis. Although a sizable literature does exist, largely devoted to examination of adult arthritic patients, unfortunately many of the studies are lacking in scientific rigor, few utilize control or comparison groups, and the methodology, procedures, and subjects employed are so varied and unsystematic that they all but preclude any comparison from one study to the next. In addition many of the studies are anecdotal, restricted to clinical observation of a single, special case with all the limitations inherent in generalizing from one possibly atypical patient. No large-scale prospective study has appeared to answer the basic question of whether any particular pattern of premorbid personality traits characterizes the potential victim of arthritis.

Despite the limitations and inadequacies found in much of the published literature on arthritis, Moos was able to conclude that a consensus did exist among certain independent investigators as to some of the common characteristics in the personality of rheumatoid arthritics. Several investigators employing appropriate control groups were in agreement that arthritics tend to be self-sacrificing, masochistic, conforming, self-conscious, shy, inhibited, and perfectionistic, and involved or interested in sports, games, and other vigorous physically active pursuits. Less agreement was found on the importance of separation trauma in the childhood history of arthritic patients, the mode of expression of anger among arthritics, or the impulsive and defiant manner among this group.

Summary of the Role of Psychological Factors in Rheumatoid Arthritis

The role of psychological factors in the etiology, development, and maintenance of arthritic symptoms can be viewed from several frames of reference. Investigators have been variously concerned with the following areas of study:

Predisposition. An assumption underlying many of the attempts to identify personality patterns characteristic of the arthritic patient is that these patterns antedate the onset of disease and in some way contribute to the development of the illness, or predispose the individual to the development of arthritic symptoms. Unfortunately, all the reported studies are retrospective, and whether the personality factors found to be unique among arthritics represent a reaction to the disease or are actually contributing to the disease is unclear. Most investigators would probably be satisfied only by a prospective study in which it was demonstrated that individuals with certain personality configurations, measured before the development of somatic illness, showed a greater tendency to develop rheumatoid arthritis than individuals with different personality characteristics.

Examples of some of the personality and behavioral characteristics identified with the known arthritic include the reported high incidence of participation in vigorous physical activity among arthritics prior to onset of the disease. As has been mentioned, several independent researchers find that adult arthritics claim a history of intense and unusually active participation in competitive athletics, physical labor, or other vigorous muscular activity for the years prior to the onset of their arthritis. However, Moos (1964) and others have pointed out that possibly this self-reported athletic investment represents a wishful distortion, a longing for lost muscular prowess, and a retrospective falsification influenced by the arthritic's present crippled and relatively immobile state. Perhaps the reported incidence of physical activity is no higher than would be found in any group of patients with chronic disease.

Adjustment to Arthritic Symptoms. Arthritic symptoms fluctuate rapidly in their intensity, and spontaneous remissions are common. Little attention has been paid to the possible role of emotional and psychological factors in facilitating remission of arthritic symptoms or in the exacerbation of symptoms in a quiescent patient. Nor has a careful personality evaluation been made of the same arthritic patients during periods of acute illness and remission. Such a study would contribute much understanding to the controversy over whether observed personality factors in arthritics represent a reaction to the illness or are contributory to symptom formation, since the same individual could be evaluated during a period of distress imposed by his painful symptoms and again during a symptom-free period when presumably the disturbing influence of the arthritic symptoms would not be operating.

Among children with arthritic symptoms and their families much of the active treatment procedure has a direct impact on both the afflicted child and other family members. For example, Cleveland et al. (1965) found that the special attention and treatment afforded the arthritic patient treated in the home according to the Home Treatment Plan devised by the Texas Children's Hospital Arthritis Clinical Research Center created problems of rivalry among healthy siblings in the home. In this same study, mothers of arthritic children tended to react to illness in their child in one of two ways, either accepting too much guilt and responsibility for having brought about the disease or denying illness altogether. It is unclear whether these attitudes on the part of the mothers were specific to arthritis, or as is more likely, whether they represented problems arising in any chronic illness.

Another aspect of the impact of a treatment program on the personality of arthritics involves the consequences of physical immobility and restraint often imposed on the arthritic child. Traditionally the treatment of arthritis in young children has involved the imposition of prolonged physical restraint through the application of body casts, bed rest, and severe limitation on physical activity. Other programs have emphasized a more permissive approach as far as physical response is concerned. No systematic studies are available to judge the relative merits of these contrasting treatment approaches in their impact on personality development.

Rehabilitation. The role of personality factors in the rehabilitation of persons with chronic disease is well documented. Individuals with crippling disease differ widely in their motivation to overcome physical handicaps, and the faithfulness with which patients adhere to their therapeutic regimen varies greatly. Research has documented the fact that by far the most important factors influencing recovery from the disability of chronic disease are the pretraumatic attitudes and outlook the patient has acquired. Often the extent or degree of actual physical disability bears little relation to the success attained by the patient in achieving rehabilitation. Of far greater importance is the desire of the individual to overcome the stigma of disability and to adopt a hopeful and constructive outlook. Research has identified some of the personality attributes associated with successful adjustment to crippling physical disability. For example, Ware et al. (1957) demonstrated that a well-defined body image among patients recovering from poliomyelitis was associated with attainment of good recovery. Similar studies with patients recovering from rheumatoid arthritis are needed to identify the factors that can predict good treatment response.

REFERENCES

Cleveland, S. E., Reitman, E. E., and Brewer, E. J.: Psychological factors in juvenile rheumatoid arthritis. Arthritis Rheum., 8:1152, 1965.
Fisher, S.: A further appraisal of the body boundary concept. J. Consult. Psychol. 27:62, 1963.
Fisher, S., and Cleveland, S. E.: Body Image and Personality. Princeton, New Jersey, D. Van Nostrand Co., Inc., 1958.
Fisher, S., and Cleveland, S. E.: A comparison of psychological characteristics and physiological reactivity in ulcer and rheumatoid arthritis groups. II. Differences in physiological reactivity. Psychosom. Med., 22:290, 1960.
Gottschalk, L. A., Serota, H. M., and Shapiro, L. B.: Psychologic conflict and neuromuscular tension. Psychosom. Med., 12:315, 1950.
Johnson, A., Shapiro, L. B., and Alexander, F.: Preliminary report on a psychosomatic study of rheumatoid arthritis. Psychosom. Med., 9:295, 1947.
Kagan, J., and Moss, H. A.: Birth to Maturity. New York, John Wiley & Sons, Inc., 1962.
Ludwig, A. O.: Psychogenic factors in rheumatoid arthritis. Bull. Rheum. Dis. 2:15, 1952.
Moos, R. H.: Personality factors associated with rheumatoid arthritis: A review. J. Chronic Dis., 17:41, 1964.
Moos, R. H., and Solomon, G. F.: Psychologic comparisons between women with rheumatoid arthritis and their nonarthritic sisters. I. Personality test and interview rating data. Psychosom. Med., 27:135, 1965.
Schilder, P.: The Image and Appearance of the Human Body. London, Regan, Paul, Trench, Trubner & Co., Ltd., 1935.
Ware, K. E., Fisher, S., and Cleveland, S. E.: Body image and boundaries and adjustment to poliomyelitis. J. Abnorm. and Soc. Psychol., 55:88, 1957.
Williams, R. L., and Krasnoff, A. G.: Body image and physiological patterns in patients with peptic ulcer and rheumatoid arthritis. Psychosom. Med., 26:701, 1964.

Chapter Seven

HOME TREATMENT PROGRAM

Elizabeth Barkley, B.S., R.N., P.T.*
and Earl J. Brewer, Jr., M.D.

Home treatment programs for chronic diseases are established to give the patient the benefits gained by performing daily routines. They are designed to fit the individual needs of the patient, particularly in the home environment. Since rheumatoid arthritis requires long-term treatment, daily appointments with a physical therapist are both costly and inconvenient. The length of time spent in a treatment center can never be adequate for good rehabilitation without continuing additional therapy in the home.

The duration of treatment for rheumatoid arthritis may range from a few weeks to several years, and the establishment of a home treatment program is essential in order to obtain the best results. The child is kept in his usual environment and fits the program into daily activities. With as few restrictions as possible, he is allowed to participate with children his own age. Too frequent visits to the hospital may tend to overemphasize the illness to the child.

With this program, both the child and the parents are made aware of the part they must play in treatment of the condition; by their assuming of this responsibility better results are obtained. Activities and exercises directed toward prevention and correction of disabilities, performed in a relaxed manner with daily routine, will prove effective. The program must be kept as simple and uncomplicated as possible or failure is certain. To have a few of the most important aspects fulfilled is better than to have a more detailed program disregarded.

EVALUATION OF THE CHILD

Evaluation of the patient is done to establish a base line to determine the areas of concentration for treatment, and to plan an overall program based on the severity of involvement. The sequence for evaluation of the child starts with the examination of each joint for swelling,

---

*Formerly Physical Therapist, Arthritis Clinical Research Center, Texas Children's Hospital, Houston, Texas

range of motion, tenderness, pain, and heat. This is followed by determination of the tightness of muscle groups, atrophy of muscles, and loss of muscle strength. Next, to evaluate posture, the child is examined while standing, and lastly the gait is observed, revealing valuable information about total involvement.

Swelling

Measurements should be taken with a narrow metal tape. The measurement of the circumference of a joint for swelling is taken at an established area. The joint is compared to its opposite member for amount of swelling, unless both are swollen. Future measurements indicate increase or decrease in involvement. The joints measured by circumference are the elbows, wrists, proximal interphalangeals, knees, ankles, and tarsal areas.

The elbow has swelling most frequently on the medial aspect of the joint and around the olecranon process. Measurement over the olecranon process and across the flexion crease is a stable guide. Major wrist swelling is usually over the dorsum of the wrist, and the measurement area is around the wrist distal to the styloid processes. The proximal interphalangeal joint circumference is measured by the use of a jeweler's ring gauge. The greatest swelling appears over the dorsum of the joint, but it may extend distally and proximally from the joint.

Swelling of the knee is seen most often over the anterior and lateral sides around the patella. A nonflexible area of measurement is at the superior border of the patella with the knee in extension. Swelling of the ankle occurs most frequently around the malleoli and over the dorsum of the joint. If the foot is placed in dorsiflexion, normally there is an indentation between the anterior tibial tendon and the medial malleolus. In performing this motion, swelling is easily detected if present. The measurement of the ankle should be taken distal to the malleolus, which is a stable point. When the tarsal area of the foot is involved, swelling appears over the dorsum of the foot. The best area for measurement is midway between the metatarsophalangeal joint and the ankle. Those joints in which circumference measurement is not practical are observed and the observations recorded: the shoulder, the cervical area, the temporomandibular, sternoclavicular, metacarpal, and distal interphalangeal joints, the hips, and the toes.

Swelling of the shoulder joint occurs usually over the anterior part, and is more easily recognized in the thin child. Swelling of the cervical area is seldom seen. The temporomandibular joint may occasionally be swollen, but this symptom is not as frequent as tenderness and limitation of motion. The sternoclavicular joint is often swollen if any involvement is present.

The metacarpophalangeal joints are frequently involved, with swelling apparent on the dorsum of the joints and filling the areas between. Swelling occurs in the distal interphalangeal joints less frequently than in the other finger joints. The swelling that does appear here is on the dorsum and the lateral sides of the joint.

Swelling of the hip is not easily detected unless the child is thin.

When such swelling is observed, it appears on the lateral side of the joint over the area of the greater trochanter. Swelling may be present in the joints of the toes, with the great toe more frequently involved.

Range of Motion

The range of motion is measured with a goniometer. (See Table 7-1 for normal ranges.) The small-sized instrument is easier to use for all joint measurements of the child. The range of finger motion is determined with an instrument designed for small joints. Measurements are taken of active and passive motion; the range of motion of the joints is most effectively determined with the child lying on a treatment table. Shoulder flexion is measured by starting at 0 degrees when the arm is at the side, and approaching 180 degrees as it is lifted. Measurements of abduction, adduction, and internal and external rotation at the shoulder are also recorded.

Elbow flexion and extension are measured with the forearm in supination. Complete extension of the elbow is set at 0 degrees, and by bringing the fingers toward the shoulder the degree of flexion is increased.

The wrist is measured for flexion, extension, and ulnar and radial deviation. The position of 0 degrees is midway between these motions. The finger joints are measured for flexion, the straight position being 0 degrees. The range of abduction of the fingers may be recorded if there is restriction.

Measurements of the hip motions of flexion, extension, internal and external rotation, abduction, and adduction are recorded. Correct ranges are measured on one hip as the other leg is stabilized in a position of 0 degrees of the hip and knee. Knee motions can be more accurately measured when the patient is in a prone position. The feet should extend over the edge of the table to allow for complete extension at the knee.

The ankle ranges of motion that are recorded are dorsiflexion and plantar flexion, inversion, and eversion. A 90 degree angle of the foot to the leg is considered as 0 degrees. Recordings of range of motion of the toes are difficult to obtain and of no great value. If desired, the range of motion of the head can be measured and recorded.

Tenderness, Heat, and Pain

The tenderness of the joints is determined at full, or near full, range of motion, or on deep palpation of the tissues around the joint. There is often increased swelling without increased tenderness.

The heat of a joint is evaluated by comparing it with that of the opposite joint or other areas of the body. The joints rarely exhibit extreme heat and the amount present is often not significant.

The evaluation of pain depends on the child's description. Unless he is moving, pain is infrequent, and it is usually associated with stiffness. Few children have described sharp excruciating pain; usually it is spoken of as a dull ache. Teen-age patients seem to complain more of severe joint pain than other age groups.

Table 7-1 Joint Motion and Range*

Joint	Movement	Normal Range of Motion (In Degrees)
Shoulder	Flexion	0–180
	Extension	0–60
	Adduction	0–75
	Abduction	0–180
	Internal rotation	0–90
	External rotation	0–90
Elbow	Extension	0
	Flexion	0–150
Wrist	Extension	0–70
	Flexion	0–80
	Ulnar deviation	0–30
	Radial deviation	0–20
Fingers	Flexion	
	Metacarpophalangeal	0–90
	Proximal interphalangeal	0–100
	Distal interphalangeal	0–80
	Extension	
	Metacarpophalangeal	0–45
	Proximal interphalangeal	0
	Distal interphalangeal	0
	Abduction	0–20
Hip	Flexion	0–120
	Extension	0–30
	Adduction in extension	0–35
	Abduction in extension	0–45
	Internal rotation in extension	0–45
	External rotation in extension	0–45
Knee	Extension	0
	Flexion	0–135
Ankle	Plantar flexion	0–50
	Dorsiflexion	0–20
Foot	Eversion	0–20
	Inversion	0–30
Spine		
Cervical	Flexion	0–38
	Extension	0–38
	Lateral bending	0–43
	Rotation	0–45
Thoracic	Flexion	0–85
	Extension	0–30
	Lateral bending	0–30
	Rotation	0–35
Lumbar	Flexion	0–85
	Extension	0–30
	Lateral bending	0–30
	Rotation	0–35

*Modified from: Method of Measuring and Recording, Bulletin, American Academy of Orthopaedic Surgeons, 1965.

Tightness of Muscle Groups

Motion can be restricted by tightness of muscle groups. It is necessary to determine the location of the tightness and to eliminate it by stretching exercises. The positions assumed for protection of the involved joint allow the muscles to be maintained in a shortened position; eventually the muscles must be lengthened by stretching. Most frequently involved are the areas of the hamstrings (preventing extension of the knee) and of the gastrocnemius-soleus (preventing plantar flexion of the foot). Any joint can be limited for this reason; in the upper extremities shoulder flexion, abduction, elbow extension, and wrist extension are the movements usually affected.

The back extensors may become tight and cause an increase in lordosis. The thoracic muscles do not usually have any great amount of tightness. Neck flexors often become tight because of the continual forward thrust of the head. The tightness of the hamstrings can be determined by having the child, while sitting with his legs extended, touch his toes with his fingers. If motion is limited, he will feel pull under the knees. Tightness in the back can be noted from this same position, if the knees are slightly flexed and the forehead is first placed on the knees and then brought to the lateral sides of the knees.

The gastrocnemius-soleus tightness is checked by placing the foot in dorsiflexion; if motion is limited, the child will feel pull in the calf of the leg. To distinguish tightness of the muscle group from joint involvement when there is limited motion, the child must be able to give the location of the greatest discomfort as the motion is performed. He will indicate either the joint or the muscle group. The tightness of other muscle groups may be evaluated by testing the full range of motion of the joints.

Atrophy of Muscles

Muscular atrophy in the lower extremities is easily detected. Involvement of one extremity becomes apparent by comparing both legs. Measurements of the circumference of the leg above and below the knee are recorded; the site of measurement is determined by the size of the patient. Below the knee it should be made at the greatest circumference of the calf muscles, and above the knee it should be made halfway between the hip and knee. The distance is established and recorded for future measurement.

Atrophy in the arm above and below the elbow may not be as apparent as in a weight-bearing extremity. The intrinsic muscles of the hand frequently show atrophy, but measurement is not possible. The thenar eminence will become atrophic rapidly when the thumb is involved and motion is limited. The deltoid muscle usually undergoes rapid atrophy. The amount of atrophy cannot be easily measured, and testing of the muscle strength is a better guide to involvement.

Muscular Strength

Detailed muscular testing is not necessary in the evaluation of the child; gross examination is adequate. Some areas do weaken more rapidly, and involved muscle groups should be tested. In planning a program for the child, concentrated exercise and activity should be directed to the areas of weakness.

Muscular strength is graded by having the child perform a motion through its entire range. Performance is graded on the ability of the child to complete the motion with the assistance of gravity, with the elimination of gravity, against gravity, and with manual resistance. The age of the child will determine the amount of resistance considered normal.

In the upper extremities, strength is rapidly lost in the areas of wrist extension and finger grip. Knee involvement of the lower extremity produces early weakness of the quadriceps. This prevents complete extension at the knee and can contribute to shortening of the hamstring muscles.

Posture

Evaluation of the child's posture is based on observation of the anterior, posterior, and lateral sides. In viewing the posterior side, several aspects are considered. Curvatures of the spine are observed for any increases that indicate scoliosis, lordosis, or kyphosis. Winging of the scapulae, uneven elevation of the shoulders and of the waistline, and unequal buttocks creases are some deviations that may be noted. Variation of leg lengths can be noted at this time by a lateral tilt of the pelvis and a difference in the level of the gluteal creases. Actual measurement of leg length is taken with the child in a supine position by recording the distance from the anterosuperior iliac spine to the medial malleolus. The posterior view of the feet will reveal any weakness in the longitudinal arch, and inversion or eversion of the foot. The lateral view of the child reveals head position (such as forward head), forward shoulder, protruding abdomen, and back knee stance. The anterior view shows general facial expression and forward flexed position of the body, if present. The equality of the rib cage is evaluated from the anterior view. The findings of the posture evaluation are recorded and used in planning the exercise program.

Gait

The child is asked to walk, and the gait is observed. The walking posture will be similar to the standing posture, but may be exaggerated. The gait may reveal areas of tenderness that were not found on non-weight-bearing motions; the location of tenderness in hips, knees, or ankles is easily determined. The position of the foot in gait sequence is of importance in demonstrating any deviation from normal overall body mechanics. All gait defects should be observed and incorporated in the training aspect of the program.

THE THERAPY PROGRAM

The physical therapy home treatment program consists of the use of moist heat, exercise, adequate rest, and proper diet. School and play activities are discussed and outlined for the child. The program is more effective if scheduled on a 24-hour basis. Consideration of all home factors is necessary in establishing this schedule. The most successful method of teaching this program is by daily sessions with the parent and child until they are well informed and have a good understanding of what to expect and how to manage the condition. This can usually be accomplished in about five one-hour sessions. The parent and child should be checked one week after the training sessions end to correct any errors and strengthen the program. They should be checked again at least once per month thereafter.

For a home treatment program to be effective there must be a well-established relationship between the family and the physical therapist. A feeling of interest and concern must be conveyed to the family by the therapist to gain their cooperation and to achieve the goals outlined. In any long-term program interest lessens and there is a tendency to become lax. The physical therapist will need to frequently reevaluate and adjust the program to hold the interest of the family and give the best care to the patient.

Heat

Moist heat gives the most satisfactory results for stiffness, swelling, and pain of joints. This type of heat is readily available in the home by utilizing the tub bath. Two warm baths are given daily, one upon arising and one at bedtime. The time in the tub should be limited to approximately ten minutes. The child usually awakens with stiffness, which will be eliminated by the warm bath, enabling him to move more easily and with less discomfort. The bath given before retiring permits the child a more restful night. While in the tub the patient should be allowed to move freely, performing some motions that assist him in alleviating stiffness. Drying and dressing also give some needed motions of exercise.

The more severely involved child may experience stiffness and pain during the night, causing restlessness and irritability. If this occurs, it is advisable to use a warm bath, which takes little time and is the simplest method of relieving the discomfort; it also creates less disturbance for the entire family than having the child awake for the remainder of the night. This same procedure can also be used following the daytime nap when necessary.

Moist heat, in the form of hot packs, is effective when a joint is severely involved. The hot pack is used in addition to warm baths. One application daily is sufficient and can be given during the day, usually in connection with the rest period. The procedure for using the hot pack should be kept very simple. It is recommended that a turkish hand towel, hot tap water, and a large piece of lightweight plastic, such as a dry-cleaning bag, be utilized for this procedure. The towel is held at each end and immersed in hot water; then it is twisted until it no longer drips. Wrap the joint with the towel and cover over with the plastic bag. The pack should be changed once and left in place not more than 15 to 20 minutes. Following this application the skin should be slightly pink and warm. A short duration of fairly intense heat gives better results than a longer period of mild heat.

Also available for home use is the Hydrocollator Steam Pack.* This is placed in a large pan filled with water, and heated till the water boils; then the heat is lowered. The pack is placed between layers of the towel and placed over the area to be treated for a period of 20 minutes. When in regular use the pack should be kept in hot water at all times; otherwise it should be stored, wrapped in plastic, in a freezer.

Heat in the form of the Therabath,† a commercial paraffin bath of minimal cost and convenient to use, is practical in the home. The Therabath contains a mixture of paraffin and oil that is kept at a properly controlled temperature at all times. Asking a parent to melt paraffin in a double-boiler daily is not practical: too much time is involved, and there is the danger of overheating. The Therabath is an excellent form of heat for the hands and feet; it gives a complete coating of wax around the small joints of the fingers and toes. The involved joints can tolerate immersion at a much higher temperature in this mixture than in water. The correct procedure is to dip the joint into the mixture and withdraw immediately; let it cool until there is no dripping, then immerse again. This is repeated until a thick coating of paraffin is formed—usually about ten to 12 times. The treated area is then wrapped in plastic and covered with a turkish towel for about ten minutes. At the end of this time, the paraffin is peeled off and replaced in the Therabath, and the involved joints are exercised. This type of heat is very penetrating and the resulting benefits are of considerable duration. This type of treatment in the home is ordered by the physician for some patients who have severe involvement of wrists, fingers, ankles, tarsal areas, and toes, and may also be used for elbows.

Another method of utilizing heat in the home is by use of electric blankets. These are useful in homes in which there is no controlled heat during the night, when the child has a greater tendency to become cold and stiff. The electric blanket provides warmth without added weight; heavy blankets restrict movement and increase stiffness.

Heat lamps or heating pads should not be used, as they do not provide moist heat and can easily cause burns. Other types of expensive equipment, such as whirlpool devices for the bathtub, are not recommended; the minimal benefits do not justify the cost of the appliance.

Children usually enjoy the use of heat, especially the tub bath. If the child does offer resistance, it is still necessary to perform this part of the treatment; fever is not an indication to discontinue baths. The joints are often more swollen, stiff, and painful during fever and need the relief of the tub bath.

Exercise

Exercise is necessary to maintain the range of motion of the joints and strength of the muscles. The range of motion is lost rapidly in

---

*Chattanooga Pharmacal Co., Chattanooga, Tennessee.
†W. R. Medical Electronics Company, St. Paul, Minnesota.

involved joints that are not exercised in a complete range daily. The child may be very active during the day but may never complete a full range of motion for joints such as shoulders, hips, and knees. The loss of range of motion precedes the loss of strength and eventual atrophy. Very early atrophy occurs in some areas, particularly in the deltoid muscles and the knee extensor muscles. The exercise program must be consistent to obtain and maintain the desired results. Patients with much joint involvement are advised to perform the prescribed exercises twice daily; those with minimal involvement, once daily. Exercises are performed more easily and better results are obtained following the application of heat. The types of movements most frequently used are active (the child performs the motion) and active assistive (the parents assist the child in performing the movement). It is important that these motions be done slowly and smoothly without any quick or jerky movements. Greater range will be obtained when the child is actively performing the motion to the best of his ability. The fear of pain from movement causes him to resist when there is an attempt at passive motion. The child should be instructed to move the joint to the point of discomfort, return to starting position, and gradually increase the range of motion with each succeeding movement.

Shortening of the muscles may occur in some areas as a result of prolonged joint involvement, and this condition will require some passive stretching by the parent. Additional exercises should be prescribed for a particular area that has a flexion contracture. The child can accomplish much of the stretching with frequent active exercise of the involved part. Each exercise should be performed five times and increased to ten times over a period of about two weeks.

Exercise should be conducted on a firm surface, table, or floor — never on a bed. A table may make it easier for the parent to assist the child; the degree of involvement and the age of the child will determine the choice.

When there is an exacerbation of the disease, with increased swelling and tenderness of joints, extra heat should be applied more frequently with shorter periods of exercise. The joint should be moved through its possible range, even if it is only a few degrees. Non-weight-bearing exercises are encouraged, and increased rest is indicated during periods of exacerbation.

Some areas with acute or prolonged involvement present special difficulties if they are not recognized and given extra care. The shoulder can lose its range of motion rapidly, with a resulting atrophy of the deltoid. Pain in this area creates difficulty in completing the range of flexion and abduction from a sitting or standing position. These motions can be performed more easily from a supine position that eliminates gravity for the motion of abduction, and also assists in the range of motion for flexion.

Range of motion in extension of the wrist is decreased if some activity is not performed many times during the day. However, wrist deviations are not common and are easy to correct by frequent exercise if recognized early. Extension of the wrist is often difficult to maintain when the child does much writing in school, and during the school months there should be added daily activities to combat this difficulty. Loss of strength in the grip of the fingers can follow rapidly when the hands are involved.

Deviations at metacarpophalangeal and proximal phalangeal joints are infrequent. Early detection and increased exercise, plus nighttime splinting, can produce good results. Involvement of the hips can cause limitation of motion in all ranges; flexion, abduction, and internal rotation are most important to maintain. There can be severe limitation of motion without major changes that are visible by x-ray, or minor tenderness and limitation with marked changes visible by x-ray. Hip involvement influences gait to an extensive degree. Improper gait can create many symptoms involving the lower extremities and back. It is important, therefore, to maintain a complete range of motion and strength with non-weight-bearing exercises.

Initially the thoracic and lumbar areas of the back are not frequently involved in arthritis. Back problems do arise, however, secondary to hip involvement, improper gait, and poor sitting and standing posture. The usual problem is muscle spasm. Non-weight-bearing exercises in addition to heat can help to relieve the condition.

Sternocostal involvement can influence the breathing pattern and chest expansion. Lower chest expansion is often difficult to maintain if proper breathing exercises are not used.

The temporomandibular joint is frequently involved. Morning stiffness is usually present as the most uncomfortable aspect of this joint involvement. Attempting to open the mouth wide increases the muscle spasm and pain; chewing gum has been found to be an effective means of relieving stiffness. In performing the small and frequent openings and closings of the mouth, the stiffness decreases, eventually enabling the mouth to open wide enough for adequate eating.

It is important to maintain correct posture at all times. Good standing posture is easily taught if the instructions are kept simple. The feet should be 6 inches apart, the toes pointing forward; tuck the buttocks under and lift the chest. Correct sitting posture, especially for the child in school, must be stressed. The feet should rest firmly on the floor, the back against the chair, and the writing level should be high enough to prevent forward thrust of the shoulders. For sleeping a firm mattress without a pillow is recommended; if a pillow is used it should be placed well under the shoulders. Improper use of a pillow increases flexion of the head and throws it forward.

An illustrated program of exercises appears in the Appendix, page 144.

Rest

Rest is very important in the home program of the child with arthritis. Children with rheumatoid arthritis tire more easily than healthy children, and they require longer rest periods at more frequent intervals. They are capable of many activities that need not be restricted if done for only short periods. It is recommended that the school child rest immediately upon coming home from school; the length of time depends on the severity of the disease. Some children must spend the greater part of their time away from school in comparative inactivity. These children have a tendency to be tense and fearful of any bodily contact, and should have a relaxed type of rest period, preferably in a room away from other children or disturbances. They often assume a flexed attitude for comfort and protection. Sitting in unusual positions, such as cross-legged or twisted, should be avoided; such positions put stress and strain on involved joints. Ten hours' sleep at night is preferable. The preschool child should have a midmorning and an afternoon rest period and a regular, early hour for bedtime.

Diet

The diet of the child with arthritis is important because he is a growing child with a chronic disease. In teaching the diet program to the parent it should be emphasized that food is unrelated to cause or cure, but a sensible, well-balanced nourishing diet is desirable as with any child. The child responds much better if meals and all activities are kept on a regular daily schedule. Many children with arthritis have poor eating habits, particularly the teen-ager whose diet consists mainly of soft drinks and candy bars. The selection of proper foods is an important aid in preventing obesity, which puts added stress on involved joints. A well-balanced diet should be maintained.

Play Activities

Play activities may be used extensively to complement the formal exercise program. The child will follow a planned program of play longer, and with more enthusiasm, than a more intensive formal exercise program. The play activities should include those that produce the range of motion desired and maintain strength, those that combine many motions at one time, and those that emphasize the finer movements of the fingers and hands. They should be designed according to the age and interests of the child.

In establishing this aspect of the home program the parents' observations of the child's interests, and their provision of games to bring about the desired motions, are most helpful. Restrictions may be few, but the length of time an activity is performed should be limited depending on the severity of the condition. All activities that cause an impact to the joints or body are restricted; these include jumping rope, volleyball, basketball, roller skating, horseback riding, trampoline jumping, and jumping from any height. Prolonged participation should be curtailed in activities that hold the wrist in one position, such as piano playing or continuous writing. Greatest value has been found with some of the pedal toys: the tractor and tricycle for the small child and the bicycle for the older child. The stationary bicycle may be necessary if the child has a fear of falling, or if there is no adequate riding area. However, if the stationary bicycle is used, resistance can be applied to obtain greater strengthening value.

Swimming is the best form of exercise for all children. The very young child will benefit from being in the water even when assisted by an adult. The time in the pool should be limited to not more than one hour. The child should not be permitted in and out, but should remain active in the water. Upon leaving, he should quickly shower and dress to avoid chilling.

Playing with a baton, bat and ball, golf club, ping-pong paddle, and paddle ball will increase the range of motion and strength of the wrist and arms. Finger movements are strengthened with writing, drawing, coloring, use of play dough or modeling clay, and cutting with scissors.

School Activities

An attempt should always be made to keep the child in school. The use of at-home teachers is necessary at times but should not be prolonged. The child does much better scholastically and socially if he can be kept in the classroom. To accomplish this some adjustments may be necessary in the high school level. The child in the lower grades will also require some special arrangements that allow him to move about. These children, who usually remain in one room, become stiff after remaining in one position for more than 30 minutes. Such a child can be permitted to perform some duty in the classroom that allows him to move about fairly frequently. Activities of play in the schoolyard should be kept to a minimum.

The child in the upper grades who changes classrooms after each period should be allowed extra time for changing rooms if his gait is slow. These children can often be enrolled in physical education classes with restricted activities and elimination of sports that produce a jolt to the body such as football, basketball, or volleyball. The length of time any one game is performed should also be limited, depending on the energy required for the activity.

In multistoried school buildings, class schedules that require changes from floor to floor may present difficulty for the child with arthritis. Often schedules may be rearranged with the aid of the counsellor. Overprotection should be avoided, but teachers and school nurses should be well informed about the child's condition and the extent of his capabilities.

APPENDIX

Exercise Program with Illustrations

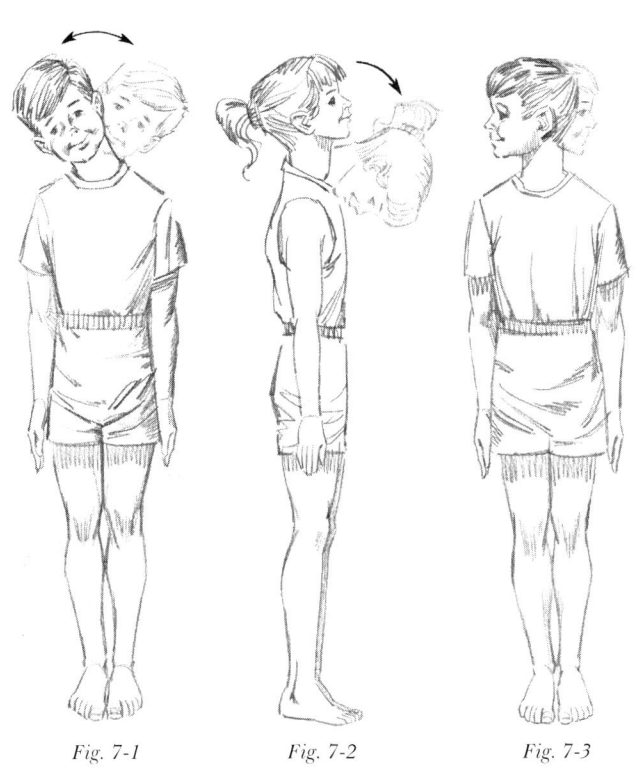

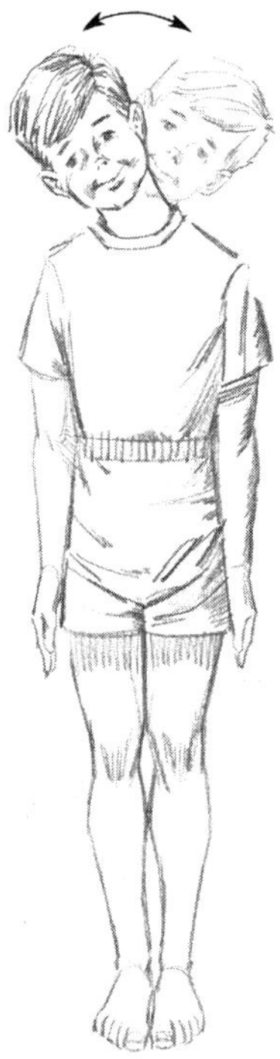

Fig. 7-1 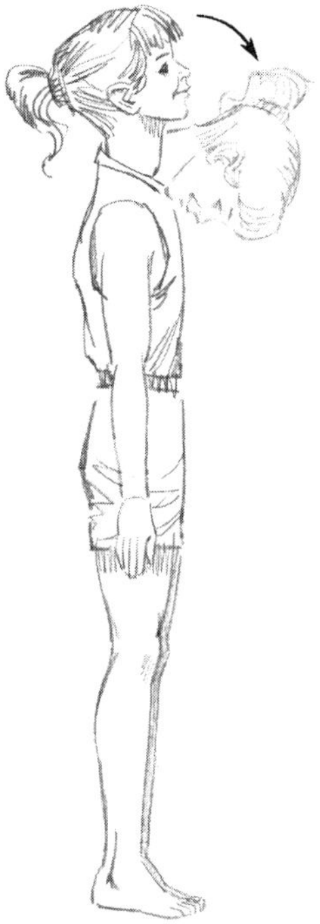   *Fig. 7-2*   *Fig. 7-3*

Figure 7-1   Lateral flexion of the head. The head is tilted laterally to each side in an attempt to touch the ear to the shoulder, without elevating the shoulder.

Figure 7-2   Extension and flexion of the head. The head is tilted backward to a 75 degree angle, then forward in an attempt to touch the chin to the chest.

Figure 7-3   Rotation of the head. The chin is moved alternately toward each shoulder.

Home Treatment Program 145

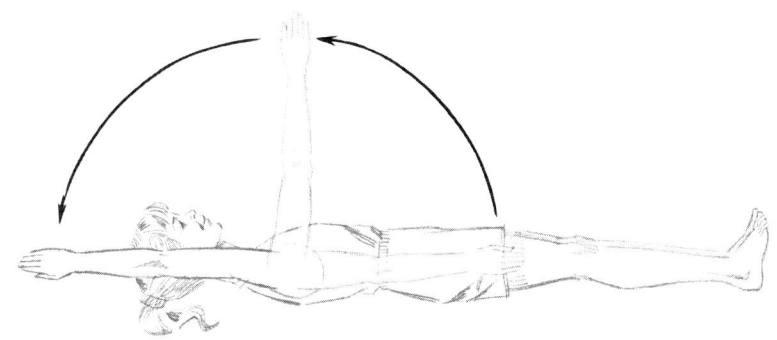

Figure 7-4 Flexion of the arm at the shoulder. Extend the arms at the sides with palms toward the body, and lift forward to a 180 degree angle.

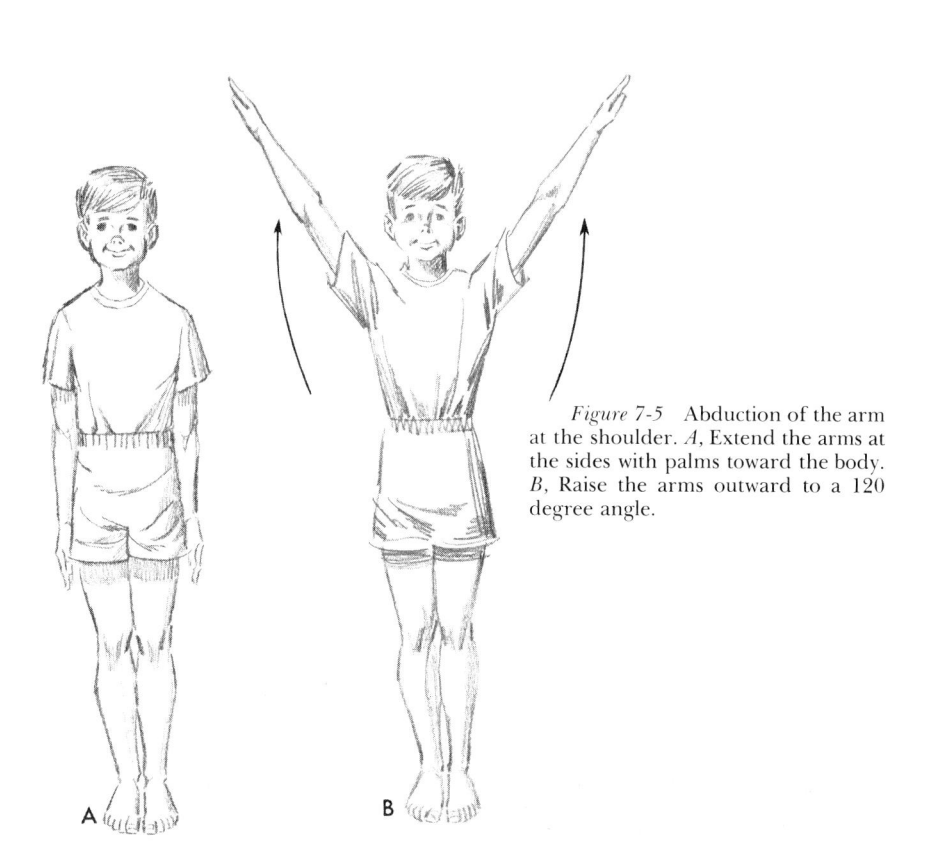

Figure 7-5 Abduction of the arm at the shoulder. *A*, Extend the arms at the sides with palms toward the body. *B*, Raise the arms outward to a 120 degree angle.

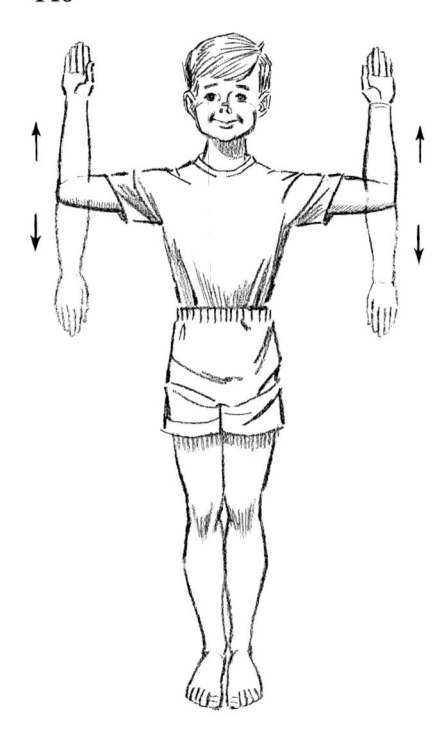

Figure 7-6 Internal and external rotation of the arm at the shoulder. Position the arms at 90 degrees abduction at the shoulders, with elbows flexed to 90 degrees. Rotate at the shoulder by moving the hands and arms upward and then downward.

Figure 7-7 Extension and flexion at the elbow with supination of the forearm. *A*, Hold the forearm in supination and extension. *B*, The elbow is flexed to touch the fingers to the shoulder, then extended.

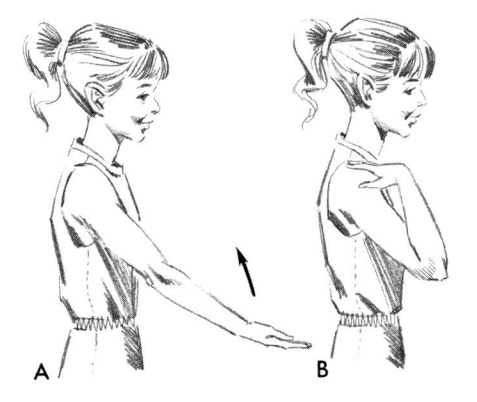

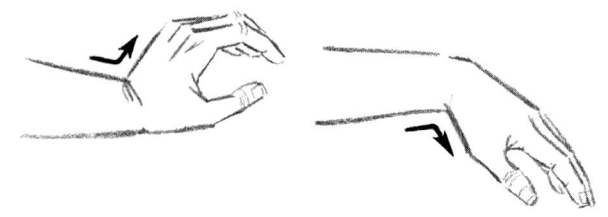

Figure 7-8 Extension and flexion of the hand. Extend the hand until deep wrinkles appear at the wrist; the fingers will be in a relaxed, slightly flexed position. Flex the hand downward; the fingers will be in an extended position.

Home Treatment Program 147

Figure 7-9 Radial and ulnar deviation of the hand. Hold the hand in a straight position; then move the hand laterally to each side.

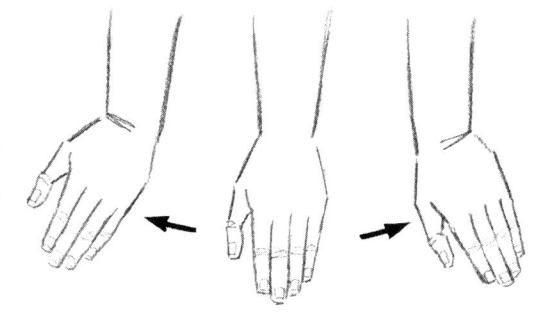

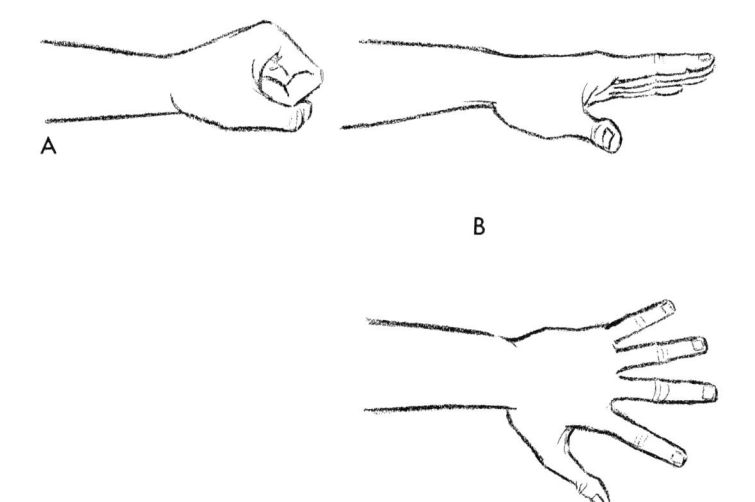

Figure 7-10 Flexion and extension of the fingers. *A*, Flex the fingers into a fist. *B*, Release and extend the fingers.

Figure 7-11 Abduction and adduction of the fingers. *A*, Hold the hand straight with the fingers together. *B*, Extend and fan fingers; then bring together again.

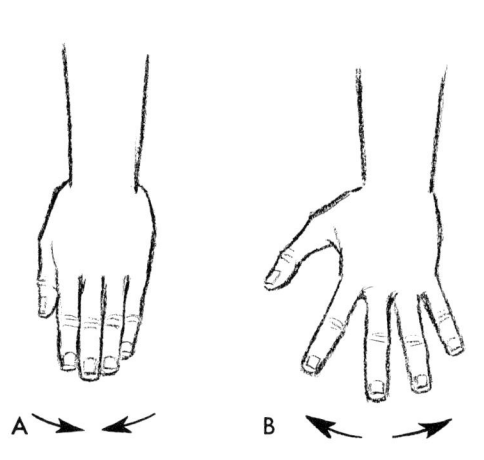

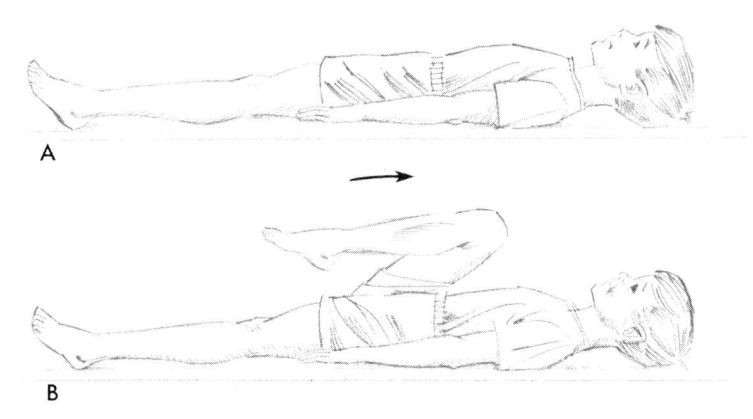

Figure 7-12 Hip and knee extension and flexion. *A*, Extend legs. *B*, Each knee is alternately flexed toward the chest, keeping the other knee straight, then lowered and extended.

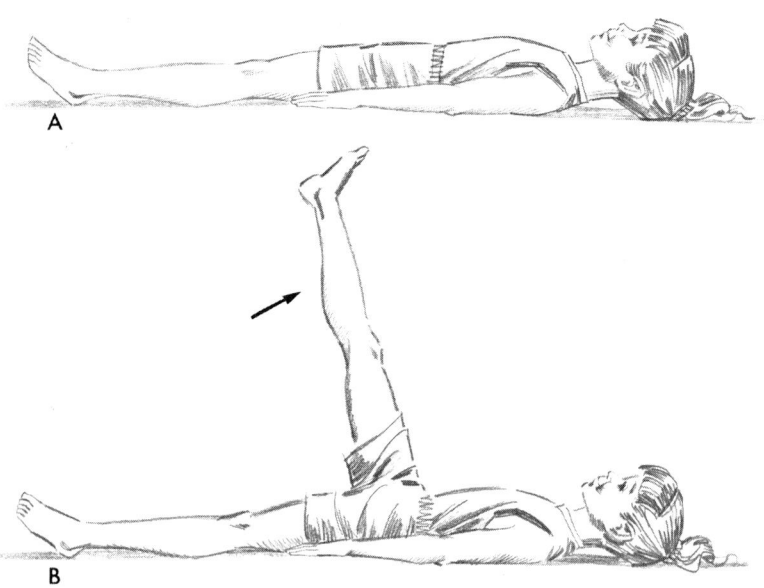

Figure 7-13 Flexion of the hip with knee extended. *A*, Extend legs. *B*, Raise each leg alternately to approximately 80 degrees.

Home Treatment Program   **149**

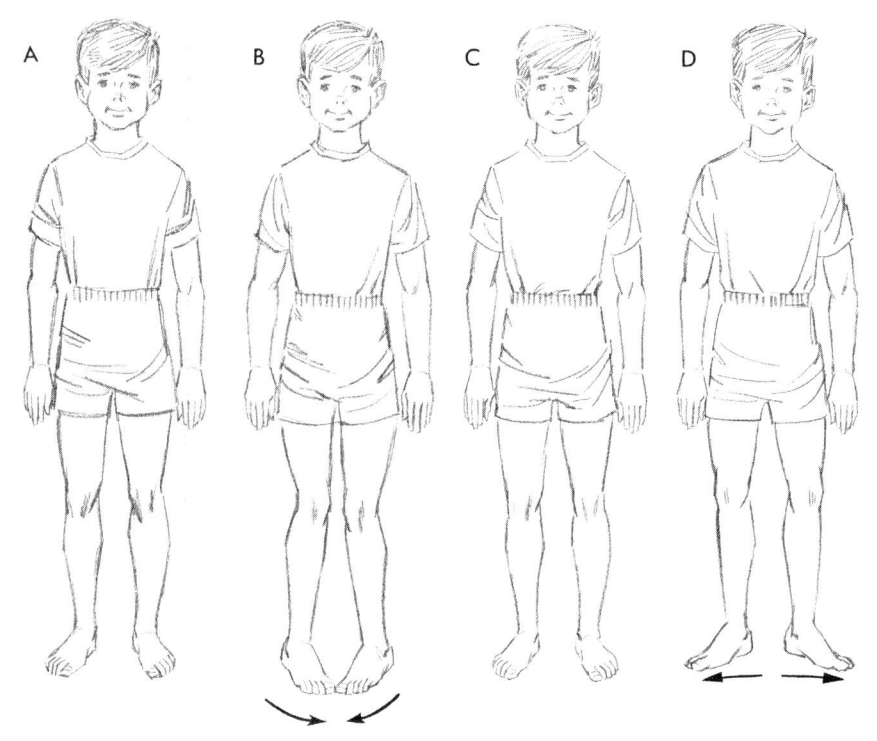

Figure 7-14 Internal and external rotation of hips. *A*, Lying supine, extend the legs and separate feet about 6 inches. *B*, Rotate the legs internally for toes to touch. *C*, Extend forward. *D*, Rotate the legs externally.

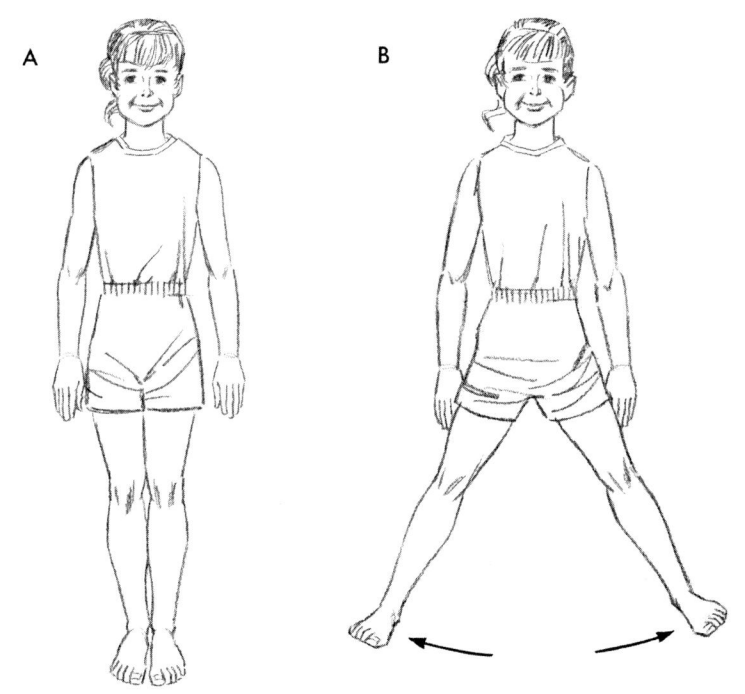

Figure 7-15 Abduction and adduction of hips. *A*, Lying supine, extend the legs together. *B*, Spread the legs; then bring together again.

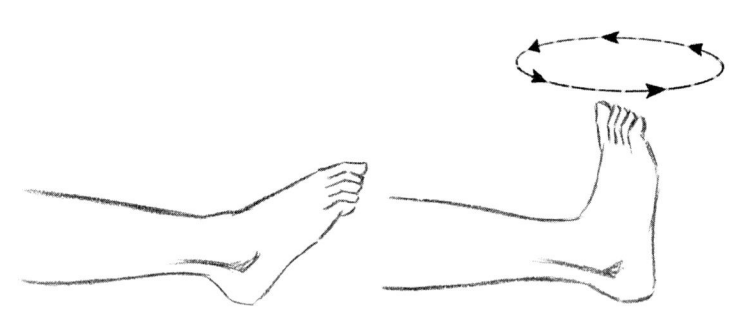

Figure 7-16 Plantar flexion and dorsiflexion of the ankle. Bend the foot upward and downward; then rotate making a circle with the toes.

HOME TREATMENT PROGRAM 151

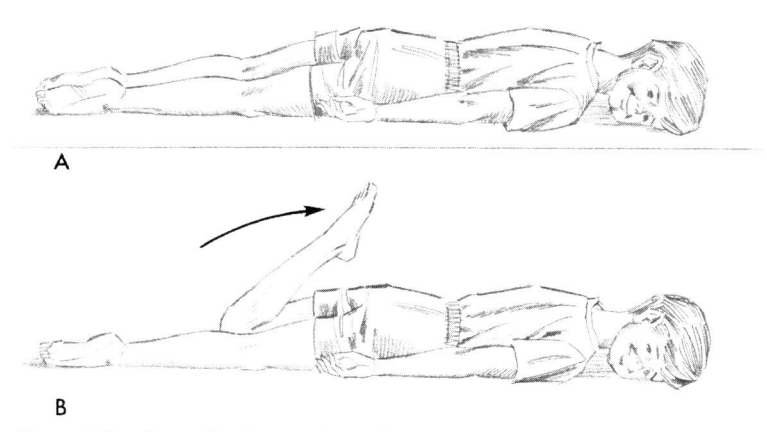

Figure 7-17 Knee Flexion. *A*, Extend the legs in prone position. *B*, Bend each knee alternately, bringing the heel toward the buttocks; then lower.

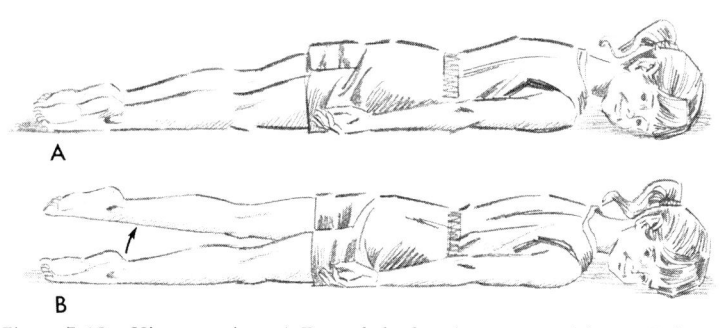

Figure 7-18 Hip extension. *A*, Extend the legs in prone position. *B*, Raise each leg alternately, keeping knee straight, to approximately 10 degrees.

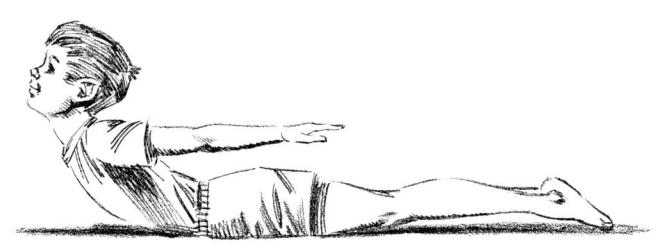

Figure 7-19 Head and shoulder extension. With arms extended at sides, raise head and upper trunk; then lower to starting position.

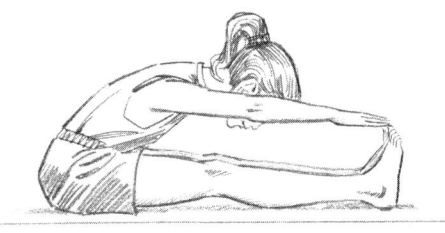

Figure 7-20 Stretching of hamstrings. Sitting with legs extended and together, touch the toes with the fingers.

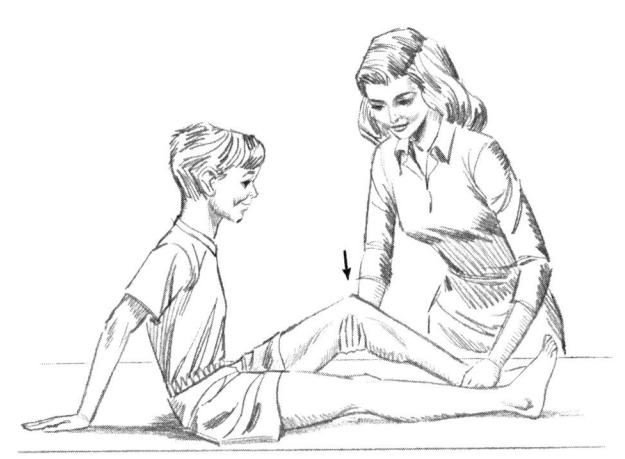

Figure 7-21 Stretching of hamstrings. With knee flexed, mother firmly places hand under knee and child pushes hand downward, straightening leg.

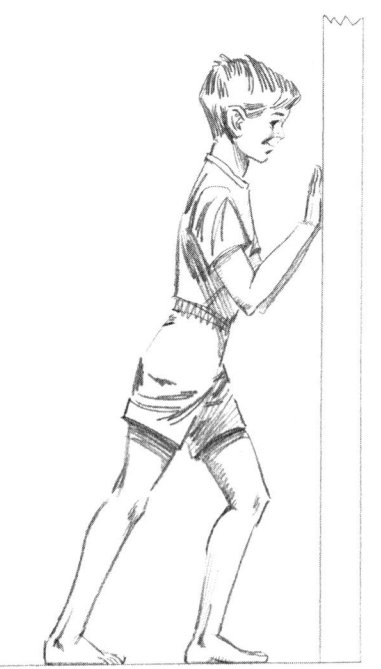

Figure 7-22 Stretching of gastrocnemius-soleus. Stand with the feet away from the wall and hands placed on the wall; one foot is moved forward with the knee flexed; the other foot is moved back, with the knee kept extended and the foot flat on the floor. Swing hips toward the wall until pull is felt in calf of leg; alternate legs.

Home Treatment Program 153

Figure 7-23 Stretching of gastrocnemius-soleus. With the patient lying down, the mother places her hand under the heel, grasping the foot with her forearm against the sole. She moves the foot in a dorsiflexed direction.

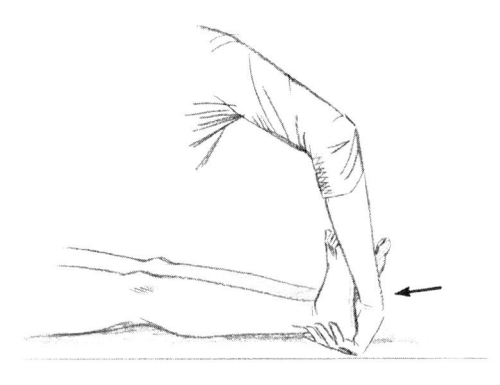

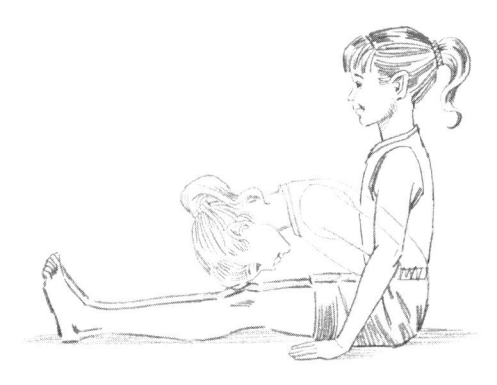

Figure 7-24 Flexion of the back. Sitting with the knees slightly flexed, bend head toward knees, then to each side of the knees.

Figure 7-25 Passive extension of the hand by using opposite hand. Grasp hands with palms together, thumb at the base of the first finger, and fingers around lateral border of the hand. Apply pressure to bring the hand in extension at the wrist.

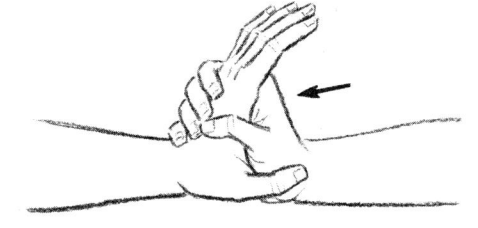

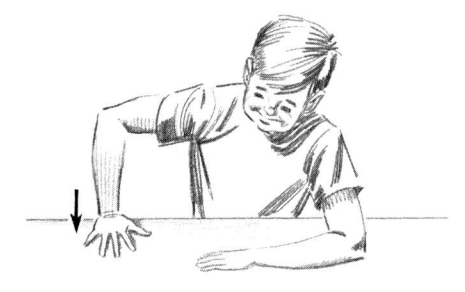

Figure 7-26 Stretching hand in extension at the wrist. Place the hand on a flat surface and raise the arm until deep wrinkles appear at the wrist.

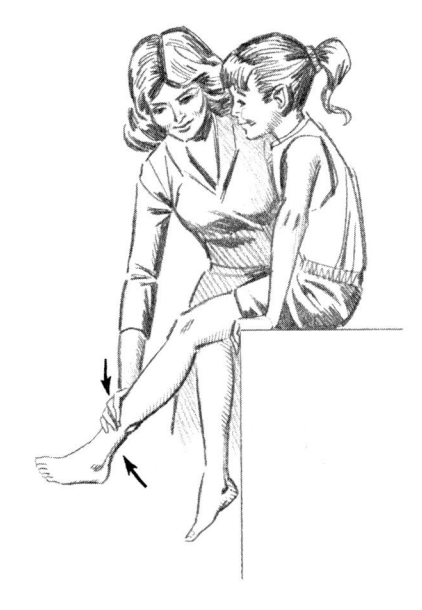

Figure 7-27 Strengthening of quadriceps. Seat the child with knees flexed over the edge of the table. With her hand just above the ankle, the mother gives resistance to the motion of straightening the leg.

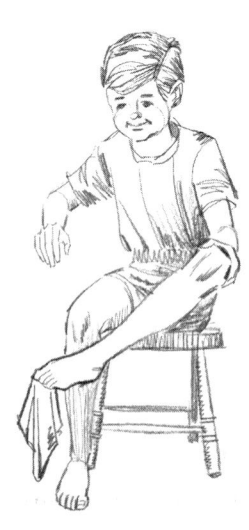

Figure 7-28 Strengthening of the legs. Sitting on a stool, pick up a washcloth with the toes and lift it to the opposite hand.

Home Treatment Program 155

Figure 7-29 Posture. Standing erect, point toes straight with the feet slightly apart, chest lifted, and buttocks tucked under.

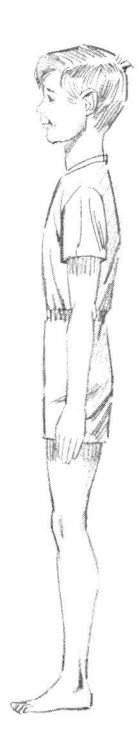

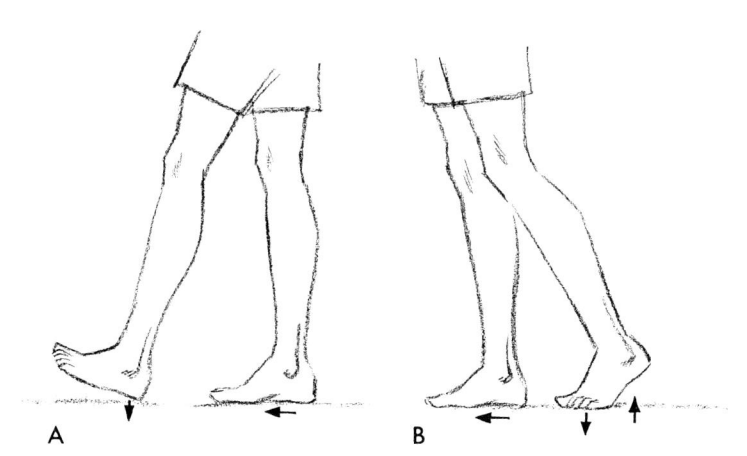

Figure 7-30 Gait. *A*, Assume correct body posture and step forward, placing heel down first. *B*, Roll on sole, pushing off with toes. This is an alternating progression of steps.

Chapter Eight

ORTHOPEDIC MANAGEMENT OF JUVENILE RHEUMATOID ARTHRITIS

W. Malcolm Granberry, M.D.*
and Earl J. Brewer, Jr., M.D.

The total management of the child with rheumatoid arthritis demands the attention of several different specialists in medicine today. The main problem in long-term chronic care centers around preserving the function and integrity of the joints. Proper organization with complete cooperation between the specialists is essential. The orthopedist must also have a rather intricate working knowledge of the field of rheumatology. The services of physical therapy, especially by a therapist who is experienced and knowledgeable in rheumatology, are also essential. Ancillary fields, such as social work and brace making, are also important. The pediatrician should also be familiar with the services of orthopedics for the child. We have found it highly beneficial to see the patient as a group, discuss the problems in the light of each field of interest, and decide upon the proper approach considering all factors.

The orthopedic management of rheumatoid arthritis in the child is approached in several ways. Nonsurgical management includes splinting, extension orthoses, braces, foot corrective devices, joint injection, and physical therapy. Surgical treatment is roughly divided into biopsy or drainage for the purpose of diagnosis, and reconstructive or corrective surgery. In recent years there has been renewed interest in attempted prevention of joint destruction by the use of early synovectomy.

ORTHOTIC APPLIANCES

The term "orthoses" or "orthotics" has come into vogue in recent years, and is used for the broad classification of splinting, bracing, and

---

*Clinical Instructor, Baylor College of Medicine; Orthopedic Consultant, Arthritis Clinical Research Center, Texas Children's Hospital, Houston, Texas.

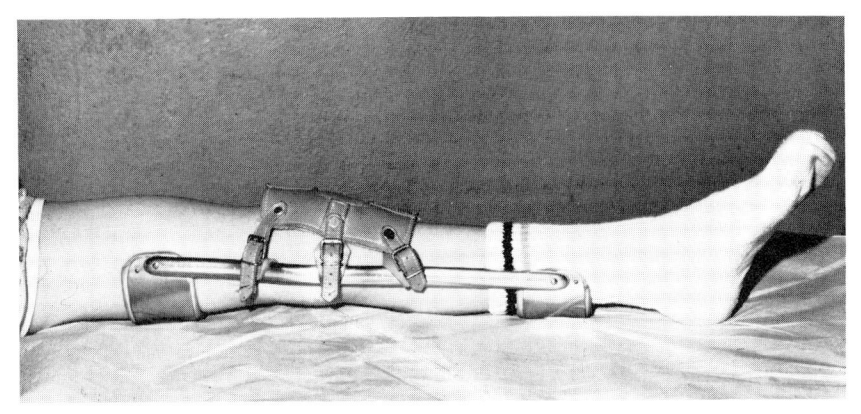

Figure 8-1 Extension orthosis for correction of flexion contracture. The device is constructed to provide pressure posteriorly at a distance above and below the joint. The bands will pivot to accommodate the correction. The anterior knee pad provides the third correcting force.

supporting of the limbs with the use of external devices. When one wishes to correct or prevent a deformity with the use of external appliance, the general principle of such a device should be clearly understood. Almost without exception devices applied to a limb should provide three points of pressure. One point should be over the apex of the deformity and two should be at a distance on opposite sides of the limb (Fig. 8-1).

If this single primary objective is kept in mind, a myriad of deformities, and even more numerous devices to correct them, can be more completely understood. A device must be so designed as to accommodate the limb in the deformed position but it must also have the ability to change as the limb is straightened or the joint is brought to extension. Improper use of these devices can do more harm than good. Frequent observation is essential in the use of orthotic devices.

Because the child's limbs are supple and growing, the effects of splinting are even more effective or destructive. This is particularly true in the case of the knee, and the general purpose of orthosis and its problems will be discussed with this joint in mind.

If the orthopedic literature is reviewed concerning the straightening of knees, numerous devices and conflicting methods are encountered (Horwitz, 1937). Many of the older devices did not embody the three-point pressure principle, and were therefore unsuccessful (Haggart, 1935). The knee is unusual in both internal and external configuration. It is the largest joint in the body and has the longest lever arms for application of pressure. It has strong external collateral ligaments, as other joints have, but it is also supplied with cruciate internal ligaments that provide anterior and posterior stability. The forces involved in the knee joint in a standard Buck's extension are shown in Figure 8-2, *A* and *B*. Buck's extension traction actually provides an anterior thrust on the proximal femur and the distal tibia.

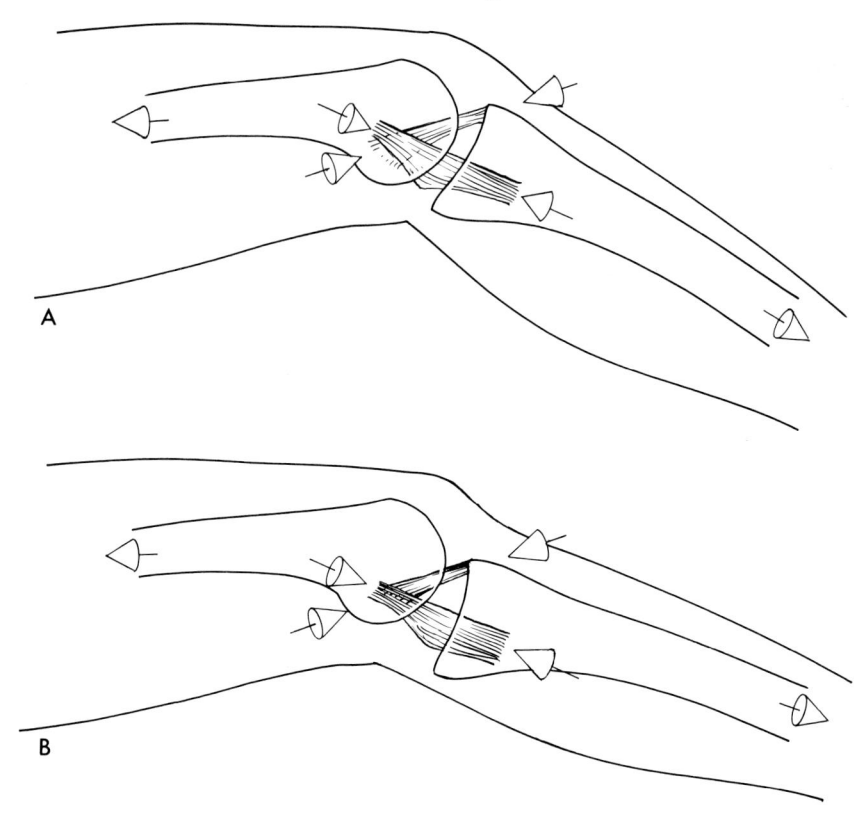

Figure 8-2, A and B This simplified diagram shows the forces produced by the standard Buck's extension traction. Axial force is provided on the tibia and opposing force is produced by the weight of the body along the femur. The posterior cruciate is relaxed in flexion and is not active. The anterior cruciate is shortened and resists extension. The medial and lateral collateral ligaments are mostly posterior to the axis center of rotation. The posterior capsule is shortened as well, but is much weaker than the collateral and cruciate ligaments. The strongest forces thus tend to slide the tibia posterior in relation to the femur.

The knee is left to stretch in between with no pressure anteriorly. Dislocation can occur and posterior subluxation of the proximal tibia can be produced with this type of traction.

The use of a wedging cast, or a cast with a hinge and outrigger for turnbuckle pressure, is demonstrated in Figure 8-3. The outrigger does not provide pressure anteriorly on the knee, and the cast must be carried quite close to the knee joint to provide such pressure. It is well known that a posterior subluxation of the tibia is produced unless the tibia is forced anteriorly with respect to the femur.

In our clinic an extension orthosis developed by Engen is used (Engen, 1961). His device, as shown in Figure 8-1, is simple but effective. As can also be seen in Figure 8-4, it provides three primary points

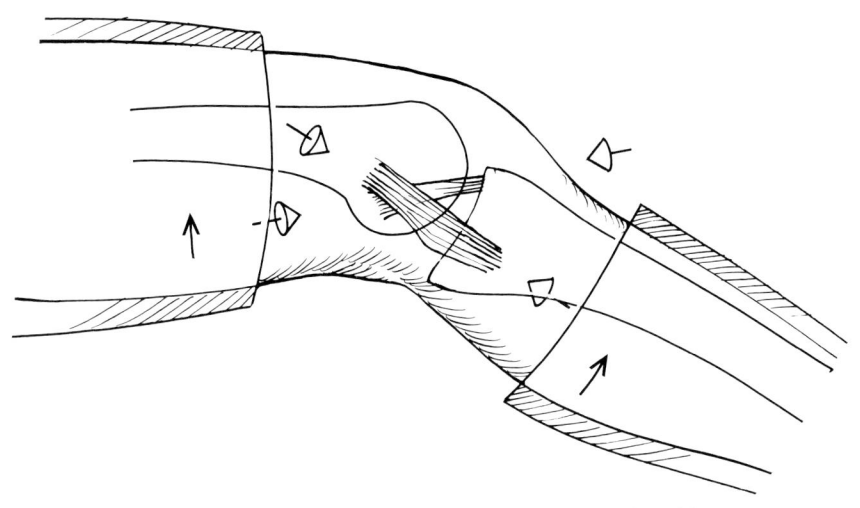

Figure 8-3 This diagram represents the major forces produced by cast pressure. The anterior cruciate and collateral ligaments tend to slide the tibia posterior. This method is effective if an anterior thrust is provided high on the tibia by proper positioning of cast hinges and wedges. This procedure is complicated and time-consuming, and we prefer the extension device seen in Figure 8-4.

of pressure. The knee joint is not a true hinge joint, and in the last 30 degrees of extension a considerable degree of sliding forward of the tibia on the femur is necessary. The downward thrust at the apex of the knee forces the femur posteriorly in respect to the tibia and stretches the posterior fibers of the collateral and the anterior cruciate

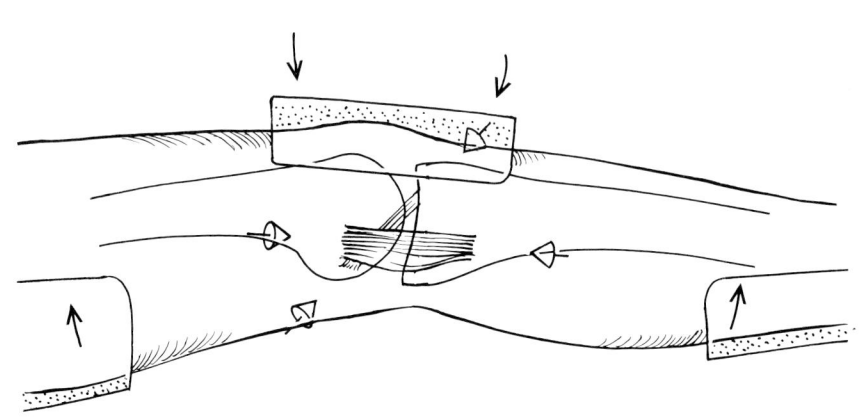

Figure 8-4 The forces shown are produced by the extension orthosis seen in Figure 8-1. Direct pressure forces both femur and tibia posteriorly, stretching not only the posterior capsule and collateral ligaments but also the anterior cruciate ligament. As the femur tends to sublux anteriorly and the tibia posteriorly, the pressure pad places relatively more pressure on the femur and less on the tibia, in effect, stretching the anterior cruciate.

ligaments, preventing posterior subluxation of the tibia. If no anterior pressure at the apex of the knee is applied, and the tibia is merely extended in respect to the femur, the tibia hinges mainly on the posterior fibers of the collateral and anterior cruciate ligaments, causing posterior subluxation.

The basic orthotic device just described can be used to correct knock-knee deformity, or knock-knee with flexion contracture at the same time. It can also be used at the elbow joint in much the same manner.

One of the oldest and still the most useful device for splinting and correcting deformities is the plaster splint. It remains the most versatile and best tolerated material the orthopedist has available. The splint is applied, either posteriorly or anteriorly, as in the leg for holding the foot at a right angle, or for holding the wrist in a neutral position. Before setting, a layer of Webril is applied over the plaster, and the limb is held in the desired position. The principle previously discussed of using three primary points of pressure must be applied. The splint is removed, covered with a piece of tubular stockinet, and applied as desired by the patient with the use of an elastic bandage. This splint is best for temporary problems such as splinting a joint acutely inflamed, maintaining position postoperatively, or as a temporary device prior to use of a definitive orthosis.

Malleable plastic has come into use in recent years. One such splint, made by the Camp Company,* is useful in maintenance of neutral position for the wrist, hand, and fingers (Fig. 8-5). Small pieces of this material can be used for appropriate areas on the smaller child where standard bracing becomes somewhat cumbersome. It can be held in place with tape or Velcro fastened to the splint. It can be

---

*S. H. Camp & Co., Jackson, Michigan.

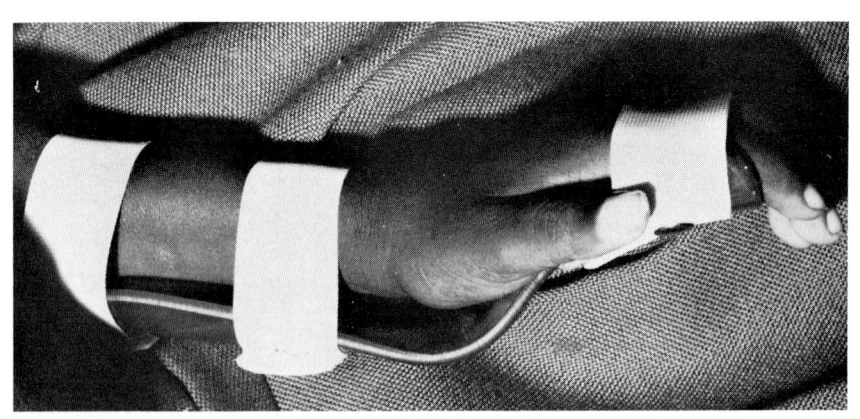

Figure 8-5 Hand and wrist splint constructed from heat-malleable plastic (polyvinyl chloride). This appliance is most useful in maintenance of neutral position for the hand, wrist, and fingers. Three points of pressure are provided for the wrist and an upward pressure is produced for the proximal phalanges.

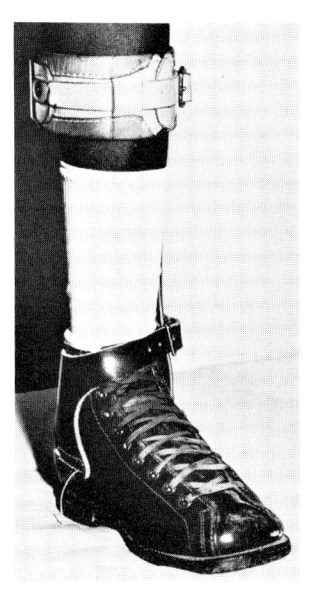

Figure 8-6 Standard below-knee brace with medial T strap, useful for severe valgus of the foot and ankle. Again, three major points of corrective pressure are produced.

altered with the use of heat as the deformity is corrected. Again, this is fashioned, fitted, and designed by the orthopedist and is usually most appropriate for the problem. The material will alter shape if left in the sun too long.

The supple arthritic foot must have adequate support to prevent deformities. A well-built shoe and standard inserts (longitudinal and metatarsal pads) are used in the child as in chronic disorders in adults. One should designate the type of last required—usually regular, but in rare instances, straight last shoes for pes cavus. The height, size, and material of the longitudinal and metatarsal pads should be designated according to needs. A wedge heel, lift, or transverse metatarsal bar should also be included on the prescription if indicated. We have found it desirable to use firm, well-constructed shoes for the child during the majority of his day, but also feel that it is perfectly all right for the child to use some of the newer tennis shoes for a portion of the time in his play and school.

Standard leg bracing is also useful for severe deformities, joint destruction or weakness (Fig. 8-6).

SURGICAL TREATMENT

Flexion Contracture Release

When a deformity becomes a hindrance to the function or use of an extremity, and the condition is rigid and unrelieved by physical therapy, orthotic devices, or exercise, then surgical release of ligaments, muscles, or tendons should be considered. Again, this is most pertinent to the knee, but the principle can be applied to any major joint. The major tendons on the side of contracture are either divided or lengthened, as the case warrants. Usually the capsular structures are divided completely across the contracted side of the joint. Care must be taken to avoid overstretching of nerves and vessels, which in severe deformities are often the only remaining structures preventing complete extension of the joint. This procedure finds its greatest usefulness in the posterior structures of the knee and ankle. It is also useful in relieving flexion contractures of the hip, wrist, and occasionally the elbow.

In some patients extensive joint release is not necessary, and simple tendon section or lengthening is sufficient. Individual judgment is necessary, and many times the final decision is made at surgery. In equinus of the ankle, lengthening of the Achilles tendon is a standard, well-recognized procedure, and it occupies a role in the treatment of rheumatoid arthritis as well. Medical treatment of flexion contracture of the wrist is sometimes helped by surgical release of the flexor carpi radialis and flexor carpi ulnaris.

Osteotomy

Osteotomy is the treatment of choice when a flexion deformity is too great or a lateral deviation is marked. It should be limited to the older age groups; we have not performed the procedure on patients younger than 11 years of age. Angular deformities of the extremities usually respond to conservative treatment in the younger age groups. Distal femoral osteotomy should be used for persistent and serious valgus deformity of the knees, a common problem in the rheumatoid patient. Again, individual judgment is necessary. If good motion and joint integrity are present, an osteotomy can correct a lateral deviation with marked help to the patient. When a joint has become fused in poor position by the rheumatoid process, as in the case of the wrist, osteotomy may be of great benefit.

Arthrodesis

Arthrodesis, or joint fusion, is a mainstay of orthopedic practice. In general, arthrodesis is reserved for extremities with only one joint involved, and is primarily indicated for the relief of persistent pain or instability. When more than one joint is involved, such as the hip and the knee, fusion should be avoided because the further loss of motion produces too much incapacitation to justify its use. In the older child, fusion of some interphalangeal deformities of the toes is an excellent procedure. One should be cautious in fusions of the immature joint to avoid damage to the adjacent epiphyseal cartilages and resultant growth disturbances.

Equalization of Lower Extremities

Monarticular arthritis, or more specifically arthritis involving one lower extremity, is quite apt to produce overgrowth rather than undergrowth. There seems to be little attention in the orthopedic literature to the amount of altered growth rate or ultimate discrepancy in leg length of the rheumatoid patient. Usually the inequality is less than 1 inch and no major surgical procedure is indicated. When the discrepancy is greater than 1 inch, the patient should be offered some type of equalization procedure. Probably the ideal procedure for this problem is stapling of the distal femoral epiphysis. Because of inability to predict growth accurately, it should be done approximately six months prior to the time indicated by the growth charts developed by Green (1963). When equalization has been accomplished, the staples can be removed and equal growth resumed. The severely damaged joint or the joint with quite active disease probably should not have this operative procedure, as further damage to the joint, and stiffness, may ensue. If possible, a synovectomy should be done as a preliminary procedure with the hope of reducing the inflammation.

After full mobilization and strength has been regained, stapling could then be considered. If a stapling procedure is not indicated it is probably better to wait until maturity, when shortening of the femur with a step-cut midshaft osteotomy and intramedullary nailing can be performed.

Manipulation of Joints

Manipulation of joints under anesthesia is occasionally indicated. With a combination of inflammatory pannus, muscle spasm, pain, and voluntary restriction of motion, a joint may have considerable intra-articular adhesions as well as periarticular arthrofibrosis. Conservative measures such as physical therapy or intra-articular injections are certainly indicated at first, but if these are not successful, manipulation under anesthesia may be helpful.

The child is given a general anesthetic and a muscle relaxant for almost total reduction of muscle tone. This is important since undue pressure may fracture the already osteoporotic bones. One should carefully grasp the bones near the joint and pull the joint around the range of motion, rather than simply bending it like a stick. In manipulation of the knee, for instance, the tibia should be pushed forward in respect to the femur in order to stretch the posterior structures without producing posterior subluxation of the tibia. Manipulation is probably best indicated in the knee, but also may be useful in the hip, shoulder, and wrist. During anesthesia for surgery of one joint, other appropriate joints may be gently manipulated with beneficial results.

It is well known that the elbow in the child responds poorly to manipulation, and here this procedure is contraindicated almost without exception in the child. This is also true of the interphalangeal joints of the fingers, but the metacarpophalangeal joints of the hand respond fairly well. The joint is usually injected at the time of manipulation.

Judicious pressure about the joint immediately after manipulation reduces swelling and postmanipulation reaction. The joint is wrapped with soft cotton material and an Ace bandage applied somewhat tighter than usual. Care should be taken to avoid excessive pressure or peripheral edema. Ice bags are then placed about the joint, and this treatment maintained for approximately eight to 12 hours. At that time, the tight bandage is removed and gentle motion is begun. Light elastic bandaging is continued until swelling has subsided.

ORTHOPEDIC TREATMENT OF SPECIFIC JOINTS

Lower Extremity

The basic dictum of orthopedics in the lower extremities is that of preservation of weight-bearing ability, form, and flexibility. Maintenance of motion is important but secondary. The lower extremity, of course, must bear weight and provide support for the body, and therefore must be kept anatomically in line, sturdy, and free from pain. If motion can be retained with these two objectives, so much the better. In general, however, flexibility is of secondary importance and is at times sacrificed for the primary objectives.

Foot. In the foot of the rheumatoid child, the tarsal and metatarsal joints are usually involved to a significant degree. These joints are difficult to examine and motion is very limited at best. Significant destruction can take place before overt clinical manifestations are evident. The ossification centers of the tarsal bones in the young child are merely circles and the cartilaginous joint surfaces are not well visualized. Severe destruction of the joint surfaces may take place without significant x-ray abnormalities.

The tarsal joints usually fuse in children with persistent arthritis. There is really little that can be done to prevent this and perhaps it is for the best; in severe cases a triple arthrodesis is allowed to occur. These bones, however, must be kept in anatomic position and alignment so that no fixed deformity is present while fusion is taking place. We have had no real problems in the metatarsophalangeal joints in children. These joints are certainly involved, but the mild toe deformities present are usually of no functional consequence. If progressive toe deformities occur, it is better to wait until the child is more mature and then advise standard adult reconstructive procedures. The most common problem is that of excessive pes valgus-planus (Fig. 8-7). This is probably an accentuation of the common problem seen in normal children. Synovitis produces relaxation of ligamentous structures and destruction of joint integrity. If there is a tendency toward valgus or loss of the longitudinal arch, this deformity is increased by weight bearing and loss of ligamentous and articular support.

Proper shoes, which fit and support, are of paramount importance in the treatment of the rheumatoid child. We find that parents and children are most cooperative if a firm, well-fitting shoe is recommended to be worn approximately 75 per cent of the time. The remainder of the time the child may use some of the newer, padded tennis shoes for play and recreation. Children who have highly variable

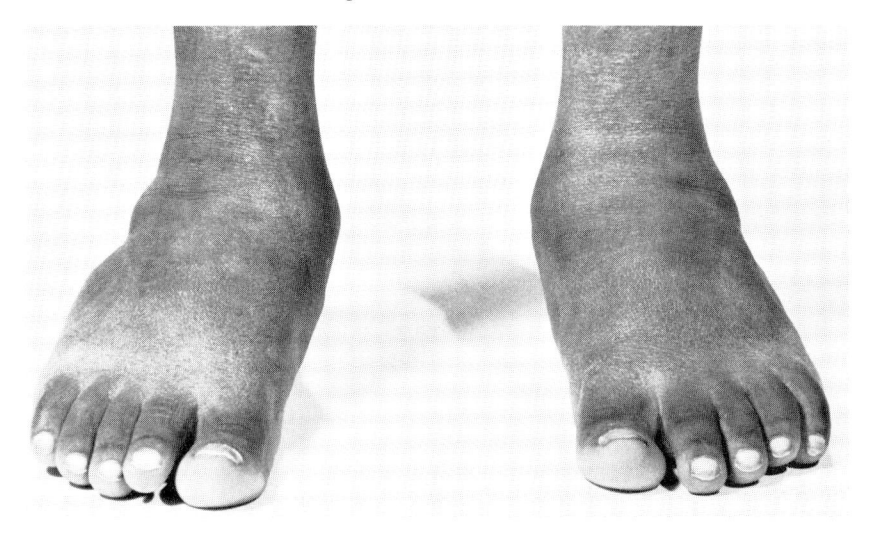

Figure 8-7 Excessive pes valgus-planus. In arthritis of the tarsal joints, the supporting capsular and ligamentous structures are weakened and the natural valgus is accentuated.

swelling of the ankles can wear only cloth-covered shoes that allow for stretch. One should not be too rigid or demanding in the treatment of these children or total rejection on the part of the child and the parents of any treatment whatsoever may occur. We aim at as nearly normal function in play and school as the disease will allow, and fit the child with as simple a shoe as possible, avoiding the heavy corrective type of shoes. The shoe, however, should have a broad, flat heel of ordinary height, with a firm counter. A small longitudinal and metatarsal pad may be prescribed, rubberized cork being the material of choice. The longitudinal pad should be between ¼ and ⅜ inch thick, and the metatarsal pad usually ¼ inch thick. Shoes with standard lasts are usually prescribed. In severe or progressive deformities a larger longitudinal support, with a ¹⁄₁₆ to ⅛ inch heel wedge, is needed. A Thomas heel and a long, rigid counter may be prescribed if desired. Periodic examination of the feet in children is essential so that early treatment of these deformities can be instituted.

We have had a few children in whom arthritis is so severe about the foot and ankle that valgus of the foot and heel cannot be controlled with shoes. A standard short leg brace with an inner T-strap is used (Fig. 8-6). The ankle joint is left free when equinus contracture is not a problem.

Several children have demonstrated mild varus and cavus of the foot, which has not been associated with clawing of the toes (Fig. 8-8). Standard straight last shoes are prescribed with a ¹⁄₁₆ inch heel wedge, in the early cases. A small longitudinal arch support is usually provided to prevent loss of the arch. With turning in of the forefoot a lateral sole wedge ⅛ inch thick is appropriate.

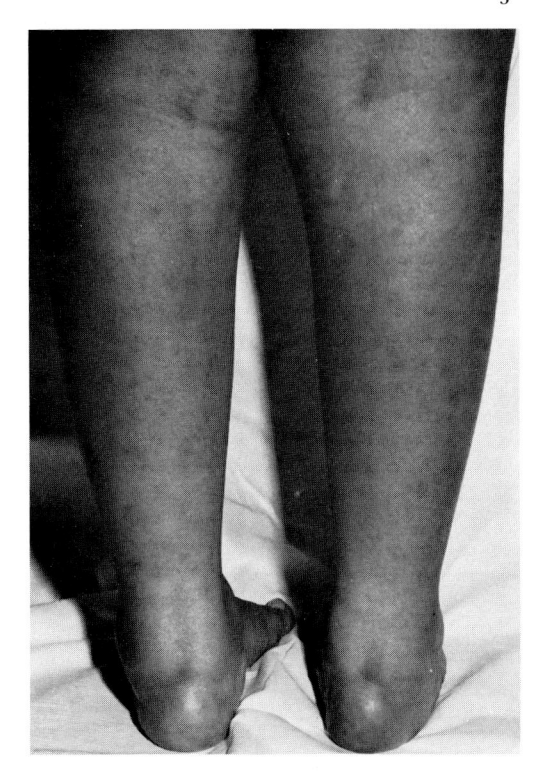

Figure 8-8 Cavo-varus, usually seen in the more severe cases, especially with tarsal involvement. Shoe wedges and stretching have been sufficient to prevent severe deformity in our patients.

With significant, prolonged arthritis about the foot, many children will demonstrate contracture of the heel cord similar to that seen in many other diseases. Stretching of the heel cord by the therapist, the mother, and the child is instituted as soon as this contracture is detected; with proper instruction, early treatment, and cooperation the contracture does not become a problem. Lengthening of the heel cord surgically has not been found necessary, but it certainly should be done if persistent, unrelieved equinus is a problem. Night splints constructed of plaster or more permanent materials can be used if equinus persists. This is a well-established method of treatment and is usually effective.

Heat-malleable plastic materials are useful in the treatment of equinus. They are somewhat springy, can easily be altered to prevent pressure spots, and are usually accepted nicely by the child. When the child is ill with generalized disease, or in the postoperative state, the foot may drop into equinus while the attention is directed to more pertinent problems; the physical therapist should see the child during this period to note range of motion of the major joints and stretching of any early contractures. One must constantly keep in mind prevention of equinus; early treatment is so much better than any surgery or late reconstruction.

Several children have been examined in the clinic who demonstrated loss of plantar flexion of the ankle. This usually is not disabling but produces a peculiar gait. Plantar flexion, on heel strike, is inadequate, and the knee is thrown forward in flexion earlier than in the normal cadence. Apparently this is due to spasm, and contracture of dorsiflexor tendons and capsular restriction occur only later. Appropriate stretching and elevated heels seem to be sufficient treatment for this problem as far as we have been able to tell. Such treatment has not produced a calcaneous foot or contracture above a 90 degree angle.

In neglected or progressively severe arthritis surgical procedures about the foot and ankle are occasionally indicated in the child. For unresolved equinus, the well-established method of lengthening the Achilles tendon is appropriate. In the ankle, when this tendon is released, the capsular and intra-articular adhesions can usually be removed by manipulation. When the problem is identified and conservative treatment yields no relief, this procedure should be done before the ankle becomes fused or badly contracted in an improper position. The earlier the procedure can be performed, the easier and more beneficial is the outcome. Somewhat earlier mobilization is probably indicated, and it is advisable to begin some early non-weight-bearing motion at about three to four weeks to prevent recurrence of intra-articular adhesions. The ankle should be injected with a corticosteroid at the time of surgery to attempt reduction of swelling and pain.

Fusions of the ankle or foot joints have not been necessary in our experience. Because of the multiarticular nature of the disease, ankle fusion is rarely indicated. In severe arthritis the tarsal joints usually undergo fusion spontaneously; triple arthrodesis, per se, is rarely performed in the child. When severe valgus or varus of the heel is present one must consider calcaneal osteotomy prior to complete fusion of the joint. This procedure, designed by Dwyer (1959), was formerly used in the treatment of idiopathic cavus feet. It has also found further usefulness in either valgus or varus of the heel resulting from many other conditions. Synovectomy of the ankle has not been attempted, and it is contraindicated in the tarsal and metatarsal joints. Occasionally an interphalangeal joint of a toe that becomes badly deformed and interferes with proper shoe fitting may be fused in the child nearing maturity. The child is not usually symptomatic, even when significant metatarsophalangeal joint destruction is present. More skeletal maturity should be present before a resection of the joint by the Hoffman procedure is attempted (Hoffman, 1911-12).

Knee. The knee deserves and has received more attention from both the orthopedist and the rheumatologist than perhaps any other joint. It is the most important joint in the lower extremity, and is more poorly constructed with regard to strength and function than either the hip or the ankle. The knee is also probably the most commonly affected joint in rheumatoid arthritis.

General measures, such as physical therapy exercises and heat, are described in another section of this book. The most common mild problem the orthopedist is called to deal with is that of valgus of the knee (Fig. 8-9). This is probably an accentuation of the common physiological valgus knee seen in usual orthopedic clinical practice. The best

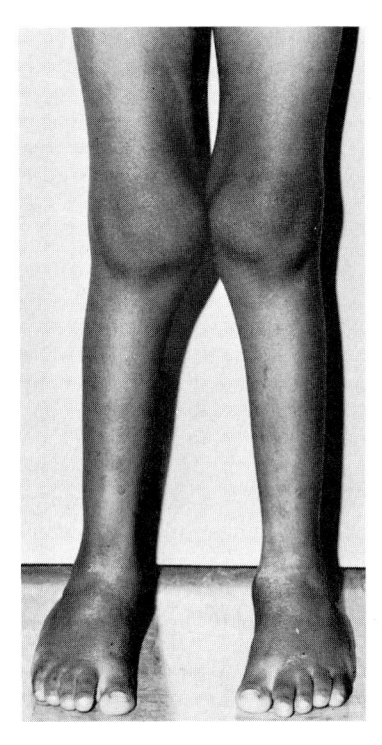

Figure 8-9 Genu valgum, probably representing accentuation of the natural valgus of the knee by the destructive effects of rheumatoid disease.

practical method of detecting the condition is by having the child stand with the knees just touching. The distance between the malleoli can be measured either in fingerbreadths or centimeters. Again, a routine examination at periodic intervals, with this in mind, would detect early deformity and render treatment much more effective.

With mild involvement (two fingerbreadths or less), a small wedge is used on the medial heel in the walking shoes and the child is observed. If the deformity progresses, or is greater than three fingerbreadths, we feel it advisable to use a night splint, since experience shows that this condition grows worse, especially when arthritis is active. One must be more aggressive than is necessary in the ordinary problem. The three point extension orthosis serves quite well in this condition (Fig. 8-1). The device is constructed so that the bands apply pressure on the lateral portion of the upper thigh and lower leg, with a cage of soft leather constructed so as to apply pressure on the medial side of the knee. With proper fit and construction, the splint need not be attached to the shoes, but if the child is small and overactive, the brace may be connected to a shoe for fixation.

Another common problem in this joint is that of mild flexion restriction or contracture. Again, early attention is necessary for a good result. A minimal contracture of 15 degrees or less that is early and not rigid can also be treated with an extension orthosis. The bands are placed posteriorly on the upper thigh and lower leg, and pressure is applied via the cage pad to push the knee directly posterior. The pressure over the knee must be on the kneecap or slightly above it. The appliance must not be allowed to slip down, as the pressure will then be applied to the tibia and invite posterior subluxation of the tibia. Simple stretching exercises are given by the therapist and the mother, and the child is carefully watched until progression or regression of the deformity can be ascertained. When proper treatment is carried out this method is quite effective and surgical intervention is rarely necessary. Some children will demonstrate valgus combined with flexion contracture. The previously described orthosis is used but the knee pad is positioned in an oblique manner to provide both posterior and lateral pressure at the knee joint.

Severe flexion deformity may be present prior to advanced destruction of the joint in the untreated or neglected child. Conservative means are used at the onset in this situation, with the hope that surgery can be avoided. If the contracture is greater than 15 degrees and rigid, more aggressive treatment is necessary. When equinus of the ankle is also present, surgical intervention is essential.

Soft tissue release of a flexion contracture is indicated when the articular surfaces are intact enough to provide a reasonably functional knee joint. If the range of motion is less than 90 degrees, arthroplasty may be more desirable. Rigid methods, such as the use of wedging casts, invite stiffness. We have found that intermittent use of the extension orthosis is much more applicable than immobilization and pressure.

When posterior soft tissue release of a flexion contracture is necessary, a modification of the method described by Wilson (1929) is quite sufficient. A lazy-S shaped incision about the lateral side of the knee is used, as it tends to leave a more cosmetic scar. The dissection is carried down to the biceps tendon, which is isolated, transected, and reflected. The peroneal nerve should be isolated and freed from its fibrous tunnel in the limits of the incision. It must be carefully watched at all times, since any amount of stretch produced by the extension may produce peroneal palsy. This is usually the limiting factor in the amount of extension that can be obtained at the time and one should rely on gradual postoperative stretching if the nerve is too tight at the time of surgery. The biceps tendon is incised in a step-cut manner and the ends reflected. The fat and areolar tissue are then separated from the posterior capsule, from lateral to medial, and the posterior capsule incised in a longitudinal manner while the knee is extended. Care should be taken to retract the posterior neurovascular structures, and the tourniquet should be released prior to closure to ascertain their integrity. Intra-articular procedures can be carried out at the same time as posterior release, and synovectomy may be done if indicated. If the medial hamstrings are contracted, they may be sectioned or lengthened through a small medial incision, although usually this is not necessary. The tibia is pushed anteriorly with respect to the femur and some of the fibers of the medial collateral ligament may be sectioned posteriorly to affect this motion. Potter (1966) reported results on release of flexion contracture of one hundred knees followed more than two years in the adult. Fourteen of these patients had practically normal extension and 75 per cent had an overall good result.

In the knee joint with severe valgus or varus deformity osteotomy must be considered (Fig. 8-9). Usually the deformity is in the supracondylar region and osteotomy is the treatment of choice. If the joint itself is severely involved one might wish to allow the child to mature, and then perform an arthroplasty with reconstruction of the joint surfaces to correct the deformity in the adult. Osteotomy is indicated only in those cases in which a deformity interferes with function and in which the knee joint is still in reasonably good condition. If valgus is present below the knee joint, a high tibial osteotomy is much better. Since it is a less traumatic procedure, earlier motion is possible.

The supracondylar osteotomy is best performed through a lateral incision with separation of the fascia lata in the midline. The quadriceps mechanism is elevated anteriorly, and the osteotomy effected in the midmetaphyseal region. An appropriate internal fixation device, such as a bone plate, is indicated because it allows the earlier motion so necessary in patients with arthritis. The high tibial osteotomy can be done through an anterior oblique incision with a dome-shaped cut through the high tibial shaft, above the attachment of the patellar tendon. A concomitant fibular osteotomy should be done at the same time. By means of a curved osteotomy the deformity can be corrected any desired amount and the bones held in place with an oblique pin that can be easily removed later. The child may be weight-bearing after this type of osteotomy, and motion started early to prevent stiffness in the knee joint.

The knee joint is perhaps the most ideal articulation for the use of prophylactic synovectomy. It has a large synovial surface, is easily palpable, and the clinical condition can be followed carefully with some degree of accuracy. X-ray examination is clearer than in most joints. Measurements of motion are accurate and reproducible, and the integrity of the joint can be ascertained easily. The knee joint lends itself well to biopsy, aspiration, and injection.

Hip. The hip is a rather small but extremely strong joint deeply situated beneath large muscular and ligamentous groups. It is relatively inaccessible for examination, treatment, or aspiration. Clinical assessment of synovitis cannot be followed accurately. The child usually does not have a great deal of pain from synovitis, and does not show symptoms until advanced destruction of the joint is present. The epiphyseal ossification center is round, and there is a large amount of cartilaginous material that forms the hip joint. X-rays, therefore, do not show the early cartilaginous destruction that precedes bony changes. Range of motion of the hip is extensive and can be tested if attention is directed toward detail. A common error in measuring such motion is failure to immobilize the pelvis and lumbar spine.

Flexion contracture, often the earliest manifestation of involvement in this joint, can be detected by performing the Thomas test. The pelvis is fixed in a neutral position by bringing the opposite thigh onto the chest, with the lumbar spine flattened against the bed. We have found it better to flex each thigh alternately until the test is completed.

One thigh is held flexed and the other allowed to extend. The amount of flexion contracture can be measured by using the table as a reference. If the thigh cannot be pushed to touch the table, a flexion contracture is present. Actually, there is no extension of the hip joint, but rather posterior rotation of the pelvis, which accomplishes the apparent extension of the hip in walking and examination.

The presence of lordosis in examination of the child may suggest flexion contracture. Also, with flexion contracture the gait shows absence of, or reduction in, posterior swing of the thigh. The patient should be examined, undressed, for the presence of adduction contracture, which is also seen in the early stages of the rheumatoid hip. With the fingers palpate the anterior superior iliac spines, and determine abduction and adduction in respect to these two points. A practical method to determine the amount of adduction is to measure the distance between the knees, both in extension and in 90 degrees of flexion. Rotation should be tested with the child lying face down, the hip in extension; the angulation of the tibia is measured from the plane of the table. Both legs can be measured at once, and small deviations can be detected quite easily. The rotation in flexion is usually greater, and should be measured with the child face up and the hips in 90 degrees of flexion. This rotation can also be tested quickly with the child sitting and rotating the tibias in and out.

The gait of the child should be checked at every clinic visit. This is an easy, quick method of determining the function in all of the major joints of the leg, but it serves best to detect problems in the hip. A description of gait patterns is difficult, but with practice one can learn to detect abnormal gaits due to stiffness or pain in the foot, ankle, knee, or hip. The Trendelenburg test can be performed either by watching the gait, or by standing behind the child and having him place his weight on one side and lift the opposite foot. The lateral abductors should stabilize the pelvis and hold it neutral or depress the side of the pelvis upon which the weight is borne. One should observe for fine deviations between one side and the other. Almost any condition causing pain or loss of function of the hip is manifested by a positive Trendelenburg sign. In the child with hip trouble one also sees a "gluteus medius gait," which is similar to the Trendelenburg. The pelvis tilts away from the involved hip because of weakness in the lateral abductors. When the condition is more severe the child will begin to lurch, or throw the body weight over the hip, in order to completely relieve the function of the lateral abductors. Any such limp in the child should lead one to carefully evaluate the function of the hip.

The treatment of arthritis in the hip includes adequate exercise, stretching, and range of motion activities on the part of the therapist, the child, and the parent. The therapist should be instructed to check range of motion and bring to the doctor's attention any tendency toward flexion or adduction contractures. With a good joint these early contractures can usually be stretched out quite well. Occasionally, as in any joint, the hip will suffer acute exacerbation, and crutches for a short period of time may be useful. The short period should be stressed and the child must not become dependent upon crutches for relief of symptoms. The joint may be injected if pain and stiffness persist, but repeated injections in the hip are contraindicated as they are apparently of no basic curative value. They do, however, help alleviate acute exacerbations and prevent muscle atrophy and stiffness resulting from pain.

The orthopedic literature contains considerable discussion concerning the stretching of hip flexion contractures for many problems (Irwin, 1940, 1947). Such stretching is extremely difficult to do because of inability to secure the pelvis. There is, of course, a long lever arm in the thigh, and extension can be accomplished with any pressure applied to the distal femur. This procedure, however, in rigid contractures merely tilts the pelvis and accentuates the lordosis. Stretching traction is useful in mild deformities that are not rigid. If rigid flexion deformity is present in the hip, and conservative measures have been of no avail, then surgical release of the flexion contracture should be undertaken, together with anterior capsulotomy and synovectomy.

Adduction contracture, which also occurs in the hip, is easier to stretch than flexion contracture. Two thigh splints, connected by turnbuckles, applied between the thighs as a night splint, can gradually stretch hip adduction contracture if the condition is detected early and treatment started before the muscles and ligaments are badly contracted. When the joint loses range of motion and there is intra-articular damage, one may not be able to accomplish a great deal of abduction. Loss of abduction is not a severe deficit and one need only provide enough to allow for proper cleansing and perineal care.

Open procedures about the hip are formidable and not to be undertaken unless the child is in good general condition. It is desirable to have a good knee and foot on the same side, since improvement of the hip in a leg with a bad knee would not be of any great benefit. If the hip joint is opened, a synovectomy should be undertaken in an attempt to reduce the progress of the disease from the inflammatory synovium. Usually, contractures due to rheumatoid arthritis produce contracture of the capsule in the adjacent anterior structures, requiring a Soutter type of procedure. The Smith-Peterson approach is used with release of structures in the anterior wing of the ilium. The anterior fibers of the gluteus medius are allowed to retract backward, and some of the anterior ilium is removed if necessary. A capsulotomy and release of the reflected head of the rectus femoris should also be done. An anterior capsulotomy is performed to allow a more thorough synovectomy. The hip should not be dislocated, as this invites aseptic necrosis of the femoral head. With flexion, abduction, and rotation, most of the contents of the joint can be removed carefully with rongeurs and sharp dissection.

Postoperatively, the patient should be placed in gentle traction with the leg completely extended and abducted. An adductor tenotomy is useful if this tendon is tight at the time of anesthesia. At about the eighth to tenth day, gentle, passive stretching and active range of motion exercises are instituted. The child and parents are again instructed in proper stretching for flexion contracture, and the child is carefully followed to see that this is being done.

If the child is near maturity one may wish to wait until growth has ceased, and then perform a cup arthroplasty for a badly damaged joint. When severe destruction of the joint is present, and the child is above ten years of age, a cup arthroplasty may be considered prior to maturation, but indications for this should be quite rare. If a cup arthroplasty is done before maturity, the child will grow but the hip joint will remain small. Revision and replacement with a larger cup may be necessary within ten years. Fairly good joint function can be present, however, even with a bad x-ray picture.

Leg Length Inequality. When a younger child has monarticular arthritis, or arthritis in several joints of one extremity, leg length inequality becomes a problem (Fig. 8-10, *A*). In our clinic we have seen only elongation in the leg due to rheumatoid arthritis. In some metacarpal and metatarsal bones epiphyseal arrest does occur, but we have not seen unilateral short legs in monarticular arthritis. The more active the disease, and the younger the child, the greater the discrepancy. Again, one must be attentive to this problem and recognition is quite important. It is useful to examine the child from behind and place the fingers on the iliac crest.

We have used wooden blocks to build up the short leg to ascertain the amount necessary to provide clinical leveling of the pelvis (Fig. 8-10, *B*). The legs may be measured in the standard way also, either way being acceptable. With more than ¼ inch of discrepancy a shoe lift is indicated for equalization. Small inequalities can be corrected by removing as much as ¼ inch from the heel of the shoe of the longer leg, and adding an appropriate amount to the heel of the opposite shoe. Most discrepancies are 1 inch or less, and the correction can be accomplished with the use of heel lifts alone. With a greater than 1 inch deviation, a heel and sole elevation is needed to prevent equinus. This elevation, of course, makes the shoe much heavier and less acceptable to the child and the parents.

Procedures for equalizing leg lengths are more fully described in the previous section on surgical treatment. However, a patient may tolerate as much as a ¾ inch discrepancy without any significant problem. The patient should be encouraged to balance the pelvis as much as possible to prevent a lumbosacral problem in later life. When the discrepancy is more than 1 inch, one may wish to offer the patient some type of bony equalization, either through epiphyseal arrest or bone shortening after maturity.

Upper Extremity

The upper extremities, in comparison to the lower extremities, require flexibility more than strength and stability. Joint destruction and laxity can be accepted if the joint maintains a useful range of motion and reasonable freedom from pain. Fusion is rarely carried out in the upper extremity, since it performs much better with deformity than the lower, and often flexibility must be maintained at the expense

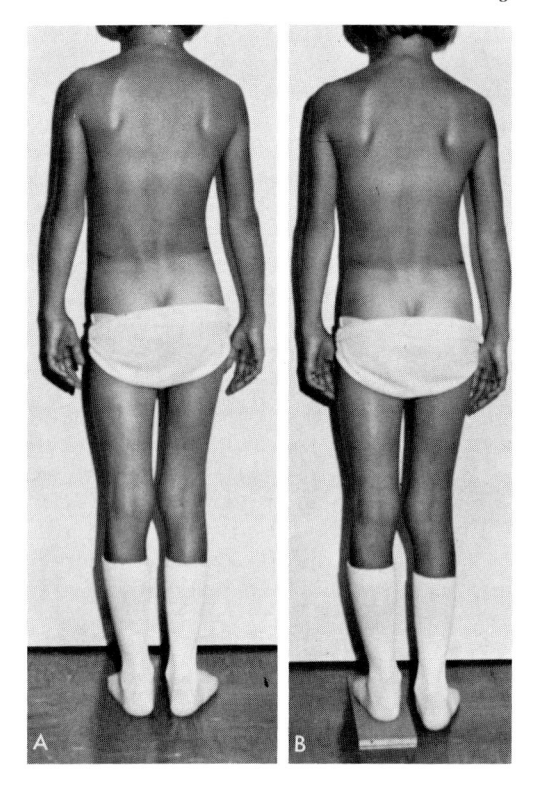

Figure 8-10 *A*, Leg length inequality of approximately 1 inch. *B*, Wooden blocks to balance the legs and pelvis are a practical measuring method to determine the lift required to be placed in the shoe. The size and weight of the shoe lift can be minimized by removing ¼ inch from the heel of the longer side and using the additional ¼ inch inside the heel on the shorter side.

of joint integrity and alignment. One must strive for all aspects of form and function, but in the upper extremity flexibility is of paramount importance.

Hand. The child with rheumatoid arthritis in the hand presents a picture different from the classic appearance of deformity in the adult. In the child interphalangeal synovitis is much more common, and ulnar deviation is almost no problem at all. The wrist joint shows early loss of motion and a tendency toward a lack of dorsiflexion. We have become accustomed to using loss of extension as a guide to involvement of the intercarpal joints. Steindler (1955) has shown that palmar flexion of the wrist takes place mostly at the radiocarpal joint, whereas dorsiflexion or extension of the wrist takes place primarily in the intercarpal region. The more complicated intercarpal joint loses range of motion first, and therefore loss of extension is seen early in children with rheumatoid arthritis.

Physical therapy, with an exercise program, is reviewed in other parts of this book. It should be noted, however, that with cooperation and diligent work, a quite flexible wrist may be maintained in spite of rather serious joint destruction seen on x-ray. If the wrist joint progresses to severe destruction or intercarpal fusion, one must strive to keep the joint in a functional position. The wrist, at times, may tend to go into ulnar deviation, or flexion and ulnar deviation. The use of heat-malleable plastic splints has proved to be a useful adjunct in maintaining a neutral position when stiffness occurs. It is used as a night splint and is usually accepted quite well by the child and parents. The exercise program is carried out during the day.

Several children have been seen with minimal radial deviation in the fingers, but this has been of no functional consequence. A prefabricated splint may be used (Fig. 8-5), or a splint can be constructed from a sheet of heat-malleable plastic (Fig. 8-11). A strap of Velcro is riveted to the splint to provide the proper pressure. With the three point pressure principle kept in mind, at least one secure strap should be placed so that direct pressure over the point of deformity is accomplished. When severe loss of motion is found, or progression of stiffness occurs in spite of treatment, alternating flexion and extension splints can be useful to regain some lost motion. Two splints are used in this situation, one forcing the wrist into flexion and the other into extension. These are worn on alternate nights in conjunction with the exercise and physical therapy program. This program has not been very satisfactory.

Injectable corticosteroids are useful in the metacarpal, interphalangeal, and carpal joints. The Hypospray Injector* (Fig. 8-12, *A*, *B*, and *C*) may be used for any of these joints, especially in the small and apprehensive child. In the older child a standard needle introduces the medicine directly, intra-articularly, and is probably better. There is some thought that the corticosteroid should be injected in the periarticular structures, but the question remains unanswered at this time.

Wrist. In a neglected or severe case of wrist flexion contracture one may be forced into operative correction. This is usually indicated in the older child, as the disease process may require several years.

---

*R. P. Scherer Corp., Detroit, Michigan.

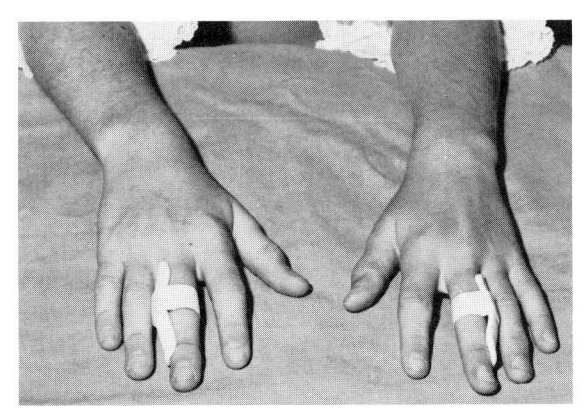

Figure 8-11 A simple splint used for mild curvature in the finger. The heat-malleable plastic is fashioned in place and held with tape. Note the three points of corrective force applied.

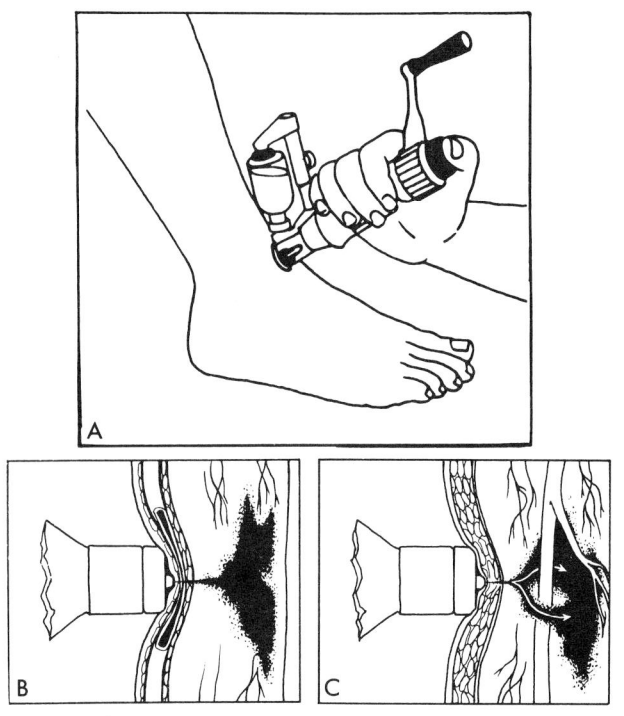

Figure 8-12 *A*, The Hypospray injector, used to inject corticosteroids in and about joints, bursae, and tendons. Ease of use and absence of a needle facilitate its use in children. *B*, Pressure of the instrument compresses superficial veins so that the medication passes through, leaving no detectable amount in the lumen. *C*, By the time it has penetrated to deep veins, the jet lacks sufficient force to enter them.

With flexion contracture only, and good articular surfaces, one can gain a lot either by lengthening or sectioning the wrist flexor tendons. These tendons have a great tendency to reattach, and in the child, section alone subcutaneously, followed by proper splinting, is the treatment of choice. When the wrist is fused in an unsuitable position, osteotomy of the distal radius should be undertaken through a dorsal curvilinear incision that allows one to resect the distal end of the ulna at the same time. The distal radio-ulnar joint is usually damaged in this situation and prevents rotation.

It is undesirable to have both wrists fused in the same anatomic position. Personal hygiene and toilet care are difficult with both wrists fused in a dorsiflexed or straight position. One should strive for one strong, stable, fused wrist in about 10 degrees of dorsiflexion, with the opposite member retaining a small amount of motion.

In the small joints of the hand we have not found it necessary to do any operative procedures. The classic appearance of the juvenile rheumatoid arthritis patient with multiple gross deformities occurs late in childhood and, to a great extent, after maturation. Only very mild ulnar deviation of the metacarpophalangeal joints has been seen; more frequently a small degree of radial deviation at the metacarpophalangeal joints occurs. We have seen several individuals with a gentle curve deformity of the fingers, either in a radial or ulnar deviation. A small molded plastic splint is quite helpful. A small piece of tape is applied about the middle joint, pushing it into the splint. This splint is used at night and usually curbs the tendency if it is noted early. The same type of splinting can be used for adduction contracture of the thumb by the use of a small V-shaped piece of plastic and appropriate taping.

In children with severe active disease in all joints of the hand and wrist, one should apply a resting splint, particularly at nighttime. There is a great deal of controversy concerning the attributes of rest or exercise. We have found it beneficial to compromise and rest the joint at nighttime, especially when the disease is active and the joints are tender and swollen. The prefabricated splint is ideal for this (Fig. 8-5). It is light, easily applied, and seemingly well tolerated by the patient. The wrist should be kept in a mild degree of dorsiflexion with neutral deviation. The metacarpophalangeal joints should rest in neutral ulnoradial deviation and a mild degree of flexion. The splint is designed to produce an upper thrust on the base of the proximal phalanges, thus preventing the tendency toward volar subluxation at this joint. The smaller child does not have this tendency to a great extent; it is more common in late childhood and in the adult patient. If there is a tendency toward deviation, the side flanges, strapping, and contour should be adjusted accordingly.

Elbow. The elbow, of course, is commonly affected in the child with rheumatoid disease, but its involvement usually occurs later, and disability and pain are less of a problem in this joint than in others. Most of the same basic principles apply in this region. The joint, however, does not respond well to forceful exercises, manipulation, or strong passive pressure. Loss of a great deal of motion in this joint is not inconsistent with a functional extremity. Flexion beyond a right angle is a more useful motion than the other motion in the joint. Usually, however, extension is lost early and treatment to retain motion of the joint can be instituted when this occurs without losing a great deal of flexion. Standard exercises and physical therapy are, of course, applied first, and usually are effective. The elbow is a true hinge joint, and most of the common splinting and extension methods are useful and not harmful to the joint. Synovitis in the elbow can be detected early by palpating the small triangle formed by the head of the radius, the olecranon, and the lateral epicondyle. At this site the synovium is closest to the skin and is more easily detectable. The elbow joint is composed of complex surfaces and has two bones articulating distally. Rotation in supination and pronation is determined at this joint, but it is also dependent upon a distal radio-ulnar articulation. The radiohumeral joint is commonly destroyed in severe arthritis of the elbow, undergoing disorganization with resultant loss of extension and rotation.

If persistent synovitis and evidence of destructive changes are noted in this joint, and no response is gained from good conservative treatment, a synovectomy should be considered. It has been our experience that this situation does not exist until the child is older. At that time a more complete débridement may be undertaken. The radiohumeral joint is usually the painful problem, and the only operation that suffices to correct this is an excision of the radial head. This must not be done in the growing child as deformity will result. In the mature child, a débridement synovectomy procedure is performed rather than a simple synovectomy. The elbow joint does not lend itself well to simple synovectomy because exposure is difficult. In débridement, a lateral exposure is used in which the extensor origin is reflected, or the lateral epicondyle is osteotomized to reflect the extensor origin. The radial head is then excised. The joint can be sprung open and the various recesses and fossae cleansed of rheumatoid tissue with sharp dissection and rongeur. The joint is quite lax, and responds to some postoperative immobilization for a period of two to three weeks. Such immobilization seems to tighten the joint, and reestablishment of motion does not become a problem. If there is severe and gross disorganization of the joint surfaces, a complete arthroplasty should be done when the child is near growth termination. Arthroplasty is more successful in the elbow than in other joints. A fascial graft from the thigh is used, opposing joint surfaces are remodeled, and the fascia is sewn over to provide interposing membrane.

Shoulder. In our experience this joint gives less trouble than any of the other major joints. It is less commonly involved, and even with marked destruction there is no great impairment of function. This joint has considerable range of motion, and the exercises and physical therapy recommended are usually effective and should be instituted as a preventive measure. We have not found the use of splinting or corrective devices necessary in treatment of the shoulder. One should consider manipulation for severe loss of abduction, as this joint responds well to this procedure. Joint injections are more beneficial here than in any other joint, and should be used if required. If there is extensive synovial proliferation synovectomy can be performed, but we have never found this necessary.

ROLE OF SYNOVECTOMY IN JUVENILE RHEUMATOID ARTHRITIS

The use of synovectomy in the adult patient is a well-established principle in modern rheumatology. It is especially useful in the knee and metacarpophalangeal joints, is effective in relieving pain in the adult patient, and has been shown to arrest the progress of the disease in a significant number of patients. Orthopedists have been reluctant to perform synovectomies about the joints of immature patients for fear of damage to the growing epiphyseal cartilage. We have employed surgical synovectomy about the knee, hip, wrist, and elbow, and have as yet seen no evidence of damage to the epiphyseal plate. The procedure is best utilized early in the disease process. The indications at the present time include unresolved, persistent, progressive synovitis that is unrelieved by physical therapy, exercise, splinting, injection, and medication. The synovitis should be present at least six months and the diagnosis established beyond a reasonable doubt before synovectomy in the child is indicated. When joint destruction has already taken place in a joint that has been involved for several years and shows x-ray changes and loss of motion, synovectomy is of very little value and may increase stiffness. However, no decrease in the range of motion after synovectomy has yet been noted, and in an occasional patient some gain in range of motion has been achieved.

At the present time we are attempting to study the benefits of synovectomy in the juvenile patient. The ultimate goal is the eradication of disease in the operable joints. The recurrence rate and the permanent status of the joint will require study over a period of several years.

REFERENCES

Dwyer, F. C.: Osteotomy of the calcaneus for pes cavus. J. Bone Joint Surg., *41B*:80, 1959.

Engen, T. J.: Adjustable knee or elbow extension orthosis: a new orthotic development. Orth. Prosth. Appl. J., March, 1961.

Green, W. H.: Growth and prediction of growth in the lower extremities. J. Bone Joint Surg., *45A*:1, 1963.

Haggart, G. E.: Knee flexion contracture treated by skeletal traction. Surg. Gynec. Obstet., *61*:239, 1935.

Hoffman, P.: An operation for severe grades of contracted or clawed toes. Amer. J. Orthop. Surg., *9*:441, 1911-12.

Horwitz, M. T.: Conservative measures of correcting flexion deformity of the knee complicated by posterior subluxation of the tibia. J. Bone Joint Surg., *19*:522-523, 1937.

Irwin, C. E.: The ilio-tibial band. Its role in producing deformity in polio. J. Bone Joint Surg., *31A*:141, 1940.

Irwin, C. E.: Subtrochanteric osteotomy in polio. J.A.M.A., *133*:231, 1947.

Potter, T. A., and Kuhns, J. G.: Correction of arthritis deformities. *In* Hollander, J. L.: Arthritis and Allied Conditions, Ed. 7. Philadelphia, Lea & Febiger, 1966, p. 435.

Steindler, A.: Kinesiology of the Human Body. Springfield, Ill., Charles C Thomas, 1955, p. 522.

Wilson, P. D.: Posterior capsulotomy in certain flexion contractures of the knee. J. Bone Joint Surg., *11*:40, 1929.

Chapter Nine

DRUG THERAPY

SALICYLATES

History

Salicylates have been used in medicine since Hippocrates prescribed the juice of poplar trees for eye diseases. Thirty-six million aspirin tablets are consumed daily in the United States, an annual total sufficient to fill four 100-car freight trains (Bayer Co.). Perhaps the first extraction of salicylate was undertaken by Celsus in the first century A.D. He prescribed an extract of willow leaves boiled in vinegar for treatment of prolapse of the uterus. The Reverend Edward Stone in 1763 discussed the antipyretic action of willow bark while seeking a substitute for Peruvian bark in the treatment of malaria. Leroux in 1830 found that salicin was the active substance of willow bark. Acetylsalicylic acid was synthesized by a German chemist, Von Gerhardt, in 1853. Over 40 years later, the father of F. Hoffman, of the Bayer Company in Germany, suffered from severe rheumatoid arthritis. Unable to tolerate impure salicylate extracts, he used acetylsalicylic acid with success. The term "aspirin" was coined by Heinrich Dreser (1899) and it soon replaced most other forms of salicylate. MacLagan (1876), in England, is often given credit for introducing salicin as the major form of therapy for the treatment of rheumatism.

Chemistry

Salicylates comprise a group of compounds with orthohydroxybenzoic acid (salicylic acid) as the base. These compounds include salicylic acid, sodium salicylate, aspirin, and methyl salicylate. The major salicylate used today is acetylsalicylic acid, or aspirin. Aspirin is often combined with various antacids or coated with gelatin to reduce gastric irritation. It is one of the most successful anti-inflammatory agents and will usually produce significant reduction of joint swelling, increased range of motion, and reduction of pain in addition to reduced synovial involvement in patients with juvenile rheumatoid arthritis.

Pharmacologic and Physiologic Effects

The exact mechanism of salicylate action on the body remains unsolved, although much knowledge has been accumulated regarding specific effects (see Table 9-1).

Absorption, Distribution, and Excretion

Salicylates are almost always administered orally and the rate and degree of absorption are affected by the chemical state (solid or liquid), with the pH of stomach and intestines and viscosity of gastrointestinal fluid all affecting the rate of dissolution. Schematically, salicylate administered in solid form must undergo:

Dissolution →Diffusion to the gastrointestinal membrane →
→Diffusion through the membrane

The dissolution step is the slowest, and therefore determines the absorption rate (Levy, 1963). A solution of salicylate would be absorbed more quickly than a tablet but salicylate is rarely administered to a patient in solution form. Sodium acetylsalicylic acid and sodium salicylate have a dissolution rate more than 100 times faster than plain acetylsalicylic acid or salicylic acid. However, the sodium and calcium salts are extremely hygroscopic and absorb moisture in usual bottles, hydrolyze, and form a highly compact cemented tablet which dissolves slowly if at all, and is extremely irritating to the gastric mucosa (Levy, 1963). As the pH increases, absorption of the dissolved drug in the gastrointestinal tract increases. Certain buffered preparations, bicarbon-

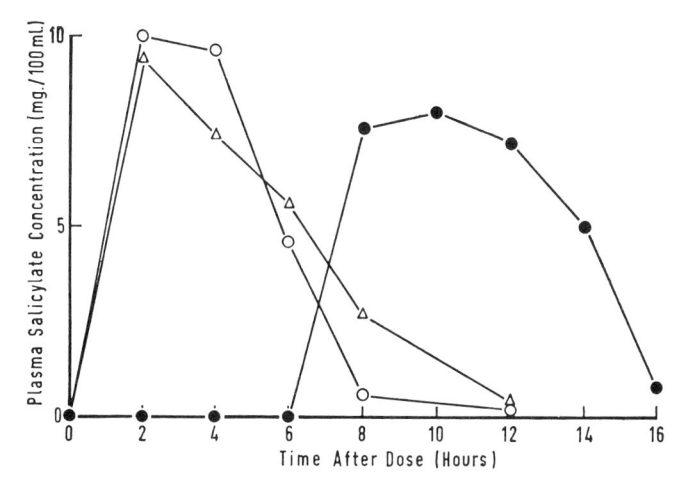

Figure 9-1 Plasma salicylate concentrations after a single dose of various aspirin preparations. 1.0 g. of an aspirin preparation was administered to the same subject in the fasting state on three occasions. Each point represents the mean of these three sets of observations. Plain aspirin is depicted by open circles, enteric-coated aspirin by closed circles, and aspirin-glycine by open triangles. The observations after buffered aspirin and soluble aspirin are not shown because they were almost identical to those after plain aspirin. (From Ansell, B. M.: Relationship of dosage and type of salicylate therapy to plasma levels in patients with juvenile rheumatoid arthritis. *In* Dixon, A. St. J., et al., [ed.]: Salicylates, an International Symposium. Boston, Little, Brown & Co., 1963, page 36. Courtesy of the Ciba Foundation.)

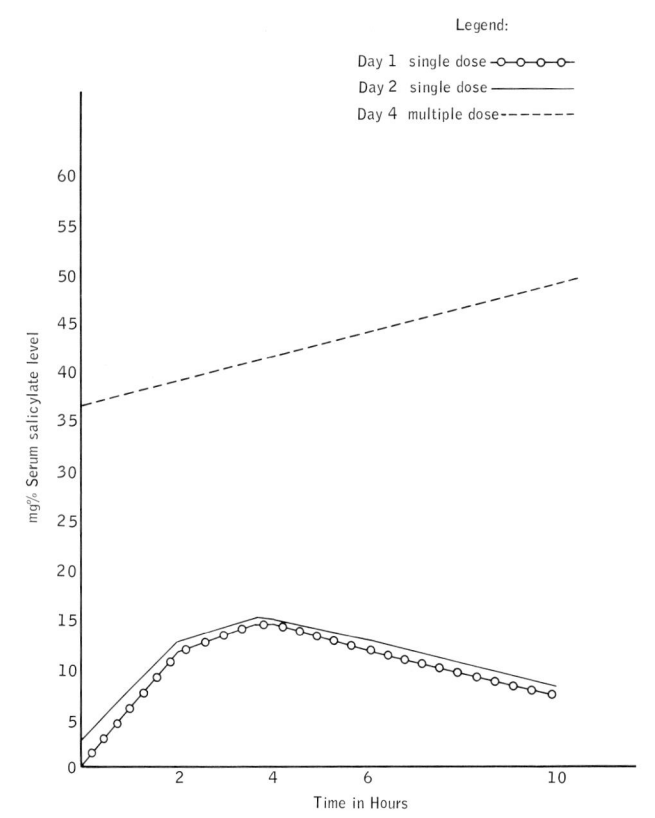

Figure 9-2 Mean serum salicylate levels following administration of acetylsalicylic acid (ASA) on a dosage basis of 800 mg./m.² of body surface area. (Day 4 is preceded by 3 days' dosage, 4 doses daily.)

ate, for example, are thought to increase the local pH around the dissolving acetylsalicylic acid and improve absorption. In addition, the buffering action is thought to reduce the gastric irritation and patients who complain of discomfort and pain after administration of ordinary acetylsalicylic acid have no further clinical complaints when using buffered preparations.

Tablet size and quality are also important in dissolution rate; highly compressed tablets are more difficult to dissolve and tend to break off in chunks, increasing gastric irritation. Acetylsalicylic acid is hydrolyzed to free salicylic acid in the stomach and small intestine with some direct absorption of acetylsalicylic acid across the mucosal membrane. Salicylate can be detected 30 minutes after ingestion, and peak blood levels are reached after about two hours in a fasting state (Fig. 9-1) and four hours in a nonfasting state (Fig. 9-2).

The rate of gastrointestinal absorption of salicylates given in solid form is limited by the dissolution process. The rate of dissolution of a salicylate is a function of its intrinsic dissolution rate, the pH, and the

Drug Therapy

Table 9-1 Salicylate Pharmacology

Type of Action	Clinical Effects	Mechanism
Analgesic	Selectively depresses central nervous system.	Poorly understood; possibly supraspinal; also peripheral.
Anti-inflammatory	Reduces swelling, erythema, and pain; antipyretic.	Unknown — may be effect of reducing capillary permeability.
Respiratory	Stimulates respiration directly and indirectly. Increases oxygen consumption.	Supramedullary?
Acid-base balance and electrolyte pattern	Respiratory alkalosis, renal compensation, then metabolic acidosis.	Increase of pH and decrease of CO_2. Excretion of bicarbonate sodium and potassium. Urine alkaline.
Cardiovascular	Flushing of skin; palpitations.	Dilatation of peripheral blood vessels with large doses by direct effect on their smooth muscle. Circulatory depressant with large doses by central vasomotor paralysis.
Gastrointestinal	Blood loss. Irritant on gastric mucosa. Peptic ulcer.	Direct effect, local ulceration.
Hepatic	Increases plasma prothrombin time.	No overt toxicity. Increase in volume output of bile. Decrease in cholate excretion.
Renal uricosuric	Increases urinary cellular element. Diuresis.	Sloughing of renal cells. Inhibits tubular reabsorption of urate and phosphate secondary to respiratory alkalosis.
Blood	Anemia	Major cause: Gastrointestinal blood loss. Minor cause: Increased erythrocyte destruction.
	Reduced ESR	Reduces plasma fibrinogen content.
Uricosuric	Increases excretion of urates. Large doses increase uricosuria and lower plasma urate levels.	
Metabolic	Undetermined	Oxidative phosphorylation; inhibition of glutamine synthesis; muscle phosphorylase activity. Stimulates adenosine triphosphatase activity in mitochondria.
Endocrine	Reduces blood sugar in diabetes.	Possibly due to uptake of glucose in peripheral tissues, muscle, etc.
	Decreases protein-bound iodine levels.	Interferes with binding of thyroxin.
	Depresses thyroid activity.	Decrease in radioiodine uptake and release.

Table 9-1 Salicylate Pharmacology *(Continued)*

Type of Action	Clinical Effects	Mechanism
Immunologic	Suppresses antibody production.	No single adequate explanation.
	Interferes with antigen-antibody aggregation.	
	Inhibits antigen-induced release of histamine (in vitro).	
	Stabilizes capillary permeability in presence of immunologic insult.	
Rare generalized side effects.	Aspirin allergy, skin rash, asthma.	

physicochemical properties of its pharmaceutical dosage form, among other factors. The absorption pattern of different salicylate compounds can be correlated with *in vitro* dissolution rate data and other physicochemical parameters. It is desirable that salicylate dosage regimes be based upon a consideration of kinetic factors, in order to prevent accumulation and to reduce the likelihood of toxicity (Levy, 1963).

Stable serum salicylate levels, however, are achieved on a multiple dosage schedule of every four hours during the day, after three days' administration (Fig. 9-2). This information is particularly important because administration every six hours is unnecessary and interferes with the patient's sleep, detracting from proper care.

Salicylate is absorbed as salicylic acid primarily, with small quantities of acetylsalicylic acid. The acetylsalicylic acid is rapidly metabolized within two hours in the serum. Salicylic acid quickly pervades the serum tissues, synovial tissues, spinal fluid, peritoneal fluid, saliva, and even milk. The placental barrier is readily crossed and there seems to be minimal secretion, if any, in sweat, bile, stool, or the intestinal tract. Varying high concentrations are found in liver, heart, lung, kidney, and synovial tissue. Of the final salicylate 50 to 80 per cent is bound to protein and the acetylsalicylic acid rapidly hydrolyzes to salicylic acid. Therapeutic levels are considered to be 15 to 30 mg. per 100 ml. However, distribution of salicylate is uneven in the body and tissue saturation is of equal importance in effect and toxicity. A serum salicylate level of 40 mg. per 100 ml. after sudden large ingestion is not as significant as the same level would be in a patient suffering from chronic salicylate toxicity with total saturation tissues at this level.

The excretion of salicylates is regulated chiefly by the glomerular filtration rate (GFR), the rate of proximal tubular secretion of salicylate, the rate of urine flow, and the pH of the urine. There are three chief metabolic products of salicylic acid: salicyluric acid, salicylic phenolic glucuronide, and salicylic acyl glucuronide, along with free salicylate and gentisic acid (Milne, 1963). Excretion is almost entirely in the urine with almost none in perspiration, bile or feces.

Of medical interest is the fact that, owing to alkalization of the urine, bicarbonate increases excretion. Almost all salicylate is eliminated in the urine within 48 hours after a single dose; in the case of prolonged multiple dosage there is a stabilization of excretion after the third day (Fig. 9-3).

Salicylates administered clinically to patients with juvenile rheumatoid arthritis are always acetylsalicylic acid in type. There are significant numbers of children who do complain of abdominal pain or other distress from uncoated aspirin. In patients who have this problem gastric distress can often be eliminated by the use of gelatin-coated preparations (Ecotrin) or a buffered preparation (Ascriptin or Bufferin). The pain is real and in spite of implications by many clinicians that relief is psychogenic, the buffered preparations do reduce or eliminate pain in a significant number of children and are worthwhile.

There is some difference in quality of aspirin tablets. Some are made in a so-called "one-press" technique that produces a tablet somewhat akin to hard brick. The author has on occasion taken a hammer to disintegrate some tablets, with little success. Absorption and dissolution of such a tablet are obviously difficult. The calcium and sodium salt salicylate preparations offer many advantages in absorption, but they are hygroscopic and absorb water ferociously, pro-

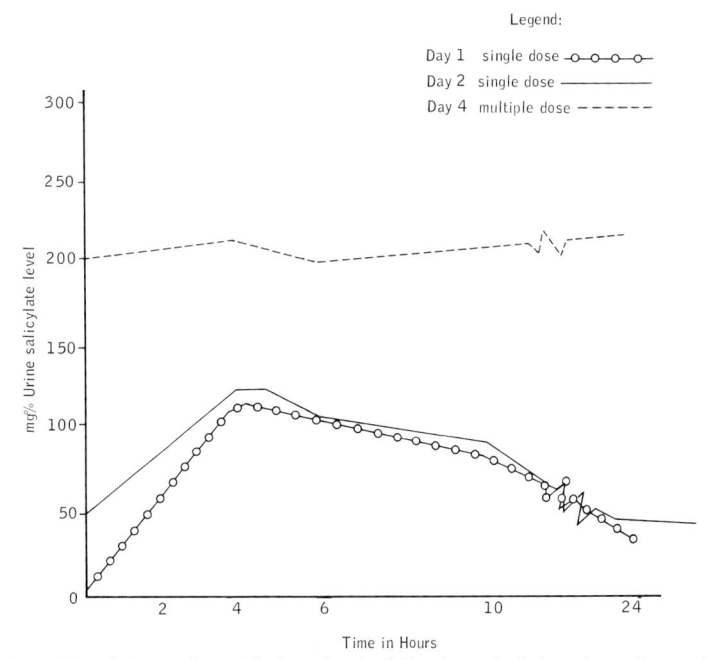

Figure 9-3 Mean urine salicylate levels following administration of acetylsalicylic acid on a dosage basis of 800 mg./m.^{2} of body surface. (Day 4 is preceded by 3 days' dosage, 4 doses daily.)

ducing a cement-glue type of substance in the bottle. Therefore, they are not as practical as plain aspirin preparations.

The dosage of salicylate is variable and the initial dosage prescribed at the Texas Children's Hospital Clinic has been 800 mg./m.^{2} per dose, four doses daily. This dosage can be reduced or increased, depending on clinical response or toxicity. In general, sufficient aspirin is given to produce satisfactory clinical effects but it is always less than the dosage that produces significant side effects such as gastric distress or other manifestations of excessive dosage. The serum salicylate level is not related to clinical response or toxicity directly. Generally, maintenance of a level 15 to 25 mg. per 100 ml. is attempted but there is wide variability (Brewer, 1966). Thirty-two patients were studied in the National Institutes of Health Clinical Research Center* at Texas Children's Hospital where a prescribed dosage of aspirin was given over a period of time. The results revealed that salicylate levels were about 36 mg. per 100 ml. on the average (Fig. 9-4). Upon discharge from hospital the same patients were continued on the same dosage of salicylate and random salicylate samples were taken in the clinic several months later. The average salicylate level in the patient now showed 15 mg. per 100 ml. The obvious implication is that patients forget to take medication at home. This is found to be the usual reason for the variability in serum salicylate levels and seemingly poor response to therapy. There are, however, occasional patients who do not absorb salicylate and no detectable salicylate levels are present in their serum despite massive dosage.

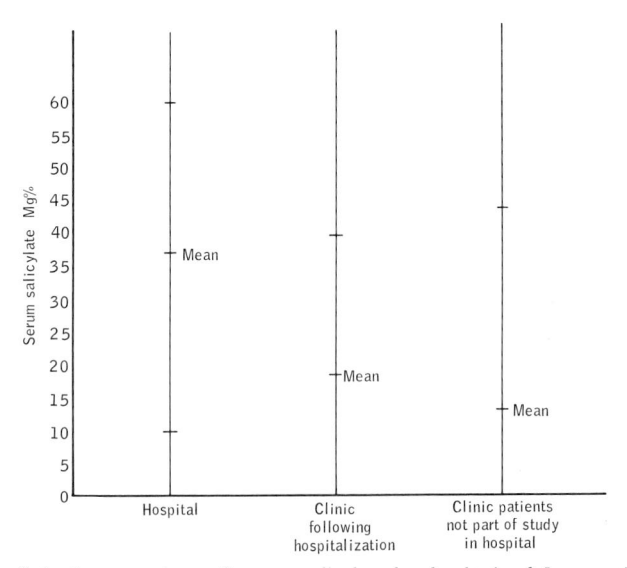

Figure 9-4 A comparison of serum salicylate levels obtained from patients in hospital, in clinic following hospitalization, and patients seen in clinic but who were not part of study.

*N.I.H. Grant FR-188.

Drug Therapy

Table 9-2 Reduction in Joint Swelling following Four Consecutive Days of Salicylates

Number of Joints Improved	Number of Patients*	Number of Joints Showing Significant Reduction	
		1/4″	1/2″
1	10	7	3
2	7	13	1
3	2	6	0
4	2	6	2
5	1	0	5
Totals	22	32	11

*Eight patients failed to exhibit any significant reduction in joint swelling.

Acetylsalicylic acid does have a significant anti-inflammatory effect that in juvenile rheumatoid arthritis can be quite striking. The usual response is some decrease in joint swelling and discomfort, and an increase in the feeling of well-being (Tables 9-2 and 9-3). However, there is certainly not the dramatic remission that occurs in rheumatic fever after several days of acetylsalicylic acid therapy.

Side Effects or Toxicity in Salicylate Administration

Gastrointestinal

1. The most striking and prominent toxicity in salicylate administration is related to the gastrointestinal tract, i.e., epigastric pain, peptic ulceration, and chronic blood loss.
2. Six ml. per day of blood may be lost in the stool during prolonged administration (see Chapter 1).

Table 9-3 Change in Range of Motion following Four Consecutive Days of Salicylates

Number of Joints Improved	Number of Patients*	Change in Range of Motion				
		5°	10°	15°	20°	35°
1	9	3	3	1	2	0
2	4	7	1	0	0	0
3	4	6	5	1	0	0
4	6	10	10	2	0	2
5	1	3	2	0	0	0
6	2	11	1	0	0	0
8	1	6	2	0	0	0
Totals	27	46	24	4	2	2

*Three patients failed to show any increase in range of motion.

3. If a piece of aspirin is placed against the buccal mucosa for ten to fifteen minutes a definite local ulcer will occur.

Acid-base Imbalance
1. The next most prominent side effect of salicylate is the disturbance in acid-base balance, resulting initially in respiratory alkylosis and later in metabolic acidosis. This condition can be controlled by eliminating salicylate administration for a day or two and reinstituting dosage at a lower level. This does not apply to acute salicylate poisoning.

Other Side Effects
1. Patients who take salicylates can develop hypersensitivity. Allergic rashes and anaphylactic shock are known to occur. However, this sort of reaction applies to any organic chemical and is quite rare.
2. Aspirin causes constipation in certain people.
3. In some children drowsiness is a rare but well delineated side effect.
4. An occasional child will have serious and significant fluid retention and edema.
5. Some children have excessive perspiration.
6. At least one or two patients have complained of palpitations that proved to be reproducible.
7. Rarely, a headache may be caused by aspirin.

STEROIDS

The introduction of adrenocorticosteroids in the treatment of rheumatoid arthritis and inflammatory disease in general in 1949 provided the single greatest impetus to lay and medical interest in rheumatic diseases. The corticosteroids have since become an accepted and needed part of the medical armamentarium but hopes for an incisive thrust against the ravages of rheumatoid arthritis have been cut short by the two-edged sword of significant toxicity. Steroid therapy continues to be a needed and useful treatment of juvenile rheumatoid arthritis when other agents fail to control clinical manifestations that either threaten life or prevent even basic activity. It is just as wrong to deny completely the use of steroids to certain patients as it is to overzealously prescribe steroids to children with minimal disease that may be satisfactorily controlled by other methods.

Advantages of Corticosteroids as Anti-inflammatory Agents in Juvenile Rheumatoid Arthritis

1. Fever is reduced.
2. Patients feel better.
3. Subjective strength is improved.
4. Appetite is better.
5. Swelling and stiffness of joints are reduced.
6. Inflammation of iridocyclitis is suppressed.

7. Size of subcutaneous nodules, enlarged liver, and spleen is decreased.
8. Polyserositis, including pericardial effusion, is suppressed.

One of the chief advantages of steroid medication in juvenile rheumatoid arthritis is the significant reduction of fever. Fever is not only a nuisance but can cause significant morbidity. Aspirin or indomethacin should be tried as antipyretic agents before corticosteroid medication is attempted (Brewer, 1968). Children often feel better and have a better appetite on corticosteroid medication, particularly at the beginning of therapy. This effect is not usually sustained but can serve a valuable purpose during the initial phases of therapy. Subjective improvement in strength is noted in children beginning corticosteroid therapy, again as an unsustained effect of the medication. A few children, however, do seem to have significant weakness, loss of appetite, and some depression.

Even though corticosteroid therapy does not cure rheumatoid arthritis, significant reduction of both swelling and stiffness of joints does occur. The degree of reduction in morbidity varies from patient to patient, but can be quite striking. In most patients there is at least some reduction in swelling and also improvement of motion.

Disadvantages of Corticosteroid Therapy in Juvenile Rheumatoid Arthritis

1. Will not prevent progression of erosive arthritis or joint destruction.
2. Toxicity is awesome.
3. Dosage must often be increased to maintain improvement.
4. Even on higher dosage, improvement often is not maintained.
5. Reduction of dosage results in temporary withdrawal symptoms.
6. Steroid addiction is a common problem (i.e., inability to remove patient from drug because of withdrawal manifestations or severe exacerbations).

Table 9-4, listing a few of the major side effects of corticosteroid administration, makes abundantly clear the need for careful consideration before committing a patient to long-term or even short-term steroid therapy. All patients with juvenile rheumatoid arthritis should have a fair trial on other modes of treatment before corticosteroids are begun. The only exception would be an acute life-threatening situation demanding immediate temporary relief of clinical manifestations. There are circumstances, however, in which corticosteroids have proved to be the only agent of benefit, in conjunction with a planned treatment program of rest, heat, and adequate exercise.

Patients in whom Steroids are Never Used

1. *Children with juvenile rheumatoid arthritis who have a mild form of peripheral articular disease,* manifested by some soft tissue swelling and minimal pain and discomfort, should never receive corticosteroid

Table 9-4 Clinical Manifestations of Pharmacologic-Physiologic Changes Caused by Corticosteroids

Pharmacologic-Physiologic Changes	Clinical Manifestations
Electrolytes	
1. ↑ Sodium retention	Hypervolemia, edema, and hypertension
2. ↑ Potassium excretion, titratable acid	Weakness and fatigue
3. ↑ Calcium excretion	Osteoporosis and pathologic fractures
4. Alkalosis	
Carbohydrate and Protein	
1. ↑ Gluconeogenesis	Loss of muscle mass
2. Hyperglycemia and glycosuria (decreased glucose tolerance, increased insulin tolerance)	"Temporary diabetes"
3. ↑ Tissue catabolism with ↓ anabolism	Wasting of muscle mass, osteoporosis, and pathologic fractures; atrophy of skin, easy bruising; striae; interruption of growth
Fat	
Redistribution of fat	Obesity with centripetal fat distribution; striae; atherosclerosis
Cardiovascular System	
Enhanced pressor effect of norepinephrine	The clinical importance of enhanced pressor effect is still unknown. May increase peripheral resistance leading to left ventricular aneurysm
Central Nervous System	
↑ Excitability	Euphoria; depression; convulsions in epileptic-prone; psychotic episodes
Lymphoid Tissue	
1. Lymphocytopenia	
2. ↓ Mass of lymphoid tissue	
Hematologic Changes	
1. ↓ Eosinophils	
2. ↑ Neutrophils	
3. ↑ RBC production	Polycythemia, intravascular thrombosis
Connective Tissue and Wound Healing	
1. ↑ Tissue catabolism and ↓ anabolism (a) fibroblasts (b) ground substance (c) granulation tissue	Impairs wound healing; masks manifestations of infection
2. ↓ Vascularization	Ulcerogenic
Androgenic Activity	
17-Ketosteroid degradation products	Acne; baldness; deepening of the voice; amenorrhea; varying degrees of enlargement of clitoris; virilization
Miscellaneous	
	Steroid addiction; posterior subcapsular cataracts; does not prevent progression of lesions; hirsutism

therapy. These patients are best controlled by salicylate therapy in appropriate dosage, along with rest, heat, and exercise. Even if these patients respond poorly to salicylates and mild articular disease persists, corticosteroid therapy must not be instituted. Steroid addiction is a real syndrome and must be avoided whenever possible.

2. *Juvenile rheumatoid arthritis patients who respond reasonably well to other agents.* Many patients who have significant peripheral articular disease with fever and perhaps anemia obtain moderate improvement with salicylate therapy and the basic conservative program of therapy. There is always a temptation on the part of the physician who is trying to do his best for his patient, to try something else to further improve the state of the patient's health. Juvenile rheumatoid arthritis patients with significant peripheral articular disease who respond well enough functionally and have no signs of continuing persistent fever should not receive corticosteroids. The adage that "a little bit is good and more is better" does not apply in this type of situation. Relief is often striking initially, as is well known, but unfortunately the need for ever-increasing dosage of steroids occurs, and when the medication is withdrawn exacerbation results. At times the patient must remain on the medication or sustain serious exacerbation of disease.

3. *Severely afflicted juvenile rheumatoid arthritis patients who have not attempted the basic conservative program of therapy and treatment with salicylates or other agents.* One of the most disconcerting manifestations of juvenile rheumatoid arthritis is high intermittent fever, occurring over a period of days, weeks, months, or even years, that is uncontrolled by salicylates or other usual antipyretics. In the past corticosteroids have performed a valuable function in reducing fever in these children and allowing them to feel well enough to carry on more normal activities. Indomethacin has been shown to be an effective agent in the control of fever, and certainly is less toxic than corticosteroid medication. For this reason the author feels that patients with high fever and a mild to moderately severe peripheral articular form of disease should have a trial on indomethacin therapy prior to institution of corticosteroid therapy (see *Indomethacin* later in this chapter).

4. *The presence of suspected or known sepsis or pyogenic arthritis* in conjunction with rheumatoid arthritis probably contraindicates the use of corticosteroids.

5. *Associated conditions that may mitigate against corticosteroid therapy* include diabetes, peptic ulcer, central nervous system disease including neuroses and psychoses, hypertension, and significant chronic renal disease.

Conditions in which Corticosteroid Therapy is Desirable

1. *Patients with iridocyclitis or uveitis* should definitely be given a course of corticosteroids, in view of the high percentage of such patients who develop blindness. Local corticosteroid eyedrops and systemic corticosteroid therapy are both indicated in this condition. Local steroid and corticosteroid eyedrops in mild iridocyclitis can often suf-

fice for remission. In many cases, however, the disease continues its dreadful progression toward blindness in spite of therapy.

2. *Patients with high fever and severe peripheral articular disease not responding to salicylates or indomethacin.* Children who have high intermittent fever (near 106° F.) usually are not able to sustain normal activity or even near normal activity. Even in the absence of severe peripheral articular disease such fever must be controlled if at all possible. A trial on salicylates, acetaminophen, and indomethacin should be given prior to the use of corticosteroids. In the absence of relief from the other agents the corticosteroids should be administered and often will provide relief. Occasionally corticosteroids must be combined with salicylates or other medications for relief. Gold and chloroquine are not effective antipyretic agents.

3. *Patients with clinically severe pericarditis.* Lietman and Bywaters (1963) have shown that in 24 patients treated for pericarditis, half of whom were given steroid therapy and half of whom were given salicylate therapy, the mortality rate was approximately the same. Patients with clinically severe pericarditis do show marked and rapid improvement in morbidity with administration of steroids. Patients with marked dyspnea and signs of serious pericardial effusion often sustain relief within twelve to 24 hours. Also, the use of steroids has reduced the need for pericardicentesis. The medication should be continued for a period of several months until the heart returns to normal size.

4. *Patients who have been committed to long periods of total immobilization.* Occasionally, patients have been seen who, for one reason or another, have been committed to total bed immobilization for one to four or five years. These patients usually have received little physical therapy, are unable to perform even basic activities out of bed, and are completely bedridden. Such patients often have fibrous ankylosis and marked weakness. During the therapeutic treatment at the hospital their strength is increased on a planned, progressive scale by the physical therapist. To overcome postural hypotension tip-table beds are used to increase the ability of the patient to sustain changes in blood pressure from the supine to the standing position. Patients who are committed to this program of ambulation require weeks, and even months, of devoted treatment by the physical therapist to increase muscular strength and the ability to maintain the standing position for walking. Corticosteroids seem to hasten the subjective improvement of the patient by increasing strength and reducing stiffness and swelling, thereby aiding mobility. In addition, corticosteroids help in elevating the blood pressure and reducing postural hypotension, enabling the physical therapist to begin ambulation sooner.

5. *Patients with severe peripheral articular disease unable to perform basic activity because of pain and limitation.* Patients who have severe rheumatoid arthritis and are unable to function in basic daily activities in spite of conservative measures and the use of salicylates or gold should probably have a trial on corticosteroid therapy. Patients on corticosteroids who sustain sufficient improvement in performing activities should probably be continued on corticosteroid therapy. As pointed

out previously, it is just as wrong to deny completely the use of steroids to certain patients as it is to prescribe steroids overzealously to children with minimal disease that can be controlled by other methods.

Administration and Dosage of Corticosteroids

Table 9-5 lists some of the large number of corticosteroid derivatives available for use in therapy. Each was developed in the hope that toxic side effects could be minimized and anti-inflammatory effects could be enhanced. Unfortunately, the development of more purified derivatives resulted essentially in a "battle of the milligrams." While each of the derivatives was shown to be more potent, a smaller amount was used in each tablet and the side effects, except for a few variations, were proved to be the same.

Prednisone has become almost a standard medication. Its sodium-retaining capacity is somewhat less than that of hydrocortisone and its anti-inflammatory potency is several times greater than that of cortisone acetate. Therefore, in the dosage prescribed, edema and cushingoid side effects are less serious than in patients treated with cortisone acetate. The other corticosteroid derivatives, while more potent with regard to anti-inflammatory activity, nevertheless have not been shown to have any significant advantages over the other corticosteroid derivatives.

Basic Principles for Use of Corticosteroid Medication

Dosage. 10 mg. prednisone or the equivalent in other derivatives is the preferred daily dosage to use at the beginning of therapy, and as therapy progresses. In the Texas Children's Hospital group of patients, peptic ulcer did not occur in those patients who received less than 10 mg. per day of corticosteroid medication.

Fisher, Panos, and Melby (1964) advocated the use of large doses

Table 9-5 Relative Anti-inflammatory Potencies of Some Corticosteroids

Compound	Relative Anti-inflammatory Potency	Relative Sodium-retaining Potency
Hydrocortisone	1	1
Cortisone	0.8	0.8
Prednisone	3.5	0.8
Prednisolone	4	0.8
Methylprednisolone	5	0
Triamcinolone	5	0
Dexamethasone	25	0
Betamethasone	25	0
Paramethasone	10	0
9a-Fluorocortisol	15	125

of corticosteroid every other day to reduce the awesome toxicity. This method has been used for many years by nephrologists in treating nephrosis and does offer considerable advantage.

The author feels that a patient who can remain off corticosteroid medication 48 hours with no exacerbation of symptoms probably does not need corticosteroid medication. The use of corticosteroid is symptomatic, as an anti-inflammatory suppressant, and other methods of treatment are preferred if the disease is so mild that a prolonged period of time may elapse between dosages of medication.

The dosage of corticosteroid varies enormously among rheumatologists and pediatricians treating juvenile rheumatoid arthritis. In general, rheumatologists trained in internal medicine use 1 to 10 mg. per day and rarely exceed this dosage; 20 mg. per day of prednisone or its equivalent is considered an extremely large dose. Pediatricians, because of their experience with the nephrotic child, often use enormous doses, in the neighborhood of 60 mg./m.^{2} daily of prednisone or its equivalent. This results in significant and serious side effects very quickly, without significant benefits over the lower dosage.

Choosing the proper dosage is much like zeroing in on target during an effective artillery barrage. The proper dosage is more than an ineffectual dose but less than a dosage causing significant toxicity such as hypertension. The patient, therefore, should be given an empirical initial dosage which can then be reduced until exacerbation of the disease is manifested.

Duration of Therapy and Reduction of Dosage. From the day corticosteroid therapy is begun, the physician begins a never-ending battle to discontinue the medication. The ideal dosage of corticosteroid is zero. The ideal duration of steroid therapy is zero, and any greater dosage or longer duration is less than perfect. If the patient is on 10 mg. per day of prednisone, in three or four divided doses, attempts should be made in a few weeks to reduce the amount of corticosteroid necessary to control the symptoms requiring institution of therapy. If the patient requires 20 mg. of corticosteroid derivatives, an attempt to reduce the dosage to 10 mg. or less is particularly imperative because the risk of peptic ulcer is vastly reduced on the reduced dosage.

In general, once the use of corticosteroid derivatives has begun in patients with severe disease, the course of therapy is considered in terms of months or years. For example, a typical course of therapy may begin with the administration of corticosteroid at a level of 10 mg. per day. The patient improves temporarily, is able to return to more normal activity, and feels subjectively better. However, improvement is only temporary, and the patient's dosage is increased to 12 or 15 mg. daily, resulting again in temporary improvement. Continuing and more frequent rounds of increased dosage follow, resulting in less and less improvement and more and more toxicity. If steroid dosage is suddenly discontinued completely, serious exacerbation of disease results and withdrawal symptoms are quite significant. This pattern fulfills the criteria for drug addiction, since more and more of the drug is required for suppression of symptoms, with less and less effect; the drug is harmful and produces significant changes within the body, and serious withdrawal effects occur upon discontinuation. Indeed, steroid addiction is very real. The problem of increased dosage and reduced response has been exaggerated, obviously, but the point cannot be emphasized too strongly that increasing dosage of prednisone above 10 to 20 mg. per day is nonproductive and can result in quite serious deleterious effects on the patient. More specifically, in the opinion of the author, nothing is to be gained by the use of 40 or 50 mg. of prednisone per day that 5 to 15 mg. per day does not offer.

In the continuing effort to reduce dosage of steroids, large reductions of medication are possible at higher dosage levels. For the patient receiving 20 mg. per day, dosage can be reduced to 15 mg. per day with reasonable ease. However, for the patient receiving 5 mg. per day dosage cannot be completely discontinued without usually producing serious exacerbation of disease. Effective reduction may be considered in terms of a percentage of the total dose rather than any specific number of milligrams.

Reduction should be carried out over a period of weeks rather than days. In general, one should not reduce the daily dosage by more than one-fourth at any given time. This means that at a level of 20 mg. per day the dosage can be reduced to 15 mg. per day, but at 5 mg. per day the dosage should be reduced only to 4 mg. per day. Clinically, in children, the most difficult time period of steroid reduction is that period when the child is receiving 2 to 5 mg. per day. Reduction by even 1 or 2 mg. per day results in significant withdrawal symptoms and, at this stage, several weeks often must elapse between such reductions. When the dosage approaches 1 or 2 mg. per day the patient often does better by retaining a dosage of 1 to 3 mg. daily but receiving the medication every other day. With this approach one may give the reduced dosage every second day, then every third day, every fourth day, and every fifth day until the administration of corticosteroids is discontinued. Another method of withdrawing corticosteroid therapy is to administer 10 to 30 units of ACTH every few days while reducing the dosage of oral prednisone or other corticosteroid derivatives.

Corticosteroid Withdrawal Symptoms

Good (1959) described pseudorheumatism, or withdrawal symptoms that occur upon reduction of corticosteroid dosage in patients with or without rheumatoid arthritis. The manifestations are particularly prominent in children with rheumatoid arthritis. The usual sequence is that, upon too rapid reduction of dosage (within one or two days), the patient develops significant exacerbation of disease with swelling and pain, or pain and tenderness, of several joints. Usually this amounts to exacerbation of peripheral articular disease, but fever also can occur if the patient has had fever with prior exacerbations. After three to five days the withdrawal symptoms disappear if the new and lower dosage of corticosteroid is effective. If symptoms persist, the patient then has to be given an increased dosage again.

If pain and discomfort were the only problems resulting from withdrawal of the drug, then the clinician would not be unduly worried and the dosage could be rather easily discontinued, with the knowledge that only a period of unpleasant symptomatology would occur. However, Dees (1959) reported the occurrence of coma following the termination of corticosteroid therapy. The coma persisted until parenteral corticosteroids were administered, and the patient responded within a few hours. Coma has also occurred in at least one of our own patients at Texas Children's Hospital. This particular child developed coma upon abrupt withdrawal of corticosteroid therapy and was thought to be near death when steroids were readministered and the patient rather miraculously became conscious and seemingly normal after only a few hours. In this patient a marked increase in cerebrospinal fluid sodium was demonstrated during the period of unconsciousness before steroid was administered again. The cerebrospinal fluid determinations were made in an indirect attempt to establish whether there had been an intracellular dehydration because of steroid withdrawal, with a sudden shift of salt from the cell to the cerebrospinal fluid.

The duration of steroid therapy is the shortest period of time necessary to help the patient. The withdrawal of steroids must be stepwise, and executed slowly if the patient has been on steroids longer than one month. Dependence on corticosteroid medication develops and steroid addiction is a difficult problem.

Steroid Toxicity

Bywaters (1965) reported 25 deaths in a group of 154 patients treated with corticosteroids for more than one month (Table 9-6). This is considerably more than the usual mortality rate of 4 to 5 per cent in juvenile rheumatoid arthritis. Significant infections occurred in about one-fourth of his patients, and gastrointestinal complications, including

Table 9-6 Toxicity in Steroid Treatment*

Complication	Number of Patients Affected†
Deaths during steroid treatment	25
Infections	40
Gastrointestinal complications	34
Vascular disorders	27
Hypertension	13
Osteoporosis	25
Osteoporosis with fractures	6
Mental disturbance	8
Glycosuria	3
No complications	43

*Bywaters, E. G. L.: The present status of steroid treatment in rheumatoid arthritis. Proc. Roy. Soc. Med., 58:650, 1965.

†Total of 154 patients (122 with rheumatoid arthritis) treated with steroids for more than one month.

peptic ulcer, occurred in over 20 per cent. Vascular disorders and hypertension occurred in over one-fourth of the patients. Significant osteoporosis, including pathologic fractures in six patients, occurred in over one-fourth of the patients treated. It should be noted, however, that all patients in Bywaters' series were adults.

Cushingoid Changes

In patients treated with significant dosage of steroids there is a redistribution of fat, leading to obesity. A centripetal fat distribution occurs and striae secondary to rapid stretching of the skin result from the change in fat distribution. Patients develop the classic puffy cushingoid facies, with a hump over the upper dorsal spine in extreme instances. Acneiform lesions on the face and shoulders also develop secondary to the androgenic activity resulting from corticosteroid medication. The acne is controlled as the acne of adolescence, with appropriate cleansing agents and astringents. Along with acneiform lesions there can occur deepening of the voice, varying degrees of clitoral enlargement, and masculinization of the female.

An interesting phenomenon in children is the marked increase in hair on the arms and legs that seems to occur with corticosteroid medication. Part of this is related to the inanition of the rheumatoid arthritis disease process. Baldness is known to occur with corticosteroid medication but is certainly not very common.

Hypertension

Significant hypertension can occur with excessive corticosteroid medication. Hypertensive encephalopathy with convulsions can be a significant problem and the convulsions can cause compression fractures of the vertebral bodies because of the accompanying osteoporosis.

Usually the hypertension, when the patient is carefully observed, will range from 140/90 to 170/110 mm./Hg, with relatively few symptoms other than headaches and possibly some visual disturbances. When the medication is decreased about one-fourth, the hypertension frequently disappears. The presence of mild hypertension does not mean the corticosteroid therapy must be terminated completely but the dosage ought to be reduced. The patient should not be allowed to persist with significant hypertension.

Edema

Edema occurs secondary to salt retention and generally is not a serious problem other than the unsightly cosmetic effect. Occasionally a patient may develop edema of the brain. A 14-year-old boy with rheumatoid arthritis had significant pericarditis and required corticosteroid derivatives over a period of years. He developed cerebral edema and papilledema secondary to steroid medication. No hypertension was present. When steroid medication was reduced an exacerbation of cardiac symptoms occurred, requiring increased steroids. When steroids were increased again, the patient again developed signs of increased intracranial pressure, and finally coma resulted. The increase in intracranial pressure was successfully reduced with intravenous injections of mannitol, and control of the rheumatologic symptoms was finally achieved with indomethacin, allowing elimination of corticosteroid medication. This patient demonstrates an idiosyncrasy of the drug, but also illustrates that edema itself, in the wrong location, can be a significant problem.

Osteoporosis

Generalized osteoporosis occurs within a month or two in most children receiving corticosteroid medication. There is increased calcium excretion and retarded anabolism of matrix, resulting not only in inadequate calcium deposition in bone but also in unusual loss of calcium. The osteoporosis can be serious and pathologic fractures can occur secondary to the weakness of the cortex caused by thinning in poor quality bone (Fig. 9-5). Fractures of this nature occur in the long bones after minimal trauma, or compression fractures of the vertebral bodies may result from convulsions or lifting activities. Tomkins and Whedon have postulated that an increased calcium intake might help prevent, or at least retard, the development of osteoporosis.

Inflammatory Suppressant Activity

Masking of Infection. The inflammatory and suppressant effects of corticosteroids definitely reduce the clinical symptoms of serious infectious disease. Mild abdominal pain in the right lower quadrant might well represent impending peritonitis secondary to a ruptured appendix. A patient with pneumonia or meningitis may feel only moderately ill because of the almost euphoric changes that can occur in some patients on corticosteroids. In general, the masking is not a serious problem, but a very real problem is the differentiation of the muscular aches and pains and vague abdominal pain present in so many children with rheumatoid arthritis who are on corticosteroid therapy.

In children receiving corticosteroid therapy respiratory infections are treated with more interest than would otherwise be necessary, and antibiotics are more freely given. The level of fever is certainly reduced in patients who are on corticosteroid therapy. Corticosteroids can prevent the fever of an infectious disease, thereby robbing the patient and physician of a valuable diagnostic tool.

Delayed Healing. Wound healing may be delayed in patients receiving corticosteroid therapy but in the author's experience surgical procedures can be safely carried out if necessary, and healing of lacerations has not presented a problem. The nutritional status of the patient is probably as important as corticosteroid medication in healing wounds.

Peptic Ulceration. Patients with rheumatoid arthritis have a greater propensity to develop peptic ulcer than the general population.

Figure 9-5 Fracture of the distal right femoral metaphysis in a child on prolonged steroid therapy. The bones are osteoporotic and there is excess subcutaneous fat. A buckle fracture of the distal femoral metaphysis is evident. The knee joint space is reduced in height and there is soft tissue swelling about the joint.

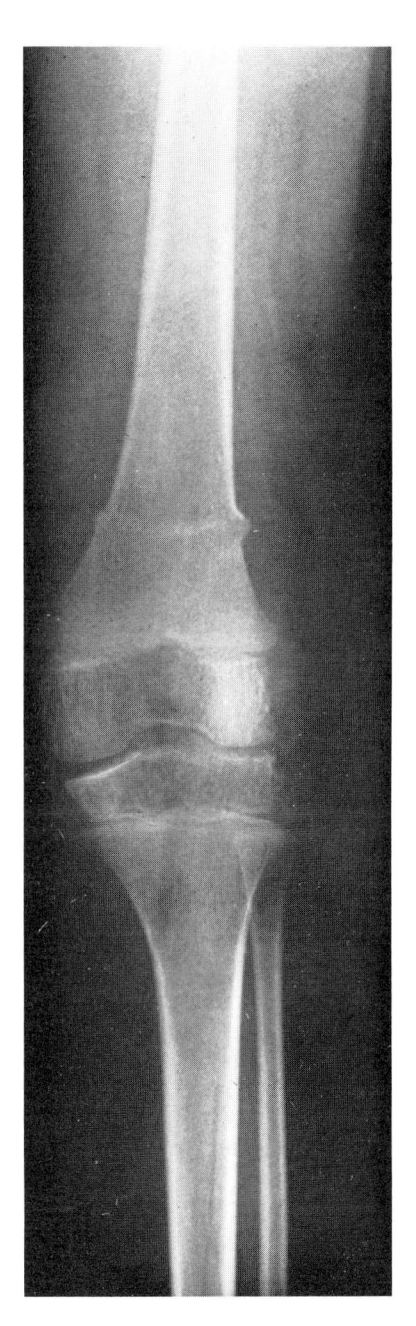

With the addition of corticosteroid medication the likelihood of peptic ulcer is increased greatly. No specific studies have been done with regard to the incidence of peptic ulcer in children receiving corticosteroid therapy, but it probably approaches 5 to 10 per cent (see Chapter 1). It is important to emphasize that peptic ulcer patients may usually be continued on corticosteroid therapy of less than 10 mg. of prednisone per day, and that healing of peptic ulcer does usually occur quite satisfactorily with appropriate medication.

Central Nervous System

Most children receiving dosage of 10 mg. prednisone or its equivalent per day have few central nervous system symptoms, and only occasional patients have problems. Euphoria is a very real manifestation and a definite side effect of prednisone administration. Children with rheumatoid arthritis who are chronically ill and depressed, with poor appetite, often show significant improvement because of this side effect alone. If it were not for the other awesome toxic manifestations steroids would have great benefit because of the euphoria produced in some patients. Unfortunately a pleasant euphoria is not always the result. Agitation, restlessness, inability to sleep, and irritability are but a few of the psychological changes that may occur.

Convulsions in epileptic-prone individuals are probably the most dramatic and terrifying side effects. Convulsions can be severe enough to cause compression fractures of vertebral bodies in patients with significant osteoporosis.

Psychotic changes in behavior, with corticosteroid derivatives in particular, are known. One patient was given dexamethasone and developed such hostile behavior that he chased his mother around the kitchen with a butcher knife. The effect wore off in a matter of a day. For obvious reasons, no attempt was made to prove the effect by a second trial.

Another patient was begun on dexamethasone, and within a three- to four-week period his weight increased from 44 pounds to 66 pounds. This represented a 50 per cent increase in body mass and was not mainly due to edema or retention of fluid. The patient would eat all the food in the refrigerator from day to day and accuse his mother of trying to starve him to death. When the patient was seen at the end of a two-week period, it was apparent that a psychic increase in appetite and an almost paranoid reaction to food denial had occurred. The patient retained the psychic disturbance for another week or so after discontinuation of the drug, but otherwise had no further trouble after withdrawal.

Posterior Subcapsular Cataracts

Posterior subcapsular cataracts in patients treated with corticosteroids were first reported by Black (1960). The incidence has varied from 9 per cent (Gordon, 1961) to over 40 per cent (Black, 1960). Posterior subcapsular cataracts occur in older adults but have not been reported in children. The author is unable to document that any child has required surgical removal of posterior subcapsular cataracts due to corticosteroid medication. Interference with vision in children must be minimal and the incidence is not yet established.

Intra-articular Corticosteroid Therapy

Cortisone acetate was first injected into a human joint by Thorn and Hollander (1951), who found that about one-fourth of the patients developed striking subjective improvement but minimal or transient reduction in swelling or temperature of the joint. Hydrocortisone was then shown to have better anti-inflammatory effect and was used by Hollander in 1951 with great success. Suppression of inflammation occurred in 90 per cent of his patients within one day after injection of 25 mg. of hydrocortisone intra-articularly. The duration of benefit was variable, ranging from a few days to many weeks. Since that time, Hollander has administered over 150,000 intrasynovial injections to more than 5000 patients with amazing results. The average duration of therapy with hydrocortisone was about six days. As newer corticosteroid derivatives appeared, the duration of significant clinical improvement was increased to an average of 14 days with prednisolone tertiary butylacetate.

Indications for intra-articular steroid therapy in pediatric subjects are the same as in adults (Table 9-7). The chief indication for use in children with rheumatoid arthritis has been for the patient with monarticular disease of weight-bearing joints. This has been proved quite often to be a satisfactory method of therapy and clinical improvement or remission lasts up to several months after a single injection. In children the response is often especially gratifying and lasts for a considerable period of time, in terms of months rather than days or weeks. Repeated injections can be limited by the hesitation of some children to subject themselves to repeated procedures. The reaction of the child is dependent upon the child's own reaction pattern of fear instilled by the

Table 9-7 Indications for Intra-articular Corticosteroid Injection*

1. When one or only a few peripheral joints are inflamed, provided specific infection has been excluded as the cause.
2. In a few actively inflamed joints, even in the presence of more generalized low-grade involvement.
3. In rheumatoid arthritis, as an adjunct to gold or other drug therapy.
4. When systemic cortisone, gold, or other therapy is contraindicated.
5. As an adjunct to systemic cortisone or other therapy for control of "resistant" joints.
6. To assist in rehabilitation and prevention of joint deformity.
7. As an adjunct to orthopedic procedures.

*From Hollander, J. L.: Intrasynovial corticosteroid therapy, in Hollander, J. L.: Arthritis and Allied Conditions, ed. 7. Philadelphia, Lea & Febiger, 1966, p. 387.

Table 9-8 Intra-articular Corticosteroid Injection

Joint	Main Indications	Injection Mixture and Quantity Used	Site and Manner of Aspiration and Injection	Failures and Pitfalls
Knee	1. Functional ankylosis 2. Monarticular arthritis 3. Marked effusion 4. Limitation of motion 5. Persistent swelling and pain	3:1 prednisolone tertiary butylacetate and 2% Xylocaine *Amount:* 20 to 30 mg.	1. Posterior-medial border of patella. Insert needle posterior to patella 2. Point of maximal effusion	If response lasts only a few days, repeated injection is not worthwhile
Hip	1. Limitation of motion 2. Persistent pain	3:1 prednisolone tertiary butylacetate and 2% Xylocaine *Amount:* 20 to 30 mg.	1. Point of imaginary line vertically, anterosuperior iliac spine, and horizontally from pubis, needle perpendicular to skin	Synovial space is difficult to find and this may cause inadequate injection
Ankle	1. Persistent monarticular arthritis 2. Difficulty in walking	3:1 prednisolone tertiary butylacetate and 2% Xylocaine *Amount:* 10 to 20 mg.	1. Point of maximal swelling 2. Site medial to extensor tendon and 1 cm. superior and lateral to medial malleolus	1. Avoid tendons and enlarged blood vessels 2. Tenosynovitis conceals amount of fluid in puffy ankle 3. Significant synovitis may cause little effusion and inadequate aspiration
Toes (Metatarsophalangeal and tarsophalangeal)	1. Rarely indicated 2. Pain and difficulty in walking	3:1 prednisolone tertiary butylacetate and 2% Xylocaine *Amount:* a few drops is maximum amount	1. Dorsolateral or medial surface 2. Use small 24 to 25 gauge needle 3. Exert pulling pressure to separate joint spaces *Manner:* Jet Hypospray injector is ideal if correctly applied	1. Bruising occurs from pressure on small joints 2. Child may be unusually disturbed if multiple injection planned 3. Fluoroscopy not recommended because of radiation exposure

Table 9-8 Intra-articular Corticosteroid Injection (Continued)

Joint	Main Indications	Injection Mixture and Quantity Used	Site and Manner of Aspiration and Injection	Failures and Pitfalls
Hands (Metacarpophalangeal and proximal interphalangeal)	1. Difficulty in writing 2. Beginning contracture 3. Pain and inflammation	3:1 prednisolone tertiary butylacetate and 2% Xylocaine or equivalent. *Amount:* a few drops is maximum amount	1. Dorsolateral or medial surface 2. Spread the joint by pulling finger *Manner:* Jet Hypospray injector	1. Bruising occurs from pressure on small joints 2. Child may be unusually disturbed if multiple injection planned 3. Fluoroscopy not recommended because of radiation exposure
Wrist	1. Limitation of motion 2. Pain and swelling	3:1 prednisolone tertiary butylacetate and 2% Xylocaine or equivalent. *Amount:* 10 to 20 mg.	1. Dorsal surface, medial and distal to radius, about in the middle	1. Multiplicity of synovial cavity 2. Tenosynovitis of extensor tendon sheath
Elbow	1. Limitation of motion 2. Difficulty in writing 3. Minimal swelling	3:1 prednisolone tertiary butylacetate and 2% Xylocaine or equivalent. *Amount:* no more than 1/2 to 1 cc. maximum	1. Elbow held flexed, inject at point of maximum bulging 2. In absence of effusion, inject lateral to olecranon, distal to lateral epicondyle of humerus, elbow partially flexed	1. Important to aspirate as much fluid as possible before injection
Shoulder	1. Inability to raise arm over head 2. Atrophy of arm and shoulder	3:1 prednisolone tertiary butylacetate and 2% Xylocaine or equivalent. *Amount:* 1/2 to 1 cc. maximum	1. Point of maximum bulging 2. In absence of effusion, inject at point inferior to coracoid process, where head of humerus articulates with glenoid fossa (*N.B.* Easily palpated in children)	1. Determine that major pain is in shoulder itself and not in bursa

situation, the parent, or the physician. The pain is actually not great when the steroid is properly injected.

The joints most readily accessible for injection are large weight-bearing joints, knee, hip, and ankle, in that order. The joints of the wrist, elbow, and shoulder are helped significantly by injection also. The metacarpophalangeal and proximal interphalangeal joints of the hands are usually involved in a multiple manner and selective injection of these joints can sometimes be helpful, but not often. Injection of the cervical spine is not practical in patients with juvenile rheumatoid arthritis.

Children who have significant peripheral rheumatoid arthritis of one or two joints, with several other joints involved minimally, often can achieve significant relief by intra-articular injection of the most seriously involved joints. Some patients with minimal peripheral articular disease may have a major exacerbation in a single weight-bearing joint such as the knee, and local steroid therapy can control the particular joint involved. Thus the patient is spared the systemic side effects of steroids or some more potent antirheumatic agent other than aspirin. Patients who are on systemic medication, such as gold therapy, often are benefited by intra-articular corticosteroid therapy in one joint that is beginning to have marked limitation of motion and uncontrolled swelling.

A valuable function of intra-articular therapy for a stiff knee or hip, is to inject the joint involved to obtain mobility to allow the physical therapist to begin the long arduous task of restoring motion to the stiffened knee or hip.

Causes of Failure of Intra-articular Corticosteroid Injection to Reduce Inflammation

1. Some joints of patients fail to respond to steroid medication for unknown reasons.
2. Failure to inject material into the joint space.
3. Local reaction to the corticosteroid crystals, producing more inflammation instead of less.
4. Local exacerbation of joint inflammation for several hours or days (2 per cent).
5. Muscular weakness of extremity injected (1 per cent).
6. Generalized weakness, fatigue, and vertigo (0.03 per cent).
7. Bacterial infection due to contamination (0.01 per cent).
8. Local urticaria at site of injection.
9. General systemic corticosteroid effects after injection of local joint.
10. Faulty dosage and administration.

One of the corticosteroid derivatives, such as prednisolone or triamcinolone, combined with a salt such as tertiary butylacetate to prolong effect, provides the best results, in the author's experience. Many patients sustain significant local pain at the time of injection but this unpleasant reaction can be avoided by mixing 1 or 2 per cent Xylocaine (lidocaine) with the prednisolone tertiary butylacetate in a 1:3 ratio (0.5 cc. Xylocaine with 1.5 cc. prednisolone tertiary butylacetate). It is important to remember that as much synovial fluid as possible must be removed from the joint prior to injection because the best results are obtained with the least dilution by synovial fluid.

Important Considerations in Joint Aspiration and Injection

1. Infection must be ruled out.
2. Sterile technique must be observed.
3. Destructiveness of pyogenic arthritis must be considered.
4. *Always* aspirate before injection.

Advantages of Joint Injection

1. May provide relief for months at a time.
2. Provides constant control by periodic injections.
3. There is ease of entry in most joints.
4. May be combined with physical therapy and night splints.
5. Provides greatest benefit in walking and writing joints.

GOLD

Harvey (1965) noted that gold in elemental form has been employed successfully for centuries as an antipruritic agent to relieve itching palm. As a therapeutic agent in the practice of medicine chrysotherapy has until recently been controversial in the treatment of rheumatoid arthritis. Koch (1890) found that growth of the tubercle bacillus was inhibited by gold salts. Lande (1927), Pick (1927), and Forestier (1929) reported clinical improvement of patients treated with gold salts over a protracted period of time (Freyberg, 1966). Since that time no fewer than 28 studies have been reported showing improvement in patients with rheumatoid arthritis, such improvement ranging from 3.6 per cent to 90 per cent (Table 9-9).

Fraser (1945) reported that of 57 patients, 24 greatly improved

Table 9-9 Efficacy of Gold Therapy in Rheumatoid Arthritis*

	Lowest Increase (%)	*Greatest Increase (%)*
Greatly Improved	3.6	84.5
Moderately Improved	10.5	90
Slightly Improved	4	35

*Adapted from Freyberg, R. H.: Gold therapy for rheumatoid arthritis. In Hollander, J. L.: *Arthritis and Allied Conditions*, ed. 7. Philadelphia, Lea & Febiger, 1966, pp. 312-313.

and 12 moderately improved. However, in the patients' own assessment of their condition, 56 per cent reported great improvement.

Merliss et al. (1951) and Brown and Currie (1953) reported chrysotherapy to be no better or worse than a placebo or salicylate alone. Merliss' study, however, used a slowly absorbed preparation, aurothioglycolanilide (Lauron), and some question arises as to the efficacy of this particular preparation. Brown and Currie (1953) used sodium aurothiomalate, as did most other investigators, and theirs constituted one of the few studies revealing no improvement with gold therapy. Sabin and Warren (1940) found that arthritis experimentally induced in rats by injection of a known strain of mycoplasma was completely prevented by prior injection of gold before such intravenous injection of mycoplasma organisms. Further, they found that the arthritis was minimal if gold was injected within ten days after intravenous injection of mycoplasma. When gold was injected after ten days, no clinical reduction or prevention was noted. Calcium aurothiomalate was used as the salt and no toxicity was encountered. In addition, in rats gold has been found to be effective in preventing arthritis due to hemolytic streptococcus and in preventing experimental arthritis produced by injecting Murphy rat sarcoma into rats (Freyberg, 1966).

Chemistry

The major gold preparation in use is sodium aurothiomalate. Several other preparations are available or have been used, but those that are soluble in water have proved to be the most effective clinically. Colloidal suspensions have been disappointing. Large amounts of the gold in oily suspension are found at the site of injection. Also, colloidal gold preparations, unlike water-soluble preparations, have been found to be concentrated in the liver.

Absorption, Distribution, and Excretion

Gold is not fully absorbed from the gastrointestinal tract; thus oral preparations are not practical. The water-soluble gold salts are readily absorbed from intramuscular sites, whereas the insoluble gold compounds are poorly absorbed and collect as intramuscular deposits at the site of injection. Plasma concentrations reach highest levels a few hours after injection and reduce to a lower level which is maintained for a prolonged period. When 25 mg. of gold sodium thiomalate are injected intramuscularly weekly an average maintenance plasma level of 330 mcg. per 100 ml. is maintained. The plasma concentration of gold depends upon the magnitude of the dose. The plasma concentration, after an average level is established, remains constant with continuing weekly dosage. Large amounts of gold are retained in the body during the period of administration (Freyberg, 1966). In fact, 76 per cent of plasma gold is loosely bound to Alpha$_1$ globulin as a gold protein complex.

The distribution of gold in tissues depends in a measure on the type of compounds administered. The water-soluble compounds have minimal muscular deposition, more constant plasma levels, and the most significant concentrations in the kidney. The liver and spleen also absorb significant amounts of gold. Lawrence (1961) found up to two and a half times the gold in inflamed joints as in normal joints (Freyberg, 1966). The chemical structure of gold in the tissues and in the urine has been fully studied. Ganz and Brucer believe that the gold present in the urine is the administered compound. In animals injected with an insoluble gold compound in oily suspension a depot of gold accumulated at the site of injection, and the gold content was reduced in the kidney and markedly increased in the liver (Freyberg, 1966). Excretion of gold is mainly by the kidney with small amounts in the feces and none in the sweat. There is apparently a limit to the amount of gold that can be excreted and dosages in excess of this limit result in significant storage. There are patients who appear to excrete abnormally large amounts of gold and attempts have been made to correlate clinical improvement in such patients with this factor.

Clinical Effectiveness

The clinical effectiveness of gold has been reported in at least 30 studies (Freyberg, 1966). Except for two or three exceptions all studies have found gold to be helpful in the therapy of rheumatoid arthritis. Perhaps the best controlled and most widely discussed study was that of the Research Subcommittee of the Empire Rheumatism Council (1960). Two hundred adult patients were studied in a "double blind-fold" trial; they were divided equally into two groups balanced for sex, age, and duration of disease. These patients had had rheumatoid arthritis for not less than one year and not more than five years. Their ages ranged from 20 to 64 years. All patients had bilateral involvement of the hands and/or wrists and an erythrocyte sedimentation rate of 20 mm. or more per hour (Westergren). No previous gold therapy was administered to the patient, nor chloroquine or systemic steroid therapy, in the three months preceding admission to the trial. Both groups were given similar supportive measures such as rest, splints, aspirin, and physical therapy. Clinical and functional assessments were made at 1, 3, 6, 12, 18, and 30 months after treatment was begun and radiological changes were determined at 18 and 30 months. The incidence of complications was recorded. Patients in the treatment group received a total of 1 gram of sodium aurothiomalate over a period of 20 weeks by intramuscular injection of 50 mg. at weekly intervals. All patients in the control group were given a total dose of 0.01 mg. of sodium aurothiomalate over 20 weeks by injection of 0.05 mcg. at weekly intervals. The control group received 1/100,000 of the quantity of gold that the treated group received. The medication was prescribed in a prearranged, random system. The following 11 assessments were made on the occasion of each examination:*

---

*From Empire Rheumatism Council, Research Subcommittee: Gold therapy in rheumatoid arthritis, report of a multicenter controlled trial. *Ann. Rheum. Dis.*, 19:95, 1960.

1. Functional capacity (physician's estimate) in five grades.
2. Subjective estimate of fitness by the patient in five grades.
3. Assessment of joints involved (42 joints were listed).
4. Strength of grip in each hand (mm. Hg).
5. Hemoglobin concentration (g. per cent).
6. Erythrocyte sedimentation rate (mm./hr. Westergren).
7. W.B.C. (total and differential counts) per cu. mm.
8. Sheep cell agglutination test (S.C.A.T.) initially and at 18 and 30 months.
9. Complications present at, or occurring between, each assessment.
10. Number and nature of analgesic tablets taken daily (assessed retrospectively at each attendance).
11. Radiological examination of hands and wrists initially and at 18 and 30 months.

Functional Capacity. Functional capacity estimated by the physician revealed a significant difference between gold-treated subjects and control subjects (Table 9-10). Subjective well-being as estimated by the patient also revealed significant differences between the gold-treated group and the control group at 6, 12, and 18 months after administration of medication (Table 9-11).

Table 9-10 Functional Capacity (Physician's Estimate) at Periodical Assessments*
(Gold 90; Controls 95)

PERCENTAGE IN EACH GRADE AT EACH ASSESSMENT

Month of Assessment	Group	1 = best	2	3	4	5	Mean Grade
0	Gold	9	53	34	3	—	2.3
	Control	12	57	32	—	—	2.2
1	Gold	9	62	26	3	—	2.2
	Control	14	54	33	—	—	2.2
3	Gold	22	57	20	1	—	2.0
	Control	15	64	20	1	—	2.1
6	Gold S	41	47	11	1	—	1.7
	Control	23	60	16	1	—	2.0
12	Gold S	40	44	12	1	2	1.8
	Control	23	55	22	—	—	2.0
18	Gold S	43	42	13	2	—	1.7
	Control	25	49	25	—	—	2.0

S = Significant difference between the distribution of the two groups.
*From Empire Rheumatism Council, Research Subcommittee: Gold therapy in rheumatoid arthritis, report of a multicenter controlled trial. Ann. Rheum. Dis., 19:95, 1960. Reproduced with the permission of the Editor and the British Medical Association.

Table 9-11 Subjective Well-being (Patients Own Estimate), Showing Percentage in Each Grade at Each Assessment*
(Gold 90; Controls 95)

Month of Assessment	Group	Functional Capacity (per cent "fit")					Mean Grade
		100	75	50	25	1	
0	Gold	3	42	44	10	—	59.5
	Control	5	40	46	8	—	60.2
1	Gold	8	40	41	9	2	60.2
	Control	5	44	42	8	—	61.2
3	Gold	20	51	26	3	—	70.6
	Control	11	54	33	2	1	67.0
6	Gold S	41	46	12	1	—	78.8
	Control	22	53	22	2	1	71.7
12	Gold S	35	47	11	4	2	74.7
	Control	18	56	24	2	—	71.1
18	Gold S	37	41	19	2	1	75.1
	Control	23	47	27	2	—	71.2

S = Significant difference between the distributions of the two groups.
*From Empire Rheumatism Council, Research Subcommittee: Gold therapy in rheumatoid arthritis, report of a multicenter controlled trial. Ann. Rheum. Dis., 19:95, 1960. Reproduced with the permission of the Editor and the British Medical Association.

Joint Involvement. This particular assessment is extremely important in that the average number of joints involved in the gold-treated group decreased from 17 to 8 joints at 18 months' assessment (Table 9-12). The number of joints involved in the control group decreased from 19 to 12. The difference is statistically significant.

Grip Strength. The mean grip strength in the gold-treated group increased from 140 to 180 mm. of mercury as compared with 145 to

Table 9-12 Mean Number of Joints Involved per Patient at Each Assessment*
(Gold 90; Controls 95)

Group	Month of Assessment					
	0	1	3	6	12	18
	Mean ± S.E.	Mean ± S.E.	Mean ± S.E.	Mean ± S.E.	Mean ± S.E.	Mean ± S.E.
Gold	17.3 ± .92	14.3 ± .86	10.5 ± .73 S	7.8 ± .67 S	7.5 ± .76 S	8.0 ± .81 S
Control	19.2 ± .95	15.6 ± .79	14.0 ± .87	12.6 ± .95	12.7 ± .91	12.5 ± .95

S = Significant difference between the two groups.
*From Empire Rheumatism Council, Research Subcommittee: Gold therapy in rheumatoid arthritis, report of a multicenter controlled trial. Ann. Rheum. Dis., 19:95, 1960. Reproduced with the permission of the Editor and the British Medical Association.

Table 9-13 Mean Strength of Grip (mm. Hg)*
(Gold 90; Controls 95)

Hand	Group	\multicolumn{6}{c}{Month of Assessment}
		0	1	3	6	12	18
Right	Gold	144 ± 6	151 ± 6	167 ± 7	184 ± 6 S	177 ± 7	180 ± 7 S
	Control	145 ± 6	151 ± 7	155 ± 6	159 ± 6	162 ± 6	159 ± 7
Left	Gold	149 ± 6	147 ± 6	172 ± 6	183 ± 6 S	181 ± 6 S	180 ± 6 S
	Control	145 ± 6	147 ± 6	155 ± 6	157 ± 6	155 ± 7	155 ± 7

S = Significant difference between the two groups.
*From Empire Rheumatism Council, Research Subcommittee: Gold therapy in rheumatoid arthritis, report of a multicenter controlled trial. Ann. Rheum. Dis., *19*:95, 1960. Reproduced with the permission of the Editor and the British Medical Association.

159 in the control group (Table 9-13). The results are significantly different and objectively indicate that strength was improved in the treated group.

Mean Hemoglobin Concentration. A statistically significant increase in hemoglobin in the gold-treated group is of particular interest, revealing that gold not only does not produce clinically significant anemia but actually improves the red cell mass of the patient (Table 9-14).

Erythrocyte Sedimentation Rate. The mean erythrocyte sedimentation rate as determined by the Westergren method declined from 42 to 27 mm. per hour in the gold-treated group and from 38 to 32 mm. per hour in the control group (Table 9-15). Significant differences occurring at the 3, 6, and 12 month assessments give some indication of a reduction in the inflammatory disease.

There were no differences in the sheep cell agglutination test, and only minimal differences in the leukocyte cell counts.

Mean Number of Analgesic Tablets Taken (per Patient). The average number of tablets taken per day decreased from 8 to 5 in the gold-treated group and from 7.7 to 7.4 in the control group (Table 9-16).

Table 9-14 Mean Hemoglobin Concentration
(g. per cent ± S.E.)*
(Gold 90; Controls 95)

Group	\multicolumn{6}{c}{Month of Assessment}
	0	1	3	6	12	18
Gold	12.4 ± 0.17	12.3 ± 0.14	12.5 ± 0.15	13.0 ± 0.13 S	13.1 ± 0.21 S	13.0 ± 0.11 S
Control	12.3 ± 0.15	12.4 ± 0.14	12.5 ± 0.14	12.6 ± 0.11	12.6 ± 0.19	12.4 ± 0.20

S = Significant difference between the two groups.
*From Empire Rheumatism Council, Research Subcommittee: Gold therapy in rheumatoid arthritis, report of a multicenter controlled trial. Ann. Rheum. Dis., *19*:95, 1960. Reproduced with the permission of the Editor and the British Medical Association.

Table 9-15 Mean Erythrocyte Sedimentation Rate
(mm./hr. Westergren)*
(Gold 90; Controls 95)

Group	Month of Assessment					
	0	1	3	6	12	18
Gold	42 ± 2	43 ± 2	28 ± 2 S	21 ± 2 S	23 ± 2 S	27 ± 2
Control	38 ± 2	37 ± 2	36 ± 3	33 ± 2	34 ± 2	32 ± 2

S = Significant difference between the two groups.
*From Empire Rheumatism Council, Research Subcommittee: Gold therapy in rheumatoid arthritis, report of a multicenter controlled trial. Ann. Rheum. Dis., *19*:95, 1960. Reproduced with the permission of the Editor and the British Medical Association.

Radiological Comparison of the Two Groups. Progression of disease in both the gold-treated group and the control group was apparently the same as measured by radiological comparison.

The author has been particularly impressed with the disappearance of morning stiffness in children after the third or fourth month of gold therapy. Results in children studied in uncontrolled observations have paralleled the findings of the Empire Rheumatism study.

Administration

The gold preparation preferred by the Arthritis Clinic at Texas Children's Hospital is sodium aurothiomalate. It is administered by the following schedule: 10 mg. intramuscularly initially, followed by weekly dosage of 25 mg. sodium aurothiomalate intramuscularly for 20 weeks. The patient then receives 25 mg. intramuscularly every two to four weeks for an indefinite period. A hemogram and urinalysis are performed one week after administration of the first dosage and then at weekly intervals for two weeks, followed by hemogram and urinalysis at monthly intervals for two to three months. If toxicity has not occurred at this time, then the hemogram and urinalysis are repeated at three-month intervals, or more frequently if indicated. After completion of

Table 9-16 Mean Number of Analgesic Tablets Taken (per Patient)*
(Gold 90; Controls 95)

Group	Month of Assessment					
	0	1	3	6	12	18
Gold	8.0 ± .46	7.4 ± .48	6.5 ± .46	5.6 ± .49	4.6 ± .48 S	5.0 ± .46 S
Control	7.7 ± .46	7.5 ± .44	7.3 ± .44	7.0 ± .48	7.1 ± .49	7.4 ± .53

S = Significant difference between the two groups.
*From Empire Rheumatism Council, Research Subcommittee: Gold therapy in rheumatoid arthritis, report of a multicenter controlled trial. Ann. Rheum. Dis., *19*:95, 1960. Reproduced with the permission of the Editor and the British Medical Association.

the 20-week course dosage is continued at intervals of two to four weeks because of the high relapse incidence following cessation of weekly gold therapy.

Toxicity

Significant toxicity to gold in children is indeed minimal and certainly less than in corticosteroid therapy. In the Empire Rheumatism Council study 35 of 100 patients treated sustained some toxic complication of gold while 16 of the patients in the control group sustained significant "toxicity." Of the former group, only 14 of 100 treated required withdrawal from medication. Of the 35 patients with toxicity 21 sustained some form of dermatitis; 14 per cent of patients sustained significant toxicity other than skin rash, and 7 per cent of the control group sustained significant "toxicity." Any patient receiving medication over a prolonged period of time may have symptoms similar to those of toxicity but not actually related to the compound in question.

Dermatitis. A drug rash is the most common toxic effect, as previously noted; usually a reduction of dosage from 2 to 5 mg. per dose results in disappearance of the rash. Only one of the initial 22 children treated in our clinic with sodium aurothiomalate sustained a significant exfoliative dermatitis. Other lesions of skin and mucous membrane reported include stomatitis, pharyngitis, vaginitis, and glossitis. Some patients report a metallic taste in the mouth preceding stomatitis (Freyberg, 1966).

Gastrointestinal Side Effects. Gastritis, colitis, and hepatitis have been reported but must be exceedingly rare. Freyberg, in 25 years of experience with gold therapy in over 1800 cases, has yet to see a single instance of important digestive disorder or liver disease.

Central Nervous System Symptoms. During the year 1940, so-called "nitrotoid" reactions characterized by vertigo, giddiness, flushing of the face, and headache were observed (Freyberg, 1966). The side effects reported probably were related to the impurities of the product during that year because these particular toxic effects have not been noted since that time.

Nephritis. Toxic nephritis as exhibited by significant hematuria or albuminuria can occur but is extremely rare. Transient albuminuria, consisting of a trace of albumin, occurs at some point during medication but is of no significance. An occasional patient will have significant hematuria and nephritis. Renal biopsy reveals membranous glomerulonephritis as well as a rare nephrotic-like syndrome.

Hematopoietic Toxicity. As with any organic salt or heavy metal, bone marrow depression may occur causing any one or all hematopoietic elements to be depressed. In particular, thrombocytopenia or leukopenia may occur. Only two or three children may have exhibited this side effect, which disappears upon discontinuation of the medication.

Exacerbation of Disease. An occasional patient experiences mild to moderately severe exacerbation of joint pain and swelling after each injection of gold. Freyberg (1966) states that such symptoms usually decrease and disappear after five or six injections, but a few children have continued to have moderately severe pain of the joints after each injection of gold, requiring withdrawal of therapy.

Toxicity in gold, therefore, is an important factor in therapy but certainly does not preclude the use of gold when indicated. In the opinion of the author, gold is less toxic than steroids, and few children have required withdrawal from therapy. In the author's personal experience, no children have died as a result of gold therapy.

Treatment of Gold Toxicity

In cases of gold toxicity evident by skin rash, reduction of the dosage of gold is all that is necessary. When more severe forms of rash occur, the use of parenteral steroid is indicated and is definitely beneficial in controlling symptoms. No patients in our experience have required Dimercaptopropanol (BAL). Penicillamine may be useful in those patients who do not respond to parenteral corticosteroids (Freyberg, 1966).

Nephritis seems to respond to discontinuation of the drug. Any irreversible changes must be rare. Thrombocytopenia seems also to respond to discontinuation of the drug. If necessary, systemic corticosteroid medication would seem indicated.

INDOMETHACIN

Indomethacin is a nonsteroidal, anti-inflammatory analgesic and antipyretic agent that was first introduced in 1961 and reported in 1963 (Katz et al, 1963; Norcross, 1963; Paul, 1963; Winter et al, 1963; Merck Sharp & Dohme Research Laboratories, 1964; Lockie and Norcross, 1966). The compound has a unique chemical structure, different from corticosteroids, salicylates, and phenylbutazone. Since introduction, reports have varied concerning its efficacy in the treatment of rheumatoid arthritis. In a survey of the literature, O'Brien (1967) reviewed 46 reports specifically dealing with the use of the drug in rheumatoid arthritis. He felt that the degree of enthusiasm for the drug varied inversely with the degree of objective measurements of improvement in the reports. In those reports that contained no objective measures of joint function, 56 per cent of 607 cases of rheumatoid arthritis were believed improved when treated by the drug, whereas in those reports that contained evidence of objective measures, only 34 per cent of 218 cases were classified as improved. At least four supposedly unexplained fatalities have been recorded in children with rheumatoid arthritis under therapy with indomethacin (Jacobs, 1967). For this reason indomethacin is not recommended at the present time for routine use in juvenile rheumatoid arthritis. The drug is not prohibited, however, and the author feels that there is a definite place for indomethacin in the treatment of juvenile rheumatoid arthritis because of its unusual and superior antipyretic effect (Brewer, 1968).

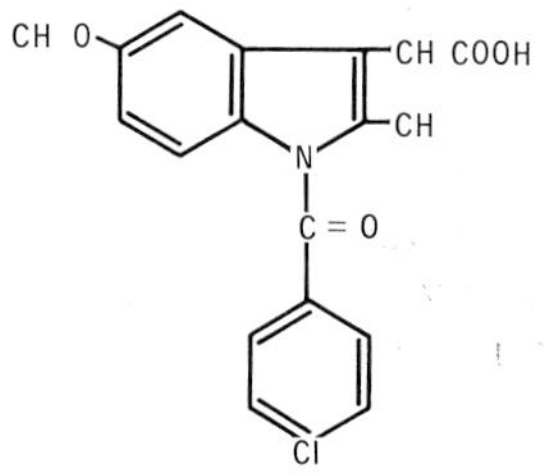

Figure 9-6 Indomethacin.

Chemistry

Indomethacin is 1-(p-chlorobenzoyl)-5-methoxy-2-methylindole-3-acetic acid, with a molecular formula of $C_{19}H_{16}NO_4Cl$ and a molecular weight of 357.8 (Figure 9-6). There is no chemical structural relationship to the other commonly used anti-inflammatory drugs and indomethacin has no effect on the pituitary or adrenal glands.

Pharmacology and Toxicology

Indomethacin has been primarily described as an anti-inflammatory agent with analgesic and antipyretic properties. Anti-inflammatory activity has been demonstrated both in the cotton pellet granuloma inhibition test and in inhibition of edema induced by subplantar injection of carrageen in rats (Winter, 1965). Antipyretic activity has been demonstrated in both rabbits and rats (Winter et al., 1963) by inhibition of fever produced by an injection of a bacterial lipoidal polysaccharide, *E. coli* endotoxin. The duration of this action was longer than that of aminopyrine and comparable to that of phenylbutazone. Indomethacin has analgesic properties at least as potent as aspirin (Winter et al., 1963).

In man, indomethacin is absorbed to a high degree rather promptly from the gastrointestinal tract (Hucker et al., 1966). No measurable quantity of the drug was found in the plasma of human subjects 24 hours after ingestion. There was no evidence of drug accumulation. Indomethacin present in the plasma is essentially unchanged and bound to a nondiffusible plasma constituent.

About two-thirds of the dosage given is recovered in the urine as indomethacin glucuronide and the remainder in the feces as free indomethacin. Thus far indomethacin in the usual dosage has been shown to have little effect on inflammatory response of bacterial infections (Merck Sharp & Dohme, 1964).

Side effects from a single dose of indomethacin occur infrequently. Administration for one or two weeks can result in morning headaches, often frontal in location and significantly severe; however, the headaches usually disappear with continued administration. As with salicylate therapy, lethargy and drowsiness have occurred (Lockie and Norcross, 1966). Peptic ulcers have developed in a few adults who have taken indomethacin for extended periods for treatment of chronic diseases.

Radioactive chromium-labeled erythrocyte studies have revealed fecal blood loss to be about 1 to 2 ml. per day in one-third of patients taking indomethacin. This amount is considerably less than that in patients receiving salicylate therapy, more than 90 per cent of whom had blood loss averaging about 6 ml. daily (Chapter 1).

Dermatologic reactions, which have been reported infrequently, are pruritus, urticaria, angioneurotic edema, angiitis, skin rashes, and loss of hair. In our clinic one patient with rheumatoid arthritis, who received the drug over a one-year period, developed alopecia accompanied by loss of eyebrows and eyelashes, with subsequent regrowth after discontinuation of therapy.

Acute respiratory distress, including sudden dyspnea and asthma, has been rarely encountered with indomethacin administration.

Recently a warning was issued (Chapman, 1966) concerning the use of indomethacin in children because unexplained deaths were reported in a few children under treatment (Jacobs, 1967; Kelsey and Sharyj, 1967). The evidence was not conclusive that any causative association existed between these deaths and the drug.

Clinical Use of Indomethacin in Children

There is considerable disagreement among rheumatologists as to the efficacy of indomethacin in providing significant relief for the adult patient with rheumatoid arthritis. Lockie and Norcross (1966) found that in most patients clinical activity was usually rapid but that exacerbation of symptoms and signs occurred within 24 to 72 hours after discontinuation of the medication or substitution with a placebo. There were some patients who required two to three weeks of administration before definitive objective evidence of improvement occurred. Of 180 patients studied 55.5 per cent did achieve progressive reduction of joint swelling and inflammation, decreased pain on palpation and motion of involved joints, increased range of motion, and improved functional capacity. Of the same 180 patients 20 had less convincing evidence of improvement and sustained relapses upon discontinuation of the drug or substitution with a placebo. When indomethacin therapy was resumed prompt improvement once again occurred. Lockie concluded that after three years of clinical experience indomethacin did produce some improvement in 66 per cent of the 180 patients studied (Lockie and Norcross, 1966).

On the other hand, the Cooperating Clinics Committee of the American Rheumatism Association in 1967 performed a 3-month, 11-clinic blindfold trial designed to study arthritic symptom changes and the frequency of nonarthritic symptoms in 71 indomethacin-treated and 65 placebo-treated adult patients with peripheral rheumatoid arthritis. Salicylates were permitted as desired in both groups and five clinically objective measures (number of clinically active joints; grip strength; morning stiffness; erythrocyte sedimentation rate; and walking time) were used to record improvement or deterioration of condition. Subjective impressions also were recorded. This study reveals there was no demonstrable difference in the frequency, extent, or rate of change of symptoms in patients treated with placebo or indomethacin. This study produced the interesting revelation, however, that the placebo group and the indomethacin-treated group sustained significant side effects such as headache, dizziness, and lightheadedness. The committee hastened to point out, however, that there is always a limited value to the subordinate and limited role of statistical significance tests. Further, there is an inevitable degree of uncertainty regarding the patients selected because of the wide previous usage of indomethacin in patients with rheumatoid arthritis. In this study patients who had previously been on indomethacin were excluded from the study and a significant number of the patients who were aided may well have been eliminated. The interval of study was significantly short.

The author feels that there are definitely selected children who have achieved significant benefits from indomethacin in reducing peripheral articular manifestations. When indomethacin is effective the reduction of joint swelling occurs within a week or two. For this reason a trial on indomethacin usually need not last longer than one month before adequate evaluation is possible. Several patients have achieved enough relief of particular manifestations to permit reduction or elimination of corticosteroid medication. This effect alone would justify a continuation of its usage in such patients because the toxicity of corticosteroids certainly exceeds that reported with indomethacin.

An even more important clinical effect of indomethacin is its effect on fever. In a study conducted by the author (Brewer, 1968) 223 infants and children under the age of 14 years with fever greater than 101° F. (rectally) were given a single dose of indomethacin suspension, placebo, or acetaminophen (Table 9-17). The medications were given in coded bottles and indomethacin suspension and placebo suspension were indistinguishable by color, consistency, or taste. Acetaminophen suspension was unchanged from the commercial product because of the Food and Drug Administration Regulations, prohibiting alteration

Table 9-17 Distribution of Treatments by Cause of Fever†

Diagnosis	Indocin	Tylenol	Placebo
Upper respiratory infection	29	19	29
Lower respiratory infection	11	15	13
Measles	17	16	19
Gastroenteritis	7	14	8
Infection, skin and lymph nodes	9	3	4
Renal tract infection	0	2	1
Other	3	3	0
Total:	76	72	74*

*One placebo patient had no admitting diagnosis.
†From Brewer, E. J.: A comparative evaluation of indomethacin, acetaminophen and placebo as antipyretic agents in children. Arthritis Rheum., 11:645, 1968.

Table 9-18 Mean and Adjusted Mean Temperature Decreases (Degrees Fahrenheit; Analysis of Covariance)*

Treatment	Patients	½ hour Mean	½ hour Adj. mean	1 hour Mean	1 hour Adj. mean	1½ hour Mean	1½ hour Adj. mean	2 hour Mean	2 hour Adj. mean	2½ hour Mean	2½ hour Adj. mean	3 hour Mean	3 hour Adj. mean
Indomethacin	76	.345	.394	1.028	1.110	1.748	1.861	2.378	2.527	2.804	2.945	3.137	3.289
Acetaminophen	72	.472	.387	1.183	1.040	1.847	1.652	2.248	1.989	2.603	2.359	2.600	2.335
Placebo	75	.023	.053	0.174	0.228	0.240	0.313	0.348	0.444	0.457	0.548	0.483	0.581

*From Brewer, E. J.: A comparative evaluation of indomethacin, acetaminophen and placebo as antipyretic agents in children. Arthritis Rheum., *11*:645, 1968.

in any manner. Indomethacin was given as a suspension of 10 mg. per 5 ml. in a dosage of approximately 1 mg. per kg. The dosage of acetaminophen was given as Tylenol Elixir, 120 mg. per 5 ml. or approximately 3 mg. per lb. The temperature was measured rectally before medication was given and again at intervals of ½ hour, 1 hour, 1½ hours, 2 hours, 2½ hours, 3 hours, and 4 hours. No additional medication was given after the initial dose during the time the temperature was being measured. The patients had fever due to a variety of causes.

In Table 9-18 the adjusted mean temperature decrease was calculated by analysis of covariance (Ostle, 1963). Statistically significant differences are at the 0.05 level of confidence, as shown in Table 9-19. Indomethacin and acetaminophen differed significantly and were statistically superior in reducing temperature from the first half hour to the end of the study. Indomethacin and acetaminophen were equally effective in reducing temperature until the 2-hour interval, when indomethacin became more effective. In Table 9-20 the mean and adjusted decrease is compared in patients with initial temperatures

Table 9-19 Significant Differences in Adjusted Mean Temperature Decreases †

Treatment	½ hour	1 hour	1½ hour	2 hour	2½ hour	3 hour
Indomethacin and acetaminophen	—	—	—	*	*	*
Indomethacin and placebo	*	*	*	*	*	*
Acetaminophen and placebo	*	*	*	*	*	*

— Not significantly different.
*Significantly different at minimum of 0.05 level.
†From Brewer, E. J.: A comparative evaluation of indomethacin, acetaminophen and placebo as antipyretic agents in children. Arthritis Rheum., *11*:645, 1968.

Table 9-20 Mean and Adjusted* Mean Temperature Decrease (Of the 103 Patients with Initial Temperature in Excess of 103° F.)†

Treatment	Patients	½ hour Mean	Adj. mean	1 hour Mean	Adj. mean	1½ hour Mean	Adj. mean	2 hour Mean	Adj. mean	2½ hour Mean	Adj. mean	3 hour Mean	Adj. mean
Indomethacin	25	.628	.636	1.592	1.603	2.464	2.478	3.324	3.339	3.852	3.860	4.380	4.386
Acetaminophen	47	.515	.485	1.251	1.209	2.068	2.016	2.261	2.566	2.853	2.823	2.902	2.879
Placebo	31	.139	.177	0.458	0.513	0.558	0.626	0.774	0.847	0.977	1.017	0.997	1.027

*Adjusted by Analysis of Covariance.
†From Brewer, E. J.: A comparative evaluation of indomethacin, acetaminophen and placebo as antipyretic agents in children. Arthritis Rheum., *11*:645, 1968.

greater than 103° F. rectally. Indomethacin produced a greater temperature decrease from the second hour until the completion of the study, by a significantly greater amount. Table 9-21 shows the statistically significant differences in the adjusted mean temperature decrease in patients with initial temperature greater than 103°. Perhaps even more significant, Table 9-22 reveals that patients with temperature of 103° or greater whose temperature was reduced at least 3° almost always responded to indomethacin with a dramatic and significant reduction of temperature. Only 60 per cent of patients receiving acetaminophen responded to this degree, while 10 per cent or fewer of patients receiving a placebo achieved significant temperature reduction spontaneously.

Patients with temperature of 104° F. or greater rectally, who sustained a greater reduction of temperature (4° or more) produced even more striking results. More than 8 of 10 patients who received in-

Table 9-21 Significant Differences in Adjusted Mean Temperature Decreases (Of the 103 Patients with Initial Temperature in Excess of 103° F.) †

		½ hour	1 hour	1½ hour	2 hour	2½ hour	3 hour
Indomethacin and Acetaminophen	(25) (47)	—	—	—	*	*	*
Indomethacin and Placebo	(25) (31)	*	*	*	*	*	*
Acetaminophen and Placebo	(47) (31)	—	*	*	*	*	*

— Not significantly different at 0.05 level.
*Significantly different at minimum of 0.05 level.
†From Brewer, E. J.: A comparative evaluation of indomethacin, acetaminophen and placebo as antipyretic agents in children. Arthritis Rheum., *11*:645, 1968.

Table 9-22 Per cent of Patients Showing Specified Temperature Reduction*

	103° + F.			103° + F.			104° + F.		
Treatment	Patients	Patients reduced 2°	Per cent reduced	Patients	Patients reduced 3°	Per cent reduced	Patients	Patients reduced 4°	Per cent reduced
Indomethacin	25	25	100	25	24	96	11	9	82
Acetaminophen	47	41	87	47	29	62	24	9	38
Placebo	31	9	29	31	3	10	12	0	0

*From Brewer, E. J.: A comparative evaluation of indomethacin, acetaminophen and placebo as antipyretic agents in children. Arthritis Rheum., 11:645, 1968.

domethacin achieved such a response while less than 40 per cent of patients receiving acetaminophen sustained the same degree of temperature change. None of the placebo group achieved these results spontaneously.

Colgan and Mintz (1957) have shown acetaminophen to be equal to acetylsalicylic acid in antipyretic activity. Their study reveals the superior ability of indomethacin to reduce fever, from whatever cause, over acetaminophen or placebo.

This particular study is of significance in the treatment of juvenile rheumatoid arthritis. At one time or another 70 per cent have significant fever lasting for weeks, months, or even years. Often the administration of corticosteroids in the past has been predicated upon the significant pyrexia in patients and the failure of acetylsalicylic acid to reduce significantly the dreadful daily spiked temperature of 105 to 106°. Children with rheumatoid arthritis who have significant pyrexia unrelieved by aspirin, in the author's opinion, probably should be given a trial on indomethacin before beginning corticosteroid therapy. Often such patients will have minimal articular disease but serious pyrexia. If these patients can be satisfactorily controlled by indomethacin therapy the drug is worthy of trial. The clinician must remember that infection is masked by effective anti-inflammatory agents. The patient must be examined and significant bacterial infection must always be considered in any illness.

While certainly one must use indomethacin with great care, a controlled multiclinic study seems not only indicated but mandatory to establish its role in the armamentarium of the physician treating rheumatoid arthritis in children.

PHENYLBUTAZONE

Phenylbutazone is an analgesic, antipyretic, and anti-inflammatory agent with a chemical structure of 3,5-dioxo-1,2-diphenyl-4-n-butyl-pyrazolidine. The compound is a pyrazolon derivative related to antipyrine and aminopyrine. All compounds mentioned are highly toxic and should be used with the greatest of caution in children with juvenile rheumatoid arthritis. Some type of side effect is noted in almost half the patients and such serious toxic effects as peptic ulcer, hypersensitivity reactions, stomatitis, hepatitis, nephritis, aplastic anemia, leukopenia, agranulocytosis, and thrombocytopenia are known. If the medication is used, constant and extremely close medical supervision is necessary and a complete hemogram and urinalysis should be performed at frequent intervals, at least during the early weeks or months of therapy.

There are occasional children with juvenile rheumatoid arthritis who do not respond well to the other modalities of treatment but who have achieved satisfactory relief of peripheral articular disease with phenylbutazone. The author feels that its use should be severely restricted to those few patients with serious articular disease who do not respond to any other form of therapy.

CHLOROQUINE

Chloroquine is 7-chloro-4(4-diethyl-amino-1-methyl-butyl-amino) quinoline. The author feels that chloroquine should not be used in children because of its known toxic ability to reduce peripheral vision in the absence of clinically observable changes in the retina (Sataline and Farmer, 1962).

CYCLOPHOSPHAMIDE

Cyclophosphamide is one of the nitrogen mustard derivatives which has not been used extensively in juvenile rheumatoid arthritis. Fosdick et al. (1968) have reported satisfactory results in the treatment of certain adult rheumatoid arthritis patients with cyclophosphamide (Cytoxan). If preliminary reports continue to be promising, a multiclinic trial should probably be performed in juvenile rheumatoid arthritis.

GENERAL PRINCIPLES OF CHEMOTHERAPY IN JUVENILE RHEUMATOID ARTHRITIS

Most patients, when initially evaluated, should be tried on a program of salicylate therapy for several months in addition to the application of basic principles of care already discussed. Exceptions would be those patients who are so seriously ill that life is thought to be threatened, as in serious pericarditis; those with peripheral articular disease so severe that total immobility is present because of pain and limitation of motion; or those with fever so significant that activity is sharply restricted. When aspirin has been given an adequate trial, with inadequate results, and the patient continues to be significantly disabled with peripheral articular disease but has no serious systemic manifestations, the author prefers to attempt a course of gold therapy in conjunction with continuing salicylate therapy. Patients who have mild peripheral articular disease, even if they show no significant improvement using salicylates, probably are as well off with no added medication.

Corticosteroid therapy should be reserved for those patients who have clinically severe pericarditis or such severe peripheral articular disease that life has become unbearable.

Children with significant pyrexia, in the author's opinion, deserve a trial on indomethacin therapy when salicylate therapy has failed, before instituting corticosteroid therapy.

These principles of chemotherapy are generalities and must not be construed as absolute guide lines to therapy.

REFERENCES

Ansell, B. M.: Relationship of dosage and type of salicylate therapy to plasma levels in patients with juvenile rheumatoid arthritis. *In* Dixon, A. St. J. et al. (eds.): Salicylates, an International Symposium, Boston, Little, Brown and Co., 1963, pp. 35-36.

Bayer Co.: Product Information Department, Division of Sterling Drug Co. and Glenbrook Laboratories.

Black, R. L., Oglesby, R. B., Sallman, L., and Bunim, J. J.: Posterior subcapsular cataracts induced by corticosteroids in patients with rheumatoid arthritis. J.A.M.A., 174:166, 1960.

Brewer, E. J., and Fahlberg, W. J.: Proceedings of the conference on effects of chronic salicylate administration, Lamont-Havers, R. W., and Wagner, B. M. (eds.). National Institutes of Health, New York, 1966, pp. 26-39.

Brewer, E. J.: A comparative evaluation of indomethacin, acetaminophen and placebo as antipyretic agents in children. Arthritis Rheum., 11:645, 1968.

Brown, R. A. P., and Currie, J. P.: Observations on Gold Therapy, British Med. J., 1:916, 1953.

Bywaters, E. G. L.: The present status of steroid treatment in rheumatoid arthritis. Proc. Roy. Soc. Med., 58:649, 1965.

Celsus, A. C.: On Medicine, Vol. 2, (Translated from Targa, L., edited by Lee, A.). London, Cox, 1836. As quoted by Gross, M., and Greenberg, L. A.: The salicylates. New Haven, Hillhouse Press, 1948, p. 1.

Chapman, R. A.: Suspected adverse reactions to indomethacin. Canad. Med. Ass. J., 95:1156, 1966.

Colgan, M. T., and Mintz, A. A.: The comparative antipyretic effect of N-acetyl-p-aminophenol and acetylsalicylic acid. J. Pediat., 50:552, 1957.

Dees, S. C., and McKay, H. W., Jr.: Occurrence of pseudotumor cerebri (benign intracranial hypertension) during treatment of children with asthma by adrenal steroids: Report of three cases. Pediatrics, 23:1143, 1959.

Dixon, A. St. J., et al. (Eds.): Salicylates, an International Symposium. Boston, Little, Brown and Co., 1962.

Empire Rheumatism Council, Research Subcommittee: Gold therapy in rheumatoid arthritis, report of a multicenter controlled trial. Ann. Rheum. Dis., 19:95, 1960.

Fisher, D. A., Panos, T. C., and Melby, J. C.: Intermittent corticosteroid therapy of juvenile rheumatoid arthritis. Arthritis Rheum., 7:413, 1964.

Forestier, J.: Bull. et mem. Soc. med. d. hop. de Paris, 53:323, 1929.

Fosdick, W. M., Parsons, J. L., and Hill, D. F.: Long-term cyclophosphamide therapy in rheumatoid arthritis. Arthritis Rheum., 11:151, 1968.

Freyberg, R. H.: Gold therapy for rheumatoid arthritis. *In* Hollander, J. L.: Arthritis and Allied Conditions, Ed. 7. Philadelphia, Lea & Febiger, 1966.

Good, T. A., Benton, J. W., and Kelley, V. C.: Symptomatology resulting from withdrawal of steroid hormone therapy. Arthritis Rheum., 2:299, 1959.

Gross, M., and Greenberg, L. A.: The Salicylates. New Haven, Hillhouse Press, 1948, p. 1.

Harvey, S. C.: Heavy metals. *In* Goodman, L. S., and Gilman, A.: The Pharmacological Basis of Therapeutics, Ed. 3. New York, The Macmillan Company, 1965.

Hollander, J. L.: Intrasynovial corticosteroid therapy. *In* Hollander, J. L.: Arthritis and Allied Conditions, Ed. 7. Philadelphia, Lea & Febiger, 1966, p. 382.

Hucker, H. B., Zacchei, A. G., Cox, S. V., Brodie, D. A., and Cantwell, N. H. R.: Studies on the absorption, distribution, and excretion of indomethacin in various species. J. Pharmacol. Exp. Ther., *153*(2):237, 1966.

Jacobs, J. C.: Sudden death in arthritic children receiving large doses of indomethacin. J.A.M.A., *199*:932, 1967.

Katz, A. M., Pearson, C. M., and Kennedy, J. J.: The antirheumatic effects of indomethacin in rheumatoid arthritis and other rheumatic diseases. Arthritis Rheum., *6*:281, 1963.

Kelsey, W. M., and Sharyj, M.: Fatal hepatitis probably due to indomethacin. J.A.M.A., *199*:586, 1967.

Levy, G.: Biopharmaceutical aspects of the gastrointestinal absorption of salicylates. *In* Salicylates, an International Symposium, edited by Dixon, A. St. J., et al. Boston, Little, Brown and Co., 1963, pp. 10-16.

Lietman, P. S., and Bywaters, E. G. L.: Pericarditis in juvenile rheumatoid arthritis. Pediatrics, *32*:855, 1963.

Lockie, L. M., and Norcross, B. M.: Salicylates, phenylbutazone, chloroquines, and indomethacin in treatment of rheumatoid arthritis. *In* Hollander, J. L.: Arthritis and Allied Conditions. Philadelphia, Lea & Febiger, 1966.

MacLagan, T.: The treatment of acute rheumatism by salicin. Lancet, *110*:342, 1876.

Merck Sharp & Dohme Research Laboratories: Informational material on Indocin (indomethacin), Rahway, N.J., 1964.

Merliss, R. R., Axelrod, B., Fineberg, J., and Melnick, M.: Clinical evaluation of aurothioglycolanilide (Lauron-Endo) in rheumatoid arthritis. Ann. Intern. Med., *35*:352, 1951.

Milne, M. D.; The excretion of salicylate and its metabolites. *In* Salicylates, an International Symposium, edited by Dixon, A. St. J., et al. Boston, Little, Brown and Company, 1963, pp. 19-22.

Norcross, B. M.: Treatment of connective tissue diseases with a new non-steroid compound (indomethacin). Arthritis Rheum., *6*:290, 1963.

Ostle, B.: Statistics in Research. Ames, Iowa, Iowa State University Press, 1963.

Paul, W. D.: Iowa Chapter Arthritis and Rheumatism Foundation, Med. Info. Bull., 4, 1963.

Sataline, L. R., and Farmer, H.: Impaired vision after prolonged chloroquine therapy. New Eng. J. Med., *266*:346, 1962.

Winter, C. A.: Anti-inflammatory testing methods: comparative evaluation of indomethacin and other agents. Excerpta Med. Intern. Conf. Series, No. *82*:190, 1965.

Winter, C. A., Risley, E. A., and Nuss, G. W.: Anti-inflammatory and antipyretic activities of indomethacin. 1-(p-chlorobenzoyl)-5-methoxy-2-methylindole-3-acetic acid. J. Pharmacol. Exp. Ther. *141*:369, 1963.

Woodbury, D. M.: Analgesics and antipyretics. *In* Goodman, L. S. and Gilman, A.: The pharmacologic basis of therapeutics, Ed. 3. New York, The Macmillan Company, 1965, pp. 312-325.

Index

Numbers in *italics* refer to illustrations; (t) refers to tables.

Abdominal pain, 25
　epigastric, 26
　in salicylate therapy, 185
Acetaminophen, 216
Acetylsalicylic acid. See *Salicylates.*
Acid-base imbalance, in salicylate therapy, 188
ACTH, reduction of corticosteroids and, 195
Adduction contracture of hip, 171
　treatment of, 172
Adrenocorticosteroids. See *Corticosteroids.*
Adrenocorticotropic hormone, reduction of corticosteroids and, 195
Agammaglobulinemia, differential diagnosis of, 103
Age, onset of rheumatoid arthritis and, 2, *3*
　patterns of response and, 13
Agglutination tests, for rheumatoid factors, 76, 77(t)
　in systemic lupus erythematosus, 90
Albumin determination, 75
Allergic reactions, differential diagnosis of, 100
　fever in, 83
Alpha-1 globulins, determination of, 75
Alpha-2 globulins, determination of, 75
Anemia, 68
　sickle cell, symptoms of, 108, 108(t)
Ankle, corticosteroid injection for, 202(t)
　equinus of, 167
　examination of, 33
　motion of, 34, 134
　　loss of plantar flexion, 167
　soft tissue calcification of, *43*
　swelling of, 33, *34, 65*
Ankylosing spondylitis, differential diagnosis of, 104, 105(t)
Ankylosis, of elbow, *42*
　of wrist, 36
Antinuclear factor, 78, 87
　in systemic lupus erythematosus, 90

Antistreptolysin O titer, 76
　polyarthritis and, 87
Arthritis, gonococcal, signs and symptoms of, 98, 99(t)
　in leukemia, 102
　in plasma cell hepatitis, 110
　in sarcoidosis, 105
　in scleroderma, 96
　infectious, 66
　meningococcal, 100
　monarticular, differential diagnosis of, 85
　pauciarticular, 13
　peripheral articular, 10
　rheumatoid. See *Rheumatoid arthritis.*
　septic, 96
　　incidence of, 97, 98(t)
　traumatic, 86, 106
　tuberculous, 66, 97
Arthrodesis, 162
Arthroplasty, cup, of hip, 173
Aseptic necrosis, of femoral epiphysis, 66
ASO titer. See *Antistreptolysin titer.*
Aspirin. See *Salicylates.*
Atrophy, muscular. See *Muscle(s), atrophy of.*

Band keratopathy, 24
Barrier score, of body image, 122
Baths, 138
　paraffin, 139
Bentonite flocculation test, 76, 77(t)
Beta globulins, determination of, 75
Biopsy, in scleroderma, 96
　joint, in differential diagnosis, 82
　liver, hepatomegaly and, 23
　muscle, in polymyositis, 94
　skin-muscle, in polyarteritis, 95
　synovial, in monarticular arthritis, 86
Blood, loss of, anemia due to, 69
　　indomethacin and, 215

223

Blood cells, red. See *Erythrocyte*.
　white. See *Leukocyte*.
Blood cultures, in fever of undetermined origin, 83
Body image, 119-125
　neurological and psychiatric contributions to, 120
　perception and, 124
　research on, 121
　scoring indices of, 122
　　arthritics and, 123
Bone formation, periosteal, radiography in, 64, *64*
Bracing, leg, 161, *161*, 165
Brain, lesions of, body image and, 120
Buck's extension traction, 157, *158*
Bursae, of ankle, 34
　of knee, 33
　swelling of, vs. subcutaneous nodules, 17, 31

Calcification, in polymyositis, 94
　metastatic, of soft tissues, 42, *43*
　radiography of, 60
Carditis, 48-58. See also *Pericarditis*.
　of rheumatic fever, 48, 49(t), 89
　types of, 48-51
Cartilage, destruction of, radiography in, 61
Casts, knee, 158, *159*
Cataracts, 24
　in corticosteroid therapy, 200
Cavo-varus, 165, *166*
Central nervous system. See *Nervous system, central*.
Cervical spine, examination of, 37
　fusion of, 38, *38*
　motion of, 37, 81
　radiography of, 65, *66*
Children, evaluation of, 132-137
　gout in, 103
　subcutaneous nodules in, 18
Chloroquine, 220
Christmas disease, differential diagnosis of, 108
Climate, rheumatoid arthritis and, 5
CNS. See *Nervous system, central*.
Coma, reduction of corticosteroid dosage and, 196
Conjunctivitis, of Reiter's syndrome, 106
Contracture, adduction, of hip, 171
　　treatment of, 172
　flexion, of hip, 170
　　treatment of, 172
　of knee, 168
　of wrist, 175
　　release of, 161
　of heel cord, 166
Convulsions, in corticosteroid therapy, 200

Corticosteroids, 188-205
　administration of, 193
　cataracts and, 200
　central nervous system symptoms and, 200
　contraindications to, 189
　cushingoid changes due to, 197
　derivatives of, 193(t)
　disadvantages of, 189
　dosage of, 193
　　reduction of, 194
　duration of therapy, 194
　edema due to, 197
　for pericarditis, 57, 192
　hypertension due to, 197
　Hypospray Injector for, *176*
　inflammatory suppressant activity of, 188, 198
　intra-articular, 201, 202-203(t)
　　failure of, 204
　　for hand, 175, *176*
　　indications for, 201, 201(t)
　osteoporosis due to, 198, *199*
　peptic ulcer and, 198
　side-effects of, 190(t)
　toxicity of, 196, *196*
　withdrawal symptoms, 195
Cortisone. See also *Corticosteroids*.
　growth disturbance and, 29
C-reactive protein test, 73
Crepitation, of joints, 32
Cultures, blood, in fever of undetermined origin, 83
Cup arthroplasty, of hip, 173
Cushingoid changes, in steroid therapy, 197
Cyclophosphamide, 220
Cytoxan, 220

Demineralization, of elbow, *42*
　radiography in, 61, *61*
Dermatitis. See also *Skin, lesions of*.
　in gold therapy, 212
Dermatomyositis, symptoms of, 92, *92, 93*
Dexamethasone. See also *Corticosteroids*.
　central nervous system symptoms of, 200
Diet, in rheumatoid arthritis, 5, 142
Drug therapy, 180-221
　allergic reaction to, 101
　vs. polyarteritis, 95
　for fever, 192
　peptic ulcer and, 26
　principles of, 220-221

ECG. See *Electrocardiogram*.
Economic factors, in rheumatoid arthritis, 5

INDEX

Edema, in corticosteroid therapy, 197
Effusion, joint, 31
    radiography of, 60
    pericardial, 50
Elbow, examination of, 41
  intra-articular corticosteroids for, 203(t)
  motion of, 41, 134
  orthopedic management of, 177
Electrocardiogram, in pericarditis, 51-57, 52-56
Electromyography, in polymyositis, 94
Emotional factors, in rheumatoid arthritis, 125
Encephalopathy, hypertensive, in corticosteroid therapy, 197
Eosinophilia, 71, 71(t)
Epiphysis, femoral, aseptic necrosis of, 66
  stapling of, 163
Equalization of lower extremities, 162
Erosions, bony, radiography of, 62, 62, 63
Erythema, 31
Erythema marginatum, differential diagnosis of, 89
Erythrocyte sedimentation rate, 72, 72(t)
  gold therapy and, 210, 211(t)
ESR. See *Erythrocyte sedimentation rate.*
Euphoria, prednisone and, 200
Exercise, 139, *144-155*
  play activities and, 142
  reaction of child to, 118
Extension traction, Buck's, 157, *158*
Extremity(ies), lower, equalization of, 162
    orthopedic management of, 164-173
  upper, orthopedic management of, 173-178
Eyes, disorders of, 24

Family history, of rheumatoid arthritis, 6-9
Femoral epiphysis, aseptic necrosis of, 66
  stapling of, 163
Fever, 20
  corticosteroids for, 189, 192
  in allergic reaction, 101
  in meningococcal arthritis, 100
  in polymyositis, 94
  indomethacin for, 216, 216-219(t)
  intermittent, differential diagnosis of, 81
    indomethacin for, 191
  lymphadenopathy, and hepatosplenomegaly, 83
  of undetermined origin, 82
  rheumatic. See *Rheumatic fever.*
  types of, *21*
Fingers, motion of, 134
  splints for, 160, *160*, 175, *175*
Flexion, plantar, loss of, 167
Flexion contracture. See under *Contracture.*

Fluid, joint, differential diagnosis and, 81
  in monarticular arthritis, 85
  synovial, in juvenile gout, 104
  in septic arthritis, 97
Foot, examination of, 35
  orthopedic management of, 164-167
  undergrowth of, *30*
Fungal diseases, differential diagnosis of, 100
Fusion, cervical spine, 38, *38*
  joint, 162
  in hip disorders, 171

Gait, evaluation of, 137
  exercise for, 141
  gluteus medius, 171
  in loss of plantar flexion, 167
Gamma globulin, determination of, 75
Gastrointestinal disturbances, in gold therapy, 212
  in salicylate therapy, 187
Genetic studies, 7, 7(t), 8(t)
Genu valgum, 167, *168*
Geographic distribution, of rheumatoid arthritis, 6
Globulins, alpha, determination of, 75
  beta, determination of, 75
  gamma, determination of, 75
"Gluteus medius gait," 171
Gold, 205-213
  absorption of, 206
  administration of, 211
  chemistry of, 206
  distribution of, 206
  effectiveness of, 205(t), 207-211, 208-211(t)
  excretion of, 206
  toxicity of, 212
    treatment of, 213
Gonococcal arthritis, signs and symptoms of, 98, 99(t)
Gout, juvenile, differential diagnosis of, 103
Growth, alterations in, 27-30. See also *Overgrowth; Undergrowth.*
  equalization for, 162
  localized, 30
  of ankle, 35
  of hip, 40
  of knee, 33
  of leg, orthopedic management of, 173

Hand, examination of, 36
  intra-articular corticosteroids for, 203(t)
  motion of, 37
  orthopedic management of, 174
  splint for, 160, *160*

Heart, inflammation of, See *Carditis.*
Heat, moist, 138
 of joint, 31, 134
 therapeutic, 139
Heat lamps, 139
Heating pads, 139
Heel, valgus or varus of, 167
Heel cord, contracture of, 166
Hemangioma, synovial, differential diagnosis of, 103
Hematocrit, 68, 69(t)
Hematological tests, 68-73, 68-72(t)
 in polymyositis, 94
 in systemic lupus erythematosus, 90
Hematopoietic toxicity, in gold therapy, 212
Hemoglobin, 68, 68(t)
 gold therapy and, 210, 210(t)
Hemoglobin C disease, differential diagnosis of, 108
Hemoglobinopathies, differential diagnosis of, 108
Hemophilia, differential diagnosis of, 102
Hemorrhage, in hemophilia, 103
Hepatic. See *Liver.*
Hepatitis, plasma cell, laboratory data in, 110, 112(t)
 signs and symptoms of, 109, 111(t)
 vs. rheumatoid arthritis, 23, 83
Hepatomegaly, 23
Hepatosplenomegaly, lymphadenopathy, and fever, 83
Hip, examination of, 39
 intra-articular corticosteroids for, 202(t)
 motion of, 39, 134
  exercise for, 141
 orthopedic management of, 170-173
 swelling of, *39*, 133
Hodgkin's disease, differential diagnosis of, 83, 102
Hot packs, 138
Humeroulnar joint, osteoporosis of, *63*
Hydrocollator Steam Pack, 139
Hydrocortisone. See also *Corticosteroids.*
 in pericarditis, 57
 intra-articular, 201
Hypertension, in corticosteroid therapy, 197
Hyperuricemia, in gout, 104
Hypogammaglobulinemia, differential diagnosis of, 103
Hypospray Injector, *176*

Immobilization, corticosteroids and, 192
Indomethacin, 213-219
 chemistry of, 214, *214*
 clinical use of, 215, 216-219(t)
 for intermittent fever, 191
 pharmacology of, 214
 toxicity of, 214

Infants, patterns of response in, 13
Infection, masking of, in corticosteroid therapy, 198
 rheumatoid arthritis and, 4
Infectious arthritis, 66
Inflammation, ocular, 24
 of heart. See *Carditis.*
 of synovium, 31
 suppression of, corticosteroids and, 188, 198
Ink blot test, arthritics and, 122
Intercarpal joint, orthopedic treatment of, 174
Interphalangeal joint, of toe, fusion of, 167
 osteoporosis of, *60, 62*
 swelling of, 60, *60*, 133
Iridocyclitis, 24, *25*
 corticosteroids for, 191
 differential diagnosis and, 80, 84
Iritis, 24, *25*
Iron deficiency anemia, 69
Iron medication, failure to respond to, 69

Joint(s). See also specific joint, i.e. *Ankle.*
 biopsy of, in differential diagnosis, 82
 effusion of, 31
  radiography of, 60
 examination of, 30-43
 fusion of, 162
 heat of, 31, 134
 in rheumatic fever, 89
 manipulation of, 163
 motion of. See *Motion.*
 pain, exacerbation of, in gold therapy, 212
 soft tissues of. See *Soft tissues.*
 swelling of. See *Swelling.*
 tenderness of, 31, 134
Joint cartilage, destruction of, radiography in, 61
Joint fluid, differential diagnosis and, 81
 examination of, in monarticular arthritis, 85
Joint space, alterations in, radiography of, 61, *61, 62*
Juvenile gout, differential diagnosis of, 103
Juvenile rheumatoid arthritis. See *Rheumatoid arthritis.*

Keratitis, *25*
Keratopathy, band, 24
Keratosis blennorrhagica, differential diagnosis of, 106
Kidneys, disorders of, in allergic reaction, 101
 in systemic lupus erythematosus, 90

INDEX

Knee, examination of, 32
  intra-articular corticosteroids for, 202(t)
  manipulation of, 163
  motion of, 33, 134
  orthopedic management of, 157, 167
    extension orthoses, *157-159*, 158, 168
  swelling of, 32, *64*, 133
  valgus of, 167, *168*
  valgus or varus of, osteotomy for, 170

Laboratory data, 68-78, 74(t)
  in allergic reaction, 101
  in gonococcal arthritis, 99(t)
  in plasma-cell hepatitis, 110, 112(t)
  in polyarteritis, 95
  in polymyositis, 94
  in septic arthritis, 97
Latex fixation test, 76, 77(t), 87
  in systemic lupus erythematosus, 90
LE cells, 78, 87
  in systemic lupus erythematosus, 90
Leg bracing, 161, *161*, 165
Leg length, inequality of, orthopedic management of, 173, *174*
Leukemia, differential diagnosis of, 82, 101
Leukocyte count, 70, 70(t)
Leukocytes, polymorphonuclear, 70, 71(t)
Leukopenia, 70
Liver, disorders of, in plasma cell hepatitis, 110
  enlargement of, 23
Liver function tests, 23
  in plasma cell hepatitis, 110, 113(t)
Lumbar spine, rheumatoid arthritis of, 39
Lupus erythematosus, systemic, differential diagnosis of, 88, 90, 91(t)
Lymphadenopathy, 21
  hepatosplenomegaly, and fever, 83
Lymphoma, differential diagnosis of, 82, 102

Medication. See *Drug therapy*.
Meningococcal arthritis, 100
Metacarpophalangeal joints, splint for, 177
Metastatic calcification, of soft tissues, 42, *43*
Metatarsal joints, orthopedic management of, 164
Moist heat, 138
Monarticular arthritis, differential diagnosis of, 85
Morning stiffness, 14, 81
Motion, ankle, 34, 134
    loss of plantar flexion, 167
  cervical spine, 37, 81
  elbow, 41, 134

Motion *(Continued)*
  finger, 134
  foot, 35
  hand, 37
  hip, 39, 134
  joint, 31, 134, 135(t)
    exercise for, 139, *144-155*
    salicylates and, 187(t)
    tightness of muscle groups and, 136
  knee, 33, 134
  shoulder, 40
    exercise for, 140
  wrist, 35, 134
    exercise for, 140
Muscle(s), atrophy of, 32
  evaluation of, 136
  exercise for, 140
  of hand, 37
  of knee, 33
  biopsy of, in polyarteritis, 95
    in polymyositis, 94
  strength of, 136
  weakness of, in polymyositis, 92
    of hand, 37
    of wrist, 35
Muscle groups, tightness of, 136
Muscle tension, chronic, 126
Mycotic disease, differential diagnosis of, 100
Myocarditis, 50

Necrosis, aseptic, of femoral epiphysis, 66
Neoplastic diseases, fever in, 82
  of synovium, differential diagnosis of, 103
Nephritis, in gold therapy, 212
Nervous system, central, dysfunction of, 104
    in corticosteroid therapy, 200
    in gold therapy, 212
Neurological problems, body image in, 120
Nodular pneumonia, radiography of, 67
Nodules, subcutaneous, 17-20. See also *Subcutaneous nodules*.
Nutrition. See *Diet*.

Ocular disorders, 24
Orthopedic management, 156-179
  of elbow, 177
  of foot, 164-167
  of hand, 174
  of hip, 170-173
  of knee, 157, 167
    extension orthoses, *157-159*, 158, 168
  of leg length inequality, 173, *174*
  of lower extremity, 164-173
  of shoulder, 178

Orthopedic management *(Continued)*
  of upper extremity, 173-178
  of wrist, 174, 175
Orthoses, 156-161
  extension, for knee, *157-159,* 158, 168
Osteochondrosis, differential diagnosis of, 66
Osteoporosis, in corticosteroid therapy, 198, *199*
  of hip, 40
  of humeroulnar joint, *63*
  of interphalangeal joints, *60, 62*
  radiography in, 61
Osteotomy, 162
  for valgus or varus deformity, of heel, 167
  of knee, 170
Overgrowth, 28, *28,* 30
  equalization for, 162
  radiography of, 64, *65*

Pain, abdominal, 35
  epigastric, 26
  in salicylate therapy, 185
  evaluation of, 134
  exacerbation of, in gold therapy, 212
  in leukemia, 102
  in pericarditis, 50
  patterns of, 13
Papules, rheumatic, 15, 16, *16*
Paraffin bath, 139
Parents, reaction of, to rheumatoid arthritis, 116, 118
Pauciarticular arthritis, 13
Penetration score, of body image, 122
Peptic ulcer, 26, *27*
  in corticosteroid therapy, 198
Perception, and body image, 124
Pericardial effusion, *50*
Pericardial friction rub, 49
Pericarditis, 48-50, *50*
  constrictive, 50, 88
  corticosteroids for, 57, 192
  course of, 57
  differential diagnosis and, 81, 88
  electrocardiograms in, 51-57, *52-56*
  of rheumatic fever, 49(t), 89
  prognosis of, 57
  therapy for, 57
Periosteal new bone formation, radiography in, 64, *64*
Personality, and rheumatoid arthritis, 125
Perthes' disease, differential diagnosis of, 66
Pes valgus-planus, orthopedic management of, 164, *165*
Phenylbutazone, 219-220
  side effects of, 220
Plantar flexion, loss of, 167

Plasma cell hepatitis, laboratory data in, 110, 112(t)
  signs and symptoms of, 109, 111(t)
  vs. rheumatoid arthritis, 23, 83
Plastic splints, heat-malleable. See *Splints, heat-malleable plastic.*
Play activities, 142
Pneumonia, nodular, radiography of, 67
Poliomyelitis, incidence of twins in, 7, 7(t)
Polyarteritis, differential diagnosis of, 95
Polyarthritis, antistreptolysin titer and, 87
  of Reiter's syndrome, 106
  of rheumatic fever, 89
  of systemic lupus erythematosus, 91
  onset of, 11, 12, 80
  pericarditis with, 88
Polymorphonuclear leukocytes, 70, 71(t)
Polymyositis, differential diagnosis of, 92
Posture, evaluation of, 137
  instructions for, 141
Prednisolone. See also *Corticosteroids.*
  intra-articular, 204
Prednisone. See also *Corticosteroids.*
  dosage of, 193, 193(t), 194
  reduction of, 194, 195
  euphoria due to, 200
  in pericarditis, 57
Protein determination, 73
Pseudocysts, destruction of joint cartilage and, 63
Pseudorheumatism, due to reduction of corticosteroid dosage, 195
Psychiatric problems, body image in, 120
Psychological aspects, of rheumatoid arthritis, 116-131
Psychological studies, in rheumatoid arthritis, 127
Psychosomatic symptomatology, Rorschach test and, 122

Radiography, 59-67
  differential diagnosis and, 66, 82
  in leukemia, 102
  in sickle cell anemia, 109
  of demineralization, 61, *61*
  of destruction of joint cartilage, 61
  of nodular pneumonia, 67
  of overgrowth and undergrowth, 64, *65*
  of soft tissues, 59
  of spine, 64
  of wrist, 36, *36*
  periosteal new bone formation and, 64, *64*
Radiology, inhibition of growth and, 28
Rash(es), 15-17
  in allergic reaction, 101
  of dermatomyositis, 92, *92, 93*
  rheumatoid, 15, *16*
    differential diagnosis of, 80, 84

Index

Red blood cell. See *Erythrocyte*.
Rehabilitation, 130
Reiter's syndrome, differential diagnosis of, 106
Renal. See *Kidneys*.
Research, in rheumatoid arthritis, 127
Respiratory disease, rheumatoid arthritis and, 4
Rest, in rheumatoid arthritis, 141
Rheumatic fever, carditis in, 89
 vs. rheumatoid arthritis, 48, 49(t)
 differential diagnosis of, 88, 91(t)
 subcutaneous nodules and, 18
Rheumatic papules, 15, 16, *16*
Rheumatism, chronic fibrous, 2
Rheumatoid arthritis, associated conditions, 4-9
 carditis with, 48-58. See also *Pericarditis*.
 clinical manifestations of, 14-27, 22(t)
 differential diagnosis of, 80-113, 91(t)
  radiographic, 66
 drug therapy for, 180-221
  principles of, 220-221
 family history of, 6-9
 functional effects of, 44(t)
 growth factors in, 27-30. See also under *Growth*.
 incidence and prevalence of, 2-3
 laboratory data in, 68-78, 74(t)
 need for research in, 127
 onset of, 9-11, *10*
  monarticular, 10, *11*
  peripheral articular, 10
  Still's type, 2
  systemic, 11
 orthopedic management of, 156-179. See also *Orthopedic management*.
 patterns of, 12-14, *12*
 predisposition to, 129
 prognosis of, 43-45
 psychological aspects of, 116-131
 psychological studies in, 127
 radiography in, 59-67. See also *Radiography*.
 reaction to, by child, 117
  by parent, 116
 rehabilitation in, 130
 steroids for, 188-205. See also *Corticosteroids* and *Steroid therapy*.
 surgery for, 161-164
 synovectomy in, 178-179
 therapeutic program for, 132-155
  evaluation of child, 132-137
  reaction to, 118
  schedule, 137-143
Rheumatoid factor, differential diagnosis and, 80
 incidence of, 9
 tests for, 76, 77(t), 86
Rheumatoid rash, 15, *16*
 differential diagnosis of, 80, 84

Roentgenography. See *Radiography*.
Rorschach test, arthritics and, 122

Sacroiliac joint, examination of, 40
Salicylates, 180-188
 absorption of, 181, *181*, *182*
 bleeding and, 69
 chemistry of, 180
 distribution of, 181, *181*, *182*
 dosage of, 186
 excretion of, 184, *185*
 for fever, 21
 history of, 180
 in pericarditis, 57
 pharmacologic and physiologic effects of, 180, 183-184(t)
 response to, differential diagnosis and, 83, 91
 side effects of, 187
Sarcoidosis, organs affected in, 107(t)
 signs and symptoms of, 105, 107(t)
School activities, 143
Scleroderma, differential diagnosis of, 96
Season, onset of rheumatoid arthritis and, 3, *3*
Septic arthritis, 96
 incidence of, 97, 98(t)
Serological tests, for syphilis, 73
Serum albumin, determination of, 75
Serum gamma globulin, determination of, 75
Serum proteins, determination of, 73
Serum uric acid, determination of, 73
 in juvenile gout, 104
Sex, incidence of rheumatoid arthritis and, 2
Sheep cell agglutination test, 76, 77(t)
 in systemic lupus erythematosus, 90
Shoes, 161, 164
 for leg length inequality, 173
Shoulder, examination of, 40
 intra-articular corticosteroids for, 203(t)
 motion of, 40
  exercise for, 140
 orthopedic management of, 178
Sickle cell anemia, symptoms of, 108, 108(t)
Skin. See also *Rash(es)*.
 lesions of, in gold therapy, 212
  in plasma-cell hepatitis, 110
  in polyarteritis, 95
  indomethacin and, 215
Slit lamp examination, 24
Social and economic factors, in rheumatoid arthritis, 5
Sodium aurothiomalate, 206. See also *Gold*.
 administration of, 211
Soft tissues, metastatic calcification of, 42, *43*
 radiography of, 59

Spine, cervical. See *Cervical spine.*
  lumbar, rheumatoid arthritis of, 39
    radiography of, 64
  thoracic, rheumatoid arthritis of, 39
Splenomegaly, 23
Splinting, 157
Splints, heat-malleable plastic, for fingers, 160, *160,* 175, *175*
  for foot, 166
  for hand, 160, *160*
  for wrist, 160, *160,* 177
  plaster, 160
Spondylitis, ankylosing, differential diagnosis of, 104, 105(t)
  rheumatoid factor and, 76
Stapling, of distal femoral epiphysis, 163
Steroid therapy, 188-205. See also *Corticosteroids.*
  growth disturbance and, 29
  peptic ulcer and, 26
  reaction to, vs. polyarteritis, 95
Stiffness, morning, 14, 81
Still, George F., 1
Still's disease, 2
Streptococcal infection, beta-hemolytic, rheumatoid arthritis and, 4
Subcutaneous nodules, 17-20
  differential diagnosis of, 81, 85
  histological features of, 18, 18(t), *19*
  prognosis with, 45
Surgery, 161-164
  onset of rheumatoid arthritis and, 5
Swelling, ankle, 33, *34, 65*
  bursal, 17, 31
  hand, 36
  hip, *39,* 133
  in sickle cell anemia, 108
  joint, evaluation of, 133
    exacerbation of, in gold therapy, 212
    in allergic reaction, 101
    periarticular, 31
    peripheral articular, 10
      differential diagnosis of, 84
      salicylates for, 187(t)
  knee, 32, *64,* 133
  of interphalangeal joints, 60, *60,* 133
  patterns of, 13
  wrist, 35, 133
Synovectomy, 178-179
  of knee joint, 170
Synovial fluid, examination of, in juvenile gout, 104
  in septic arthritis, 97
Synovitis, of hip, 170
Synovium, biopsy of, in monarticular arthritis, 86
  hemangioma of, differential diagnosis of, 103
  inflammation of, 31
Syphilis, serological tests for, 73
Systemic lupus erythematosus, differential diagnosis of, 88, 90, 91(t)

Talipes cavo-varus, 165, *166*
Talipes equinus, splints for, 166
  surgery for, 167
Tarsal joints, orthopedic treatment of, 164
Teen-agers, patterns of response in, 14, 119
  plasma cell hepatitis in, 109
Temporomandibular joint, examination of, 40
  exercise for, 141
Tenderness, 31
  evaluation of, 134
  patterns of, 13
Tenosynovitis, 81
  of ankle, 34
  of wrist, 35
Testosterone, growth disturbance and, 30
Tests. See name of specific test.
Therabath, 139
Therapeutic program, 132-155
  evaluation of child, 132-137
  reaction to, 118
  schedule, 137-143
Thomas test, 170
Thoracic spine, rheumatoid arthritis of, 39
Tissues, soft, metastatic calcification of, 42, *43*
  radiography of, 59
Titers, antistreptolysin O, 76
  polyarthritis and, 87
Toe, interphalangeal joint of, fusion of, 167
  intra-articular corticosteroids for, 202(t)
Traction, Buck's extension, 157, *158*
  stretching, of hip, 172
Trauma, rheumatoid arthritis and, 4, 86
Traumatic arthritis, 86, 106
Trendelenburg test, for hip disorders, 171
Tuberculous arthritis, 66, 97
Twin studies, 7, 7(t), 8(t)

Ulcer, peptic, 26, *27*
  in corticosteroid therapy, 198
Undergrowth, 28, *29,* 30, *30*
  equalization for, 162
  radiograph of, 64
Urethritis, of Reiter's syndrome, 106
Uric acid, determination of, 73
  metabolism of, disorder of, 104
Uveitis, corticosteroids for, 191
  differential diagnosis and, 84

Valgus deformity, of heel, osteotomy for, 167
  of knee, 167, *168*
  osteotomy for, 170
Valvulitis, 51

INDEX **231**

Varus deformity, of foot, 165, *166*
  of heel, osteotomy for, 167
  of knee, osteotomy for, 170
Viral diseases, differential diagnosis of, 100
Vision, disturbance of, 24

Westergren erythrocyte sedimentation rate, 72
White blood cells. See *Leukocyte*.
Wintrobe erythrocyte sedimentation rate, 72, 72(t)

Wounds, delayed healing of, in corticosteroid therapy, 198
Wrist, examination of, 35
  intra-articular corticosteroids for, 203(t)
  motion of, 35, 134
    exercise for, 140
  orthopedic management of, 174, 175
  splints for, 160, *160*, 177
  swelling of, 35, 133

X-ray. See *Radiography*.